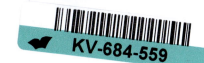
Portrait of the Psychiatrist as a Young Man

The Early Writing and Work of R.D. Laing, 1927–1960

Allan Beveridge

Consultant Psychiatrist,
Queen Margaret Hospital,
Dunfermline,
Scotland

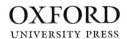

OXFORD
UNIVERSITY PRESS

OXFORD

UNIVERSITY PRESS

Great Clarendon Street, Oxford OX2 6DP

Oxford University Press is a department of the University of Oxford.
It furthers the University's objective of excellence in research, scholarship,
and education by publishing worldwide in

Oxford New York

Athens Auckland Bangkok Bogotá Buenos Aires Cape Town
Chennai Dar es Salaam Delhi Florence Hong Kong Istanbul Karachi
Kolkata Kuala Lumpur Madrid Melbourne Mexico City Mumbai Nairobi
Paris São Paulo Shanghai Singapore Taipei Tokyo Toronto Warsaw

with associated companies in Berlin Ibadan

Oxford is a registered trade mark of Oxford University Press
in the UK and in certain other countries

Published in the United States
by Oxford University Press Inc., New York

© Oxford University Press, 2011

The moral rights of the author have been asserted

Database right Oxford University Press (maker)

First published 2011

British Library Cataloguing in Publication
Data available

Library of Congress Cataloging in Publicati
Data available

Typeset in Minion by Cenveo, Bangalore, Ir
Printed in Great Britain
on acid-free paper by
CPI Antony Rowe, Chippenham, Wiltshire

ISBN 978–0–19–958357–7

10 9 8 7 6 5 4 3 2 1

Whilst every effort has been made to ensure that the contents of this book are as complete, accurate, and
up-to-date as possible at the date of writing, Oxford University Press is not able to give any guarantee or
assurance that such is the case. Readers are urged to take appropriately qualified medical advice in all cases.
The information in this book is intended to be useful to the general reader, but should not be used as a
means of self-diagnosis or for the prescription of medication.

Portrait of the Psychiatrist as

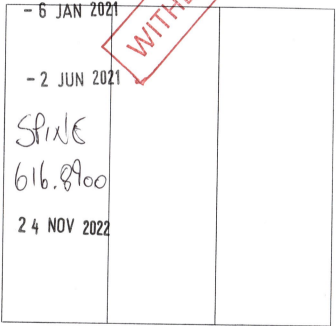

International Perspectives in Philosophy and Psychiatry

Series editors: Bill (K.W.M.) Fulford, Katherine Morris, John Z. Sadler, and Giovanni Stanghellini

Volumes in the series:

To Margaret, Rebecca, and Francis

Acknowledgements

I would like to thank Adrian and Karen Laing for their encouragement with this project and to the R.D. Laing Estate for permission to use R.D. Laing materials. These materials are held at Glasgow University Library Special Collections and include the extensive MS Laing archive and Laing's Library. I am grateful to David Weston and his staff at Special Collections for all their help over the years while I was studying the Laing archives. I would like to thank Professor Sir Michael Bond for generously giving me full access to the Southern General Hospital case conference records and to Iain Smith for telling me of their existence. I am also grateful to Iain, a consultant psychiatrist at Gartnavel, for sharing his extensive knowledge of the Glasgow institution, for providing me with access to little-known personnel papers regarding Laing, and for reading drafts of this book. I also acknowledge the help of the Wellcome Trust who awarded me a three month Clinical Research Leave grant in order to pursue my research on Laing. I'd like to thank Malcolm Nicolson who provided a great deal of help with the application to the Wellcome Trust and for his continuous support during my period of research at the Centre for the History of Medicine at Glasgow University. Thanks also to Martin Baum and Charlotte Green at Oxford University Press for their very helpful advice over the course of the writing of this book.

I am grateful to Daniel Burston and Gavin Miller, two of the world's leading Laing scholars for reading drafts of this book and for their informed and helpful comments. I am also grateful to Mike Barfoot, who also read this book in draft form and who provided a range of valuable suggestions. I would also like to thank Eric Matthews, Pat Bracken, and Phil Thomas for reading my chapter on existential phenomenology and for generously sharing their considerable expertise with me. I would like to thank Mark Evans for reading the chapter on religion. Others who have helped with this project include: Jonathan Andrews, whose pioneering work on Laing's time at Gartnavel proved to be very helpful to me in understanding this crucial period in Laing's career; Gayle Davis for our many discussions on the history of psychiatry and for her support in the process of writing this book; Charles Pickles for our discussions about philosophy and for sharing his wide knowledge of the literature in the field; Edgar Jones for providing me with information about Laing's time in the Army; my colleagues at the Queen Margaret Hospital who supported my clinical leave and Fiona Murray who worked as my locum; my secretary, Mary Westwater, who has provided technical expertise in the writing of this book as well as unstinting support; staff at the Queen Margaret Hospital Library for obtaining a great number of publications and books, many of them obscure. Finally, and most importantly, I would like to thank my wife Margaret for not only discussing early drafts, but also for remaining positive and encouraging about this book over the years of its gestation.

Contents

Introduction

For a period in the 1960s, Ronald Laing was the most famous psychiatrist in the world. His books sold in millions and were translated into many languages. In his most celebrated work, *The Divided Self*, published in 1960, he argued that madness was understandable. Laing's reputation subsequently went into serious decline, but in recent years there has been renewed interest in him and a number of biographies and books have been published. This interest has been fuelled by a disenchantment with the claims of the neurosciences and an unease about biotechnology.[1] Laing's existential approach of treating the patient as a person rather than a malfunctioning mechanism has new-found appeal.

Laing's place in the history of psychiatry and the significance of his contribution, however, remain contested.[2] One view, mainly held by psychiatrists, is that he enjoyed a fashionable notoriety in the 1960s when peddling anti-establishment opinions was very much in vogue, but that his views on schizophrenia were dangerous nonsense. They encouraged patients to stop their medication and created the impression that the family was somehow to blame for the condition. The recent triumphal march of biological psychiatry with its emphasis on genetics and physical treatment is seen as rendering his writing largely irrelevant. In tandem, the spectacular alcohol- and drug-fuelled decline of his later years is taken as confirmation that his work was, all along, the product of an unstable charlatan.

The alternative view, mainly held by non-psychiatrists, is that Laing championed the cause of the mentally ill. In opposition to the impersonal empire of orthodox psychiatry, with its drugs and ECT, its large and forbidding mental hospitals, and its belief that the mad were incomprehensible, Laing brought humanity to the subject. He demonstrated that the mad were people too, and that their utterances could be understood. His subsequent demonization by traditional psychiatry is taken as evidence that psychiatry is irredeemably wedded to a biological model of mental illness and to the unyielding defence of its power.

What are we to make of these conflicting views? Should we even spend time reassessing Laing? There are a number of reasons why Laing deserves our attention. First, Laing's early career from the 1940s to 1960 spanned an extraordinarily eventful period in psychiatry's history. It was a period that witnessed the crisis of over-crowded psychiatric hospitals, the emergence of community approaches to mental illness, the introduction of new and apparently effective drugs, and the debate as to whether

---

[1] For an extended discussion of the limitations of the neurosciences in fully explaining psychiatric illness, see Broome, M.R., Borlotti (eds) (2009). *Psychiatry as Cognitive Neuroscience. Philosophical Perspectives.* Oxford University Press, Oxford.

[2] Beveridge, A. (1996). 'R.D. Laing revisited'. *Psychiatric Bulletin*, **22**, 452–6.

physical or psychological therapies were the more successful in the treatment of schiz-ophrenia. The period also saw the rise and decline of psychoanalysis, the development of object relations theory, and attempts to develop an existential psychotherapy. Laing's early career saw him exposed to a wide variety of arenas in which psychiatry and related disciplines were enacted. Thus his first clinical attachment in 1950 was concerned with the care of patients with encephalitis lethargica, a condition that left the victim, in Laing's words, 'demented, drooling, contorted and paralysed'.[3] His next post was in a neurosurgical unit at Killearn where he witnessed the effects of loboto-mies and trauma on patients and where he pondered the relationship between mind and body, self and brain. Laing served time in the British Army as a psychiatrist, pro-viding reports and opinions on the calibre and mental stability of conscripted soldiers. He witnessed how society processed its citizens and rejected those that it deemed unfit.

In the mid-1950s Laing worked in a large, over-crowded mental hospital in Glasgow, at a time when there was a lively international debate as to whether the institution actually made patients worse. It was also at a time when the first batches of chlorpro-mazine tablets were being given to patients and its effects were observed with great interest by hospital staff. By the end of the 1950s Laing was training in London at the Institute of Psychoanalysis, which was the setting for acrimonious battles between the followers of Melanie Klein and Anna Freud as to who was the rightful bearer of the torch of Freudianism. In the clinics of the Tavistock in London, Laing was seeing a markedly different type of patient than the severely mentally ill ones he had been see-ing in Glasgow—or, as he put it, he was working in 'a sort of dilettante outpost of an organisation that dealt with normal people'.[4]

A second reason for re-considering Laing is that his private papers have recently been acquired by Glasgow University Library Special Collections.[5] These are a rela-tively unexplored source which sheds much light on Laing's intellectual development and the psychiatric context in which he worked. Laing kept extensive records of his intellectual preoccupations and he made copious notes about his clinical experiences, including detailed accounts of his interactions with patients. He kept minutes of staff conferences, educational meetings, psychotherapy groups, seminars on religion and psychiatry, and classes for the parents of disturbed children. All these provide an invaluable social history of the period. Thus, even if Laing had not become an iconic figure in psychiatry, these documents would be a rich source for historians. The fact that he did achieve fame and intellectual status makes them all the more interesting.

---

[3] Laing, R.D. (1985). *Wisdom, Madness and Folly. The Making of a Psychiatrist 1927–1957*. Canongate, Edinburgh, 1998 reprint, p. 88.

[4] Mullan, B. (1995). *Mad to be Normal. Conversations with R. D. Laing*. Free Association Books, London, p. 148.

[5] Glasgow University Library Special Collections, MS Laing. This extensive archive contains records of Laing's correspondence, drafts of work, press-cuttings relating to Laing, financial papers, certificates and curriculum vitae of Laing, and audiovisual material. The archive cov-ers the entirety of Laing's career. The present book focuses on the comparatively neglected early part of Laing's career up until 1960.

We are afforded a window into the 1950s world of Scottish and English psychiatry, and we see through it with the eyes of a psychiatrist whose testimony provides an astute, informed, intellectually probing, and at times humorous account of this world.

Thirdly, Laing asked fundamental questions about the nature of madness and of the role of psychiatry. While we do not have to agree with the answers he gave, these questions are still relevant today:

Is psychosis understandable?

Does psychiatric language serve to distance clinicians from patients and turn their experiences into abstract concepts?

Are the principles of the physical sciences applicable to the study of human beings?

Do the humanities, such as history, literature, and philosophy, contribute to our understanding of mental illness?

Should spiritual aspects be disregarded or are they of crucial importance?

What is the relationship between madness and society?

If we agree that Laing is worth re-assessing, we then have to acknowledge the pitfalls in undertaking such a project. We cannot view Laing with an innocent eye. As well as the extensive commentaries and biographical accounts of him, we have Laing's own version of his life and work; or rather, we have several of Laing's versions as he had a tendency to modify his story over the years, at times emphasizing his radical credentials, at others his orthodoxy. Laing can be seen in the context of the hero myth and he certainly made attempts to foster the view of himself as a hero. Like Freud, he did on occasions minimize the contributions of colleagues and other writers. Henri Ellenberger,[6] in his consideration of the 'Freudian legend', describes two aspects of the hero myth in relation to Freud. First, there is 'the solitary hero struggling against a host of enemies, suffering "the slings and arrows of outrageous fortune" but triumphing in the end'. Second, there is the obliteration of the scientific and cultural context in which Freud developed psychoanalysis in order to emphasize the absolute originality of his achievements and to attribute to him the ideas developed by a host of others. Some aspects of the hero myth apply to Laing, but to a lesser extent. He did have a tendency to portray himself as a lone figure whose sensitivity to the suffering of the mentally ill contrasted with the apparent indifference of others. His contention that the utterances of the mad were potentially meaningful was not original: psychoanalysts and existential therapists had been expressing such a notion several years before Laing wrote his first book, *The Divided Self*. Ingleby[7] takes a severe view of Laing and maintains that his attempt to portray himself as a lone hero struggling to liberate the mad from the clutches of psychiatry failed to acknowledge that others within the profession were trying to do the same. Jonathan Andrews, who has examined Laing's

---

[6] Ellenberger, F.H. (1970). *The Discovery of the Unconscious. The History and Evolution of Dynamic Psychiatry*. Basic Books, New York, pp. 547–8.

[7] Ingleby, D. (1998). 'The view from the North Sea'. In Gijswijt-Hofstra, M. and Porter, R. (eds), *Cultures of Psychiatry and Mental Health Care in Postwar Britain and the Netherlands*. Rodopi, Amsterdam, pp. 295–314.

time at Gartnavel Royal Mental Hospital in Glasgow, takes a less condemnatory view, but also concluded that Laing rather underplayed the contribution of his colleagues.[8]

To be fair to Laing, there were times when he did acknowledge the work of others and their influence on him. However, biographers have often amplified what was original in Laing's work and minimized the intellectual and cultural traditions upon which he drew. Laing has provided such a compelling and entertaining account of his activities that later commentators have sometimes been seduced by them and uncritically taken him at his word. Laing was a skilled story teller and he had a great ability to manipulate the emotions of his readers. For example, in perhaps his most famous set-piece—the depiction of the eminent German alienist, Emil Kraepelin, interviewing a patient before a lecture class, which appeared in the opening pages of *The Divided Self*—the reader cannot help but side with the patient against the insensitive and dehumanizing doctor. Likewise, in the passages where he wrote about himself, the reader wants to be on the side of the 'good' in the shape of the sensitive and humanitarian Dr Laing, rather than in the company of the 'bad' as represented by a cast of uncaring and uncomprehending clinicians and relatives. Laing was, of course, aware of the mythology surrounding him. As he told his would-be biographer, Bob Mullan: 'So I'm playing a part now, Ronnie Laing is playing a part in the mythologizing of R.D. Laing'.[9]

This book is based on Laing's early years, from his birth in 1927 to the publication of his first book, *The Divided Self* in 1960. The main focus is on his intellectual background and his development as a psychiatrist. As well as seeing Laing in the context of his time, it is also profitable to consider him in the light of more long-standing traditions. Thus his interrogation of the natural sciences as an appropriate method to study humanity can be traced back to the nineteenth century and to German thinkers, such as Max Weber and Wilhelm Dilthey. They made a distinction between the natural sciences, which they saw as seeking *explanations* for physical phenomena, and the human sciences, which were concerned with *understanding*. They drew on hermeneutics, which was originally a method of interpreting biblical texts, but which they applied to such subjects as history and psychology. The Personalist thinkers, such as the Scottish philosopher John Macmurray, also held that the methods of the physical sciences were inappropriate to the study of human beings.

The origins of Laing's thinking can be traced even further back: to the Enlightenment, which heralded the birth pangs of psychiatry. Reason, not tradition, superstition, or divine intervention, would unlock the cage of unreason. Although it would be a simplification to portray the development of psychiatry as an entirely secular enterprise, it nevertheless emphasized human reason over appeals to religious authority. The ravings of the madman were to be understood, not in spiritual terms, but as a form of medical malady. This conflict between Enlightenment and pre-Enlightenment approaches to mental distress was to be of fundamental importance to Laing and

---

[8] Andrews, J. (1998). 'R.D. Laing in Scotland: facts and fictions of the "Rumpus Room" and interpersonal psychiatry'. In Gijswijt-Hofstra, M., Porter, R. (eds) *Culture of Psychiatry and Mental Health Care in Postwar Britain and the Netherlands*. Rodopi, Amsterdam, pp. 121–50.

[9] Mullan, *Mad to be Normal*, p. 37.

preoccupied and disturbed him throughout his life. He asked himself: was religion just a primitive left-over from an earlier, unsophisticated age, or did it reveal essential truths about other realities beyond the reach of science. Did psychiatry represent another triumphant step forward in the onward march of human reason, or was it incapable of comprehending the spiritual dimension of life? Did it misconstrue spiritual experience as evidence of insanity?

As well as considering Laing in the context of medical and psychiatric thought, we should also see him in the wider culture generally. In fact it is important that he should be considered in this wider context because he was greatly influenced by it. In the generalist spirit which the philosopher George Davie claims is characteristic of the Scottish tradition, Laing viewed the different branches of knowledge as interconnected.[10] History, literature, philosophy, religion, music, and art all informed what he thought and what he wrote. He read extensively in European literature, taking in Dostoyevsky, Tolstoy, Strindberg, Malarme, Baudelaire, Kafka, Camus, Sartre, Genet, Beckett, Canetti, Rilke, and Thomas Mann. He was also a Classical scholar and was well-versed in the poetry of Homer and the plays of Aeschylus, Euripides, and Sophocles. In Laing's writing we see how his reading of the humanities informed his approach to the mentally ill.

Outline of book

The first chapter of the book sketches Laing's early life. Although this has been covered in previous biographies, Laing's private papers help to expand and, in some instances, modify the received narrative of his life story. Thereafter, the book is divided into a theoretical and a clinical section. In the initial theoretical section we look at Laing's immersion in the world of ideas and literature. Laing roamed widely across different intellectual disciplines and held that knowledge derived from individual fields was interconnected. Thus dividing Laing's intellectual activities into chapters dealing with distinct subjects such as psychiatric theory, philosophy, religion, and the arts, is somewhat artificial, but it is also necessary in order to provide a structured and coherent account of his thought. What unites these different areas is that Laing considered that each of them made a vital contribution to understanding madness.

The second chapter sets the scene for Laing's intellectual journey by examining how he planned his project to become an eminent thinker. It looks at his notebooks and examines his personal library to reveal what books he was reading. This chapter also looks at Laing's early intellectual productions from his talk as a second year medical student, through his undergraduate essays, to his first publications in medical journals. Following this, we look at Laing's engagement with theoretical and cultural matters. We begin in Chapter 3 with psychiatric theory. Laing was interested in the history of his discipline and read many of the classic texts by the likes of William Battie, William Pargeter, and John Conolly. These men expressed notions about madness and its treatment that Laing was subsequently to adopt and articulate in his own work.

---

[10] Davie, G.E. (1961). *The Democratic Intellect. Scotland and her Universities in the Nineteenth Century.* Edinburgh University Press, Edinburgh.

In this chapter we also look at Laing's response to the different traditions in psychiatry as exemplified, at one pole, by the psychodynamic approach of Freud and, at the other, by the somaticist perspective of Kraepelin. Laing was also interested in American clinicians such as Harry Stack Sullivan and Frieda Fromm-Reichmann, who advocated a broadly psychotherapeutic approach to patients with schizophrenia. Laing studied object relations theory and was to meet its leading proponents, such as Melanie Klein and Donald Winnicott, when he trained at the Institute of Psychoanalysis in London. This chapter examines the influence of these different theories on Laing's thinking and how he worked out his own approach to psychiatry.

Chapter 4 looks at existentialism, phenomenology, and existential psychiatry: subjects fundamental to Laing's work. It attempts to see the subjects through Laing's eyes and in the context of the time in which he was living. It looks at the leading thinkers associated with the existential tradition, such as Kierkegaard, Nietzsche, Heidegger, and Sartre, and examines what Laing took from them. This chapter also looks at the associated subject of phenomenology, before considering the work of existential psychiatrists such as Binswanger, Boss, and Minkowski. We look at how Laing drew on their writing to develop his own version of existential psychiatry. Chapter 5 describes Laing's attitude to religion and his anguished struggle with issues of belief and unbelief. It considers the influence of his Scottish Presbyterian upbringing on his development and how he responded to the many contemporary scientific and philosophical critiques of faith. We examine how Laing's religious outlook informed his approach to psychiatry and the way he conceived of mental disturbance. Chapter 6 completes the non-clinical part of the book by analysing Laing's engagement with the arts. He was particularly interested in William Blake, Gerard Manley Hopkins, and Dostoyevsky, and planned to write books about each of them. This chapter considers how Laing drew on their work and that of many other writers to articulate and enrich his views on madness.

The clinical section, which forms the second half of the book, follows Laing's medical career chronologically. Laing left extensive medical notes about his contact with patients. These have never previously been examined and they do much to enlarge our understanding of him and his work. We are able to identify patients who appeared in his later books and we are able to see how he made use of their original case histories in his published writing. We begin with Laing as an Army psychiatrist and consider his medical reports on soldiers' mental fitness for military service. In the treatment of soldier patients, Laing frequently adopted a psychoanalytic approach and, in certain cases, he engaged in dream therapy. In Laing's Army notes, we encounter the patient who would become 'David' in *The Divided Self*. The following two chapters consider Laing's time at Gartnavel, arguably the most significant experience of his clinical career. The first of these chapters looks at the psychiatric culture of 1950s Glasgow and Laing's first attempts at applying the principles of social psychiatry to the treatment of people with severe mental disorder. This was a project that he undertook with his Gartnavel colleagues and which came to be known as the 'Rumpus Room' experiment.

It was to occupy an important place in biographical and self-penned accounts of Laing's psychiatric development. The following chapter depicts Laing's work with individual patients at Gartnavel. It includes a consideration of the patient who would become 'Julie' in *The Divided Self* and the young mother described in 'The coldness of death' chapter of *The Self and Others*. There are also clinical notes on many other patients who were not subsequently discussed in his published books. These illustrate how Laing tried to apply psychoanalytic techniques to the treatment of people with psychotic illnesses.

Chapter 10 examines Laing's time as a senior registrar at Glasgow's Southern General Hospital. We are particularly fortunate in having access to the records of the psychiatric case conferences that were held regularly in the Department of Psychological Medicine. They report the verbatim statements of staff as they discuss individual case presentations. We are able to place Laing in his immediate professional context and see how much he resembled or differed from his peers in his approach to psychiatry. We also meet the patient who was to become 'Peter' in *The Divided Self* and the young boy who became 'Phillip' in *Wisdom, Madness and Folly*. At the Southern General Hospital, Laing made his early forays into group psychotherapy and was guided by the principles laid down by Wilfred Bion and Henry Ezriel. Chapter 11 looks at Laing's move to London and the patients he saw at the Tavistock. We witness him conducting individual and group psychoanalysis, as well as interviewing families in the clinic and at home. We see Laing adopting orthodox analytic techniques and then adapting them as he becomes more experienced in psychotherapy.

The final chapter examines *The Divided Self*. This brings together the many strands of the preceding chapters. We look at how Laing's wide reading in psychiatry, philosophy, religion, and the arts combined with his clinical observation and experience to shape his theories about the schizoid personality and schizophrenia. This chapter offers a critique of Laing's first book and looks at how it was received on its publication and thereafter. Laing's place in Scottish culture is considered and his subsequent career following the publication of *The Divided Self* is briefly examined.

This book aims to illuminate the early intellectual career of one of psychiatry's most challenging thinkers and to consider the strengths and weaknesses of his thought. By virtue of having access to Laing's original clinical notes, we are able to compare these with his published theoretical writings. We are thus able to compare what he *said* he did in clinical practice with what he *actually* did. This is in the spirit of the medical historian, Erwin Ackerknecht, who maintained that we need to distinguish medical theory from practice: or, in other words, 'what a doctor thought and wrote', from 'what a doctor did'.[11]

---

[11] Ackerknecht, E.H. (1967). 'A plea for a "Behaviourist" approach in writing the history of medicine'. *Journal of the History of Medicine and Allied Sciences*, **22**, 211–14.

Part I

Laing and theory

Chapter 1

Portrait of the psychiatrist as a young man 1927–1960

. . . the business of distorting the Past. Forgetting, distorting, glamorizing, glorifying, idealizing, belittling, romanticizing—how obliging, how malleable the Past is.[1]

This comment is taken from a letter that Laing wrote to his then girlfriend, Marcelle Vincent on 29 September 1949 and it alerts us to the slipperiness of grasping the past, especially Laing's past, and especially as told by Laing. Laing's private papers contain many and sometimes contradictory accounts of his life experiences. His official published autobiography, *Wisdom, Madness and Folly*, which only goes as far as his thirtieth year, was written when he was in his fifties. Here Laing is taking stock of his career, seeking to clarify his message where he thinks it has been misunderstood, revising his opinions, or even backtracking on them. Details about his subsequent career, as well as further comments, about his early days are contained in a series of illuminating interviews he gave to Bob Mullan and which were published in *Mad to be Normal: Conversations with R.D. Laing*.[2] Further biographical information about Laing is also to be found in his books, *The Politics of Experience and the Bird of Paradise* and *The Facts of Life*, as well as in the numerous interviews that he gave throughout his career. In addition to Laing's autobiography, *Wisdom, Madness and Folly*,[3] there are three book-length biographies: *R.D. Laing: A Biography* by his son, Adrian;[4] *R.D. Laing: A Divided Self* by John Clay;[5] and *The Wing of Madness* by Daniel Burston.[6] Each volume provides valuable insights into the life of Laing, although, inevitably, they differ in the degree to which they go along with the subject's account of himself and his self-mythologizing. This chapter will examine the received historical narrative of Laing's life and draw on archival material to expand and revise it. It will also examine Laing's own narratives of self-construction and how they, in turn, influenced subsequent biographers and commentators.

---

[1] Laing in a letter to Marcelle Vincent, 29 September 1949. Quoted in Mullan, B. (1997). *R.D. Laing: Creative Destroyer*. Cassell, London, p. 72.

[2] Mullan, B. (1995). *Mad to be Normal: Conversations with R.D. Laing*. Free Association Books, London. Mullan also provided his own account of Laing in Mullan, B. (1999). *R.D. Laing: A Personal View*. Duckworth, London.

[3] Laing, R.D. (1985). *Wisdom, Madness and Folly* (1998 new edition). Canongate, Edinburgh.

[4] Laing, A. (1994). *R.D. Laing: A Biography*. Peter Owen, London. Also Laing, A. (2006). *R.D. Laing: A Life* (second edition with new introduction). Sutton Publishing, Thrupp.

[5] Clay, J. (1996). *R.D. Laing: A Divided Self*. Hodder & Stoughton, London.

[6] Burston, D. (1996). *The Wing of Madness*. Harvard University Press, Cambridge, Massachusetts.

Early years

Ronald David Laing was born on 7 October 1927 at 21 Ardbeg Street in a respectable lower middle class neighbourhood of the city,[7] though the feminist literary critic Elaine Showalter[8] claims that this was 'the roughest, darkest, and most depressed district of Glasgow'. Showalter also maintains that Laing's upbringing was a 'drab mixture of sexual repression, sodden respectability, and masculine violence'.[9]

As befits the narrative of a Hero, Laing claimed he could remember being born and the 'searing pain' of his delivery.[10] This is reminiscent of the account of the birth of the nineteenth-century French poet, Arthur Rimbaud, whose work Laing admired. Legend has it that Rimbaud was born a prodigy and that by his second day he was able to talk and read to his astonished mother.[11] Laing, of course, was aware of such mythology and was to write about this subject in his 1976 book, *The Facts of Life*,[12] in which he quoted with approval Otto Rank's *The Myth of the Birth of the Hero*. Ronald was an only child, born some ten years after his parents married, and, so they very curiously claimed, long after they had stopped having sexual intercourse. Significantly, Otto Rank had written that the Hero's origins were preceded by difficulties such as 'continence, or prolonged barrenness, or secret intercourse of the parents'.[13] Laing's story has parallels with the birth of another Hero, this time, Jesus Christ, whose parents, the Bible tells us, did not 'know' each other sexually prior to his arrival. Ronald's mother, Amelia, in a peculiar parody of the Virgin Mary, managed to conceal her pregnancy until the very day of delivery. Burston speculates that this type of behaviour reflected prudery, shame, or a perverse need to keep others in the dark.[14]

Amelia decided to call the baby Ronald after the matinee idol Ronald Colman. Laing had a troubled relationship with his mother, who seems to have lacked affection for him. She made up stories to provoke discord in the family, and was prone to extravagant suspicions and bouts of jealousy. 'Everyone in the street knew she was mad', remembers Walter Fyfe, a next door neighbour and school friend.[15] Two of Laing's medical colleagues told the biographer Daniel Burston that they thought his mother had a psychotic illness.[16] Laing relates that his mother felt that her mind had been 'frozen' at the age of 11 and that consequently she could not think clearly. When she

---

[7] Laing, A. (1991). 'R.D. Laing The first five years'. *Journal of the Society for Existential Analysis*. 2, 24–9.

[8] Showalter, E. (1987). *The Female Malady: Women, Madness and English Culture, 1830–1980*. Virago Press, London, pp. 224–6.

[9] Showalter, *The Female Malady*, p. 224.

[10] Quoted in Clay, *R.D. Laing*, p. 4.

[11] Starkie, E. (1961). *Arthur Rimbaud*. Faber & Faber, London.

[12] Laing, R.D. (1976). *The Facts of Life*. Penguin, London, pp. 38–40.

[13] Rank, O. (1959). *The Myth of the Birth of the Hero and Other Writings*. Alfred A. Knopf, New York, p. 85.

[14] Burston, *The Wing of Madness*, p. 10.

[15] Quoted in Clay, *R.D. Laing*, p. 7.

[16] Burston, *The Wing of Madness*, p. 12.

was 11 her father had made a remark which made her realize that he did not love her.[17] Laing remembers other episodes that suggest a degree of oddness in his mother. When she was admitted to hospital, she would not tell the admitting doctor her address because it was 'none of his business'.[18] His mother also destroyed all the photographs of herself and refused to be photographed, though Laing felt that his mother was actually 'very beautiful', especially when she was young.[19] He remembered that his mother rarely left the house and, as the years went by, she became a virtual recluse:

> By the time I was 19 or 20, she would go out only furtively, claiming that all the neighbours were talking about 'the life I was leading'. I later learned that this was that I was a homosexual . . .[20]

He also observed that she was anti-Semitic.[21] He recalled that his mother had informed him that her sister, Mysie, was not her 'real' sister but had been adopted by the family. His mother forbade him to touch Mysie. She claimed that her sister had poison inside her and pus coming out her ears. This unhappy state had resulted, she stated, because, at the age of eight, her sister had gone into the house of a 'Jew' and picked up a 'germ'. It was only years later that Laing discovered that none of this was true and that it was, as Mysie told him, just 'another of your mother's stories'.[22] In *Wisdom, Madness and Folly*, Laing located his mother's anti-Semitism in the context of the Glasgow of the times, when negative attitudes to Jewish people were commonplace.[23] Laing wondered if she was actually partly Jewish, as he, himself, was sometimes taken for being Jewish.[24] Perhaps his mother's anti-Semitism was a reaction to being a Jew? Despite these early anti-Semitic influences, in later life Laing was to engage whole-heartedly with the Jewish philosophical and religious tradition, both through books and personal friendships.

Laing thought his mother could be a 'very tricky person' in the way she communicated with him.[25] Years later, in *The Self and Others*, when discussing how parents could give their offspring contradictory messages—the so-called 'double bind'—he used an actual childhood encounter with his mother as an example of this phenomenon, though at this stage he rendered it anonymously.[26] William James and Sigmund Freud had both given anonymized accounts of their personal experiences in their books, so Laing was participating in an established tradition.

Laing's relationship with his father, whom he was to describe as 'one of the purest spirits I have ever come across', was more positive.[27] David Laing was an electrical engineer with Glasgow Corporation, and he and Ronald shared a passion for music.

[17] MS Laing K1. Elements for an Autobiography, p. 64.

[18] Ibid., p. 11.

[19] Ibid., p. 28.

[20] Ibid., p. 29.

[21] Ibid., p. 28.

[22] Ibid., p. 9.

[23] Laing, *Wisdom, Madness and Folly*, pp. 65–6.

[24] MS Laing K1. Elements for an Autobiography, p. 28.

[25] Laing, *Wisdom, Madness and Folly*, p. 42.

[26] Laing, R.D. (1961). *The Self and Others*. Tavistock, London, pp. 160–2.

[27] Laing, *Wisdom, Madness and Folly*, p. 83.

Laing remembered as a school boy showing all his homework essays to his father and receiving 'constructive criticism'.[28] He also records having many discussions with his father about religion and music. When Laing was in his late adolescence, his father suffered a nervous breakdown, brought on by worries about his work.[29] His superior, a man named Inglis, was about to retire and David was in line for his post. However, he started to think that Inglis would block his promotion and constantly spoke about him in a critical manner. Laing said to him that he thought he was really talking about his father, 'Old Pa', rather than his colleague. Laing observed: '*He's* the one you've always said prevented you getting on.'[30] Laing recalled that this was probably his first 'interpretation' and that his father was later to thank him for helping to 'clear his fevered brain'.[31] In *Wisdom, Madness and Folly*, Laing gave a more elaborate account. Here he stated that his father considered that Inglis, who was a Christian Scientist, was hostile because he thought David was an atheist. In his autobiography Laing expanded on his 'interpretation'. As well as making reference to David's 'Old Pa', he also referred to the 'Old Pa in the sky', i.e. God.[32] Laing commented that his father was his first 'patient'. He portrays himself as instinctively grasping the psychoanalytic notion of transference, whereby an individual displaces on to another person ideas and emotions derived from previous figures in their life.[33] Not only this, but his first 'patient' improved and was able to return to work and gain promotion. Laing states that he was in his last year of school when his father had his breakdown,[34] whereas Burston maintains it occurred a little later when Laing was in his first year at medical school.[35] Whatever the exact date of the episode, Laing emerges from his account as precocious, sensitive, and therapeutically effective. However, elsewhere in his autobiography he claims that he was familiar with Freud by his mid-teens,[36] which rather undermines his picture of himself as stumbling upon psychoanalytic techniques intuitively rather than by reading about them.

Laing recalled that neither of his parents were great readers. His mother read nothing and the only book he could recall his father reading was *Religion without Revelation* by Julian Huxley.[37] Laing remembered his early years, during which he spent his time indoors, looking at his grandmother's encyclopaedia. It had many reproductions of paintings of historic events. It gave him a 'pictorial map of world history'. He also learnt that 'the early inhabitants of the British Isles were represented as civilised . . . tho North of the border, they were pretty uncouth'.[38] Laing vividly remembered *The*

[28] MS Laing K1, p. 34.

[29] Ibid., p. 63. Laing, *Wisdom, Madness and Folly*, pp. 83–4.

[30] MS Laing K1, p. 63.

[31] Ibid., p. 63.

[32] Laing, *Wisdom, Madness and Folly*, pp. 83–4.

[33] Rycroft, C. (1995). *Critical Dictionary of Psychoanalysis*. Penguin Books, London, pp. 185–6.

[34] Laing, *Wisdom, Madness and Folly*, p. 82.

[35] Burston, *The Wing of Madness*, p. 17.

[36] Laing, *Wisdom, Madness and Folly*, p. 71.

[37] MS Laing K1. Elements for an Autobiography, p. 52.

[38] Ibid., p. 24.

World's Library of Best Books, which contained extracts from literature from different countries:

> By no means world literature, but it gave me my first and still vivid impression of the face of Tolstoy, Raskolnikov being surprised in the street by 'Murderer' hissed in his ear, a wild heath, the Trojan Horse, Hansel and Gretel before an oven, Ondine, The Water Babies, The Mad Hatter's Tea Party, Excalibur disappearing back into the lake, The death of Chatterton, Rolland blowing his horn, Cyrano de Bergerac with long nose and sword drawn, the face of Voltaire, blind Homer, Socrates drinking hemlock—all these before I was 5 . . . I got my father and mother to tell me what the scenes were, but I could read a little by the time I was four.[39]

The World's Library of Best Books obviously made a profound impact on Laing, as he kept at least three of the volumes of the series for the rest of his life and they are to be found in his personal library, now housed at Glasgow University.[40] The extract mentions many literary characters and themes that were to be important to Laing in his later life. Thus we find reference to Raskolnikov, the anti-hero of Dostoyevsky's *Crime and Punishment*, a novel that Laing was to draw on in his second book, *The Self and Others*. There is reference to Greek history, literature, and philosophy, all of which shaped Laing's later development. For example, Laing set up the Socratic debating club when he was at university and he himself was to be compared to a Socratic 'gladfly' by his colleague, Leon Redler.[41] Laing used Homer's depiction of Hades to evoke the plight of the 1950s psychiatric patient stranded in a back ward of a Glasgow asylum. The stories of *Hansel and Gretel* and *The Water Babies* may have represented to Laing early versions of how children could be subjected to the cruelty of adults. He himself was to complain of the emotional abuse he experienced as a child and, as a clinician, he was alive to the torments of family life. The Mad Hatter's Tea Party, of course, would have interested a man who was to devote his life to trying to understand disturbed mental states, and indeed a copy of Lewis Carroll's two *Alice* books are to be found in Laing's library. Carroll's fascination with language and its power to mislead was also a subject with which the adult Laing was to wrestle during his psychiatric career. The image by Henry Wallis of the suicide of the teenage poet, Thomas Chatterton, prefigured Laing's later interest in the Romantic concept of the tortured artist whose sensitivity rendered him too precious for this world. Laing also mentioned other Romantic heroes: the doomed Roland, whose pride prevented him sounding his horn in time to be rescued; Cyrano de Bergerac, whose appearance made him an outsider; King Alfred, whose superiority was symbolized by his sword, Excalibur, which only he could use; and King Lear whose madness was enacted on a 'wild heath'. Voltaire, the Enlightenment thinker and merciless critic of the abuses of the *ancien regime*, and Tolstoy, who wrote about his moral and spiritual crisis, completed Laing's list.

---

[39] Ibid., p. 25.

[40] Glasgow University Library Special Collections 1892–1894. Whitten, W. (ed.) (1924–1925). *The World's Library of Best Books*. G. Newnes, London.

[41] Quoted in Mullan, B. (1999). *R.D. Laing: A Personal View*. Duckworth, London, p. 196. Bill Fulford has also compared Laing to a Socratic gadfly.

Laing's 'first existential crisis' occurred when he was a child and his parents told him that Santa Claus did not exist.[42] Laing returned to this event repeatedly in his writing and it is obvious that it had a deep effect on him. Why did this event, which most children from Laing's background would have experienced and which is often viewed as a minor rite of passage, have such an effect on him? He comments:

> I had loved an illusion, a delusion, a near hallucination I had been induced to believe by them . . . In how many other ways is my mind still under the spell of my own unnoticed socially conditioned assumptions? The ferocious dedication to the Truth bred on sheer fear, as much as love of a truth. I was terrified by being deceived, of deceiving myself. For, if I was, I could only feel, I was wasting my time.[43]

But Laing was also to discover that he, too, could lie. In *The Divided Self*, in an eloquent passage that greatly impressed Elaine Showalter[44] because of its unemphatic allusions to Kierkegaard and Defoe, he writes:

> We may remember how, in childhood, adults at first were able to look right through us, and into us, and what an accomplishment it was when we, in fear and trembling, could tell our first lie, and make, for ourselves, the discovery that we are irredeemably alone in certain respects, and know that within the territory of ourselves there can be only our footprints.[45]

School days

On 2 May 1932 Laing started attending Sir John Neilson Cuthbertson Public School.[46] Laing admitted that from the first day of school he was 'intensely competitive', though he calculated from the start in which fields to be competitive.[47] The six best pupils were identified and rewarded by being allowed to sit in the front row of the class. Laing learnt an early lesson in elitism which fuelled his innate tendencies in that direction. He observed that only the top six pupils 'really counted', while the rest of the class were 'largely ignored' by the teachers.[48] He recalled: 'I was still the youngest in the class, and all thro' school, was always very proud of being in the top six in class, and the youngest.'[49] Being the youngest continued to be important to Laing well into his adult life, for example in his autobiography he emphasizes that he was the youngest person to be appointed as a senior registrar.[50] And, as part of this race with time, Laing was determined to have his first book published before he was 30 years old.

---

[42] Laing, A., *A Biography*, p. 24.
[43] MS Laing A662. Draft notes.
[44] Showalter, *The Female Malady*, p. 228.
[45] Laing, R.D. (1960). *The Divided Self: A Study of Sanity and Madness*. Tavistock Publications, London, p. 38.
[46] Laing, A., *A Biography*, p. 25.
[47] MS Laing K1, Elements for an Autobiography, p. 41.
[48] Ibid., p. 41.
[49] Ibid., pp. 25–6.
[50] Laing, *Wisdom, Madness and Folly*, p. 135.

Laing was a clever child, and his parents were ambitious that he do well. On 26 June 1936 he left Cuthbertson's[51] and was enrolled at Hutchesons' Grammar School, an experience upon which he looked back with affection.[52] Laing studied English, mathematics, Greek, Latin, geography, history, drawing, and gymnastics. According to his son, Adrian, 'The curriculum included the pre-Socratic philosophers, Homer, Sophocles, Euripides, Aeschylus, Ovid, St Augustine, St Francis of Assisi, Plato, Aristotle, the lives of the Roman emperors, the Cynics and Sceptics, Plotinus and the fathers of Catholic and Protestant thought.'[53] Laing's best subjects were Greek, Latin, English, and history.[54] Laing was later to complain that modern literature with the exception of T.S. Eliot's 'The Wasteland' was not mentioned at school.[55] His competitive spirit continued at Hutchesons'. He admitted that two of his friends at the time found his need to win or be top of the class rather demeaning.[56]

A precocious youth, Laing extended his knowledge by voraciously reading through the collection of the local Govanhill public library. He claimed that he had worked his way from A to Z of the library collection and that, by the age of 15 he had read Voltaire, Marx, Nietzsche, Kierkegaard, and Freud.[57] In this boast, Laing was presenting himself as a Hero, but this time with a Scottish colouring. In Scottish culture there is the myth of the 'lad o' pairts', an individual from a lowly background who betters himself through hard work and education.[58] A complementary Glaswegian version, and one rooted in the working-class socialist movement, is the phenomenon of the 'autodidact' who receives little in the way of formal education but who, nevertheless, acquires intellectual knowledge through his own reading. Laing, of course, received formal education, but, by virtue of his reading, he roamed far outside the official curricula of school and, later, university. The down side to being an autodidact is intellectual isolation: although such an individual may bring an original and fresh approach to a subject, he or she may be vulnerable to misunderstanding it. Academic discipline may stifle thought, but it may also guide and enlarge it. Some have claimed that Laing would have benefited from academic instruction in philosophy.[59]

During his time at Hutchesons', Laing joined the school debating society and he also became involved in Christian meetings. In 1940 an alliance of Christian organizations, the Crusaders, Scripture Union, and Covenanters, started up at the school. Three years later, half of Laing's form had been converted, leaving only, as he put it, 'the hardened sinners, degenerates, Jews, unredeemed, unsaved'.[60] Laing wryly observed that the Grace of God operated most intensely through the summer camps that ran for two

[51] Laing, A., *A Biography*, p. 26.
[52] MS Laing K1. Elements for an Autobiography, p. 33.
[53] Laing, A., *A Biography*, p. 29.
[54] Ibid., p. 32.
[55] MS Laing K1. Elements for an Autobiography, p. 53.
[56] Ibid., p. 42.
[57] Laing, *Wisdom, Madness and Folly*, p. 71.
[58] Lynch, M. (ed.) (2001). *The Oxford Companion to Scottish History*. Oxford University Press, Oxford, pp. 612–14.
[59] His friend Walter Fyfe is quoted as saying this in Laing, A., *A Biography*, p. 34.
[60] MS Laing K1, p. 43.

weeks. These involved prayer meetings, bible study, and gathering every evening to sing hymns and listen to an account of the life of Jesus. The evening gathering was taken by a Mr Meiklejohn, whom Laing remembers as 'a fat little bachelor of about 30'.[61] In his sermon he tried to convert the boys. Laing remembers his words:

> He died to save you. You may realize that, or not. Even if you do, it is exclusively by the Grace of God. You may give thanks, and in giving thanks, realize that it is by God's Grace alone, that you are giving thanks, that you have realized that you, a sinner . . . search your heart, and you *know* you are—think of your parents, what they have done for you, and what have *you* done for *them*—they sent you to school, you didn't—God gave you your brain, you didn't—nothing you have is yours, it is given you, as a sacred trust, for God, to glorify him, praise the Lord—that you, a sinner have been saved, WASHED clean . . .[62]

Laing was 'converted' in the second year. He read his Scripture Union literature each day, attended bible class, and prayed night and morn. He didn't feel 'saved' but wanted to believe he was. He began to have doubts and a Christian circular sent to the 'older boys' about the perils of dancing increased his unease. Laing recounts the contents of the circular:

> As for dancing, some boys may argue that it was a healthy innocent pleasure. But any boy, if honest, must admit that 'modern' dancing, if not Scottish Country Dancing, was under-taken, *partly at least,* to achieve physical closeness, if not actual bodily contact, with a *girl.* In all forms of modern dancing, the right arm is placed by the boy round the girl, and this may lead . . . to the upper part of the girl's chest coming into contact with that of the boy. Other parts of the body may also, even inadvertently, on a crowded dance floor, or at a party, be brought into physical contact. Can any Christian, who knows that Jesus Christ hung on the Cross for his sins, still engage in the practice of ballroom dancing?[63]

Unsurprisingly, and despite the admonitions of Christian authority, Laing was desperate to find out about 'the facts of life'. He recalled:

> I tried looking up the Encyclopedia Britannica in the local library under Sex, with extreme embarrassment, and sat so that no one would see what page I was reading. When I got there I discovered the page which I wanted to read had been so worn that it was thinned down and worn down and was illegible.[64]

Laing eventually left the Christian organization when he was 16.

As a child Laing had showed great musical ability and, from the age of ten, was thought to have perfect pitch. He practised the piano every evening, and one of his biographers, John Clay imagines Laing playing Chopin and Liszt, the music drifting through the open window down into the street, where homeward workers would pause 'in their dirty clothes, listening almost shamefaced to the exquisite music coming from above'.[65] Laing was elected a Licentiate of the Royal Academy of Music in 1944

---

[61] Ibid., p. 43.

[62] Ibid., p. 44.

[63] Ibid., pp. 48–9.

[64] MS Laing A343. A Diary: A Personal Journey: Conception to Birth, page A.

[65] Clay, *R.D. Laing*, p. 16.

and was made an Associate of the Royal College of Music the following year.[66] There was even some debate that he might follow a career in music, but his parents felt it offered an uncertain future.

Laing decided to study medicine. This crucial decision was based on a variety of factors and Laing typically gave more than one account of the thinking behind it. For example, in one version, Laing recalled:

> When I was 14 I remember being asked, at my grandfather's birthday party, what I wanted to be and I said I wanted to be a Theologian, a Psychologist and a Philosopher. When I was asked what these terms meant I was extremely embarrassed because I wasn't able to say what they meant . . .[67]

In another account of the factors behind his choice of medicine, Laing emphasized the mystical tradition of Christianity and the equation of knowledge with spiritual development:

> I suppose I was in love with knowledge. I was reading Plato then for the first time and realised that this love of knowledge could be a means of liberating the soul. I guess at the time it took the form of a sort of Neoplatonic Christianity . . . I decided to do medicine because it would give me access to birth and death.[68]

He made these comments in 1972 and Burston has been struck that when Laing returned to this subject in his 1985 autobiography, he did not mention Neoplatonic Christianity. Of course Laing made these comments at the height of his guru-hood when gurus were expected to make references to hidden knowledge. That is not to say that Laing was being insincere. His early writings do indeed demonstrate his acquaintance with the work of Plato and his followers, and throughout his life he remained preoccupied and perturbed by spiritual matters. Perhaps a simpler explanation is that there were many factors that led to Laing's choice of medicine as a career. For example, in yet another account of the subject, Laing contrasted the study of medicine, which required attendance at university, with that of philosophy and psychology, which he felt demanded a 'personal apprenticeship'. He wrote:

> It was one of the things approved by my parents, and to me it offered entry into the secret rituals of birth, and death, and would give me access to sexual knowledge. Besides there seemed no point in studying anything that was really important like philosophy or psychology in a University curriculum. These things were matters of personal apprenticeship and I did not know of any master philosopher or psychologist teaching at a University in Britain, and my personal horizons had not stretched beyond the shores of the British Isles . . . I couldn't imagine Dostoyevsky studying literature at a University, or any great writer. But I could imagine such a person studying medicine.[69]

---

[66] Laing, A., *A Biography*, p. 33.
[67] MS Laing A343. A Diary: A Personal Journey: Conception to Birth.
[68] Mezan, P. (1972) After Freud and Jung, Now Comes R.D. Laing. *Esquire*, **77**, 92–7, 160–78.
[69] MS Laing K1. Elements for an Autobiography, p. 65.

Medical school

In his autobiography, Laing wrote:

> Medicine fell into place. If I went into medicine I would learn to be scientific. I would be addressing myself to real physical, material reality—birth, death, disease, pain—and to real social realities—poverty and pestilence—and within the warps in the brain I might find the cause of the warps in the mind.[70]

Laing left Hutchesons' in 1945 to study medicine at Glasgow University. There were over 200 students in each year, of whom about a fifth were female.[71] He remembered that he was disconcerted that some of the students came from the fifth form and were therefore younger than him, as he had left after sixth year. He was used to being one of the youngest and did not like this change in his situation. However he consoled himself that, by this stage, he had 'developed a time table for my life, which was on quite a different level'.[72] Professor Stanley Alstead, who was Regius Professor of Materia Medica at Glasgow University during Laing's time there, remembers being struck by the philosophical attitude of the teachers. They had a tendency to question and discuss issues rather than make authoritarian pronouncements.[73]

Eighteen months after becoming a medical student, Laing observed: 'I, like many others, came to the varsity with no grounding whatsoever in science. I've been learning as it were the grammar of science. So the most fundamental facts & theories of biology were largely new to me . . . and their impact on me . . . was sharp and challenging'.[74] Crossley has suggested that Laing was unique amongst his peers in not being exposed to science subjects at school, though, in fact, many other medical students in Scotland were in a similar position.[75] In his second year Laing attended meetings organized by Professor Hamilton of the Anatomy Department. Students were invited to present a short 'scientific' paper. Laing presented two papers.[76] One was an account of Joseph Needham's early contributions to embryology, with some of his own thoughts on the theory of 'organizers'. Laing remembered that the theory 'excited' him 'enormously' as it seemed to provide a 'genuine systemic approach to hard biological experimentation'.[77]

He recalled that Professor Hamilton complimented him on his presentation and Laing asked him if he thought that he had the makings of a scientist. Hamilton replied

---

[70] Laing, *Wisdom, Madness and Folly*, p. 72.

[71] Hunter-Brown, I. (2007). *R.D. Laing and Psychodynamic Psychiatry in 1950s Glasgow: A Reappraisal*. Free Association Books, London, p. 59.

[72] MS Laing K1, Elements for an Autobiography, pp. 25–6.

[73] Greater Glasgow Health Board Archive HB74/1/1. Professor Stanley Alstead interviewed by Dr McKenzie.

[74] MS Laing A519. Impressions of a second-year medical student: a paper delivered to the Glasgow University Medico-Chirurgical Society, January 1947.

[75] Crossley, N. (1998). 'R.D. Laing and the British anti-psychiatry movement: a socio-historical analysis'. *Social Science and Medicine*, **47**, 877–89.

[76] MS Laing A662, Draft Notes.

[77] Ibid.

that he thought that Laing had but that his chosen field of psychiatry would provide him with many difficulties. In a retrospective comment on this episode, Laing, in somewhat melodramatic language, wrote: '. . . at the time I did not know what agonies my scientific soul was going to go through in the purgatory awaiting it'.[78] On a more prosaic but pressing matter, Professor Hamilton pointed out to Laing that although he had scored 95% in embryology, he had only scored 48% in gross adult anatomy. He advised Laing to improve his performance. In the event, Laing failed his anatomy, physiology, and biochemistry second year examinations.[79] He recalled that he worked hard in first year studying physics, botany, zoology, and chemistry, even though he had no interest in them. He blamed his failure on not having studied science at school.[80] He also admitted that he had miscalculated how much he needed to study in order to pass. His parents were very upset. They said he had been living an 'irregular life' and staying up too late. His mother couldn't face the neighbours and his father was ashamed to go to the office.

Laing recalls:

> For the first time, as I sat listening to and looking at their reactions to the terrible news, they sickened me. I realized that to a great extent that I had been miserable for years, not just passing those endless bloody exams, but trying to be first, or get a distinction. Why? So that they would be proud of me. Or, as in running, to hear the cheers of the crowd. I hadn't been interested in Greek irregular verbs, Plutarch's bloody lives, the divisions of the brachial complex, or whether nerve impulses went forward or backward. Or whatever interest, I had been and was being well throttled, suffocated under the fear of failing, this need to succeed, in order to get thro that little wicket gate. And then into what? I had been a willing lamb trundling along into the pen, for my own slaughter. When would it end?[81]

Laing repeatedly referred back to his medical days in his later writing. In *The Bird of Paradise*, he described an episode in the anatomy dissecting room which may or may not have been apocryphal. On the last day, having completed the dissection of the bodies, the students began to throw the dissected organs about. They were seen by the professor who condemned them: 'You should be ashamed of yourselves,' he thundered; 'how do you expect them to sort themselves out on the Day of Judgement?'[82]

In *The Bird of Paradise*,[83] Laing mentions a young mother of two who was dying of cancer. He describes the desensitized nature of the clinicians and medical students who were intent on finding a diagnosis rather than on how the condition was affecting the patient. They were disappointed that she died before they could make a definitive diagnosis but were cheered that there was always the post-mortem to look forward to. Laing also comments that the time spent on the patient had made them miss their lunch. Laing described his gruesome experiences in the maternity unit in Dublin. One birth

---

[78] Ibid.

[79] MS Laing R34. University of Glasgow, Faculty of Medicine. Certificate on Laing.

[80] MS Laing K1. Elements for an Autobiography, p. 64.

[81] Ibid., p. 66.

[82] Laing, R.D. (1967). *The Politics of Experience and The Bird of Paradise*. Penguin, Harmondsworth, pp. 144–5.

[83] Ibid., pp. 142–4.

gave rise to 'an anencephalic monster, no neck, no head, with eyes, nose, froggy mouth, long arms'.[84] Laing continues the story:

> Maybe it was slightly alive. We didn't want to know. We wrapped it in newspaper—and with this bundle under my arm to take back to the pathology lab., that seemed to cry out for all the answerable answers that I ever asked. I walked along O'Connell Street two hours later.
>
> I needed a drink. I went into a pub, put the bundle on the bar. Suddenly the desire, to unwrap it, hold it up for all to see, a ghastly Gorgon's head, to turn the world to stone.[85]

In *Wisdom, Madness and Folly*, Laing described a surgical operation—a mid-thigh amputation—performed without anaesthetic. It left the patient screaming and he subsequently died. Laing records: 'However shocking such things are, I could "take" them. Life has to go on'.[86] But there were other types of suffering which Laing felt 'went beyond all reason and struck terror right into my bone marrow'.[87] He described the case of a man with myositis ossificans progressiva, whose muscles were slowly turning to bone. He was slowly asphyxiating as his respiratory muscles turned to bone. Laing records:

> I was horrified and terrified. It was a genetic condition. It could not be put down to human error, in any obvious way to human evil. These terrible diseases I saw turned me totally against any God who was supposed to be omnipotent and good. If He were omnipotent how could He be good if He were responsible for the creation of such suffering? I could tell myself that only through the very spirit of love, our Holy Spirit, or in John Wycliffe's translation our Healthy Spirit, God incarnate in us, could I feel such outrage. Maybe God couldn't help it. But then how could He be omnipotent? I told myself that this was all human reasoning: that God, if He existed, must be infinitely beyond the paltry projections of my idealized conception of my own ideals. I was terrified of Him if He existed, and terrified if He did not. Life was a ghastly joke. We were the joke, but I could not see it. Or else it signified nothing. I could not forget, or go beyond the conflict. And it would not somehow or other melt away.[88]

At the end of first year, medical students paid a traditional visit to the Royal Gartnavel Mental Hospital. In *Wisdom, Madness and Folly*, Laing recalls seeing Dr Angus MacNiven, the Medical Superintendent, interviewing a patient in the main hall.[89] Laing was later to work under MacNiven as a junior doctor, and the older psychiatrist was to prove to be a great support to him and also a great influence. Here Laing describes his first impressions of MacNiven:

> I came in late. There were two men on the stage sitting on chairs, having a chat. One of them, in impeccable dress, with a cheerful flower in his buttonhole, sat with composure and assurance, talked fluently with the other man, who had his legs twisted round each

---

84 Ibid., p. 146.

85 Ibid., pp. 146–7.

86 Laing, *Wisdom, Madness and Folly*, p. 81.

87 Ibid., p. 81.

88 Ibid., p. 81.

89 Ibid., pp. 81–2.

other, grimaced, stammered, fidgeted, all but picked his nose, and wriggled around in his chair.

It was not until that interview ended, when the patient got up, gave a bow and left the stage that I realized that Dr MacNiven was the man I had taken to be the patient.[90]

Laing was in fact very impressed with the interview as it seemed to him that it was conducted on an equal footing. He commented: 'It was a very decent interview. It sounded like two old friends talking about the hospital, the changes they had seen.' This event gave Laing an early demonstration of how the patient could be treated as a person, or, as he put it, a 'companion'.[91] He later told the anecdote to MacNiven who found it very amusing.

In his fourth year, Laing attended his first psychiatric 'clinical demonstration', an event which he writes about in *The Facts of Life*.[92] This was to be a much less positive experience than that at Gartnavel. He remembers sitting with about two dozen medical students on the tiered benches of a small amphitheatre in the Glasgow Western Infirmary. Below them, the consultant interviewed a series of patients. The first patient was a 'thin, pale, bespectacled chap of seventeen, with marked acne'. He had been referred by his general practitioner for 'psychosomatic' treatment of his skin condition. Laing was clearly appalled at the manner in which the consultant interviewed him. Within minutes he was asking the patient very personal questions, as Laing records:

Consultant and what is your complaint, apart from your acne, which we can all see?
Patient I'm afraid people are looking at me in the street
Consultant you are afraid they know you masturbate
Patient (His white face turned scarlet, and his red pimples went white) yes
Consultant how often do you masturbate?
Patient two or three times a week

Laing recalls that this was the first time he had heard the word 'masturbate' used in public. He 'cringed in terror' at the prospect of the consultant asking the medical students the same questions that he had asked the patient. Whether or not this was an entirely accurate account of events, such 'clinical demonstrations' were a common method of teaching, and they were certainly a source of discomfort and distress to the unfortunate patient on display. Laing was very sensitive to the perspective of the patient, and in *The Divided Self*, he exposed what he saw as the essential inhumanity of such a procedure when he described the eminent German professor, Emil Kraepelin giving a clinical demonstration to a class of students. Interestingly in his second book, *The Self and Others*, Laing devoted a whole chapter to the subject of masturbation and noted that psychiatric textbooks used to advise that it led to mental illness.

---

[90] Ibid., p. 82.
[91] Ibid., p. 126.
[92] Laing, *The Facts of Life*, pp. 84–5.

Laing's first encounter with actually interviewing psychiatric patients himself was in the wards of the Psychiatric Unit in Duke Street Hospital under Dr Sclare.[93] In his autobiography, Laing describes only one patient he met as a student.[94] He does not present the event in dramatic terms. It does not seem to have been a Road to Damascus experience that suddenly made him decide to become a psychiatrist; nor did the patient have exotic symptomatology. Rather, it was the fact that the case was 'so typical'. For Laing, it encapsulated the 'nuclear problems of psychiatry': it was an everyday clinical problem, but it was, nevertheless, perplexing. He describes the case of a thin, middle-aged, married man, who presented in a state of 'catatonic immobility'. While conceding that such conditions were no longer common, Laing describes the patient's presentation in such a way to suggest that there was no easy explanation for it. He asks rhetorically if it was the result of disordered neurochemistry; but he also asks if there was a religious explanation, or was the patient just pretending? In this, Laing reveals three themes that preoccupied him throughout his psychiatric career: the limitations of exclusively biological explanations of disturbed mental states; the role of spiritual factors; and the phenomenon of lying or malingering and whether it was possible to detect it when it happened. Laing was awarded a first class merit certificate in mental diseases.[95] The only other certificate he gained during his student days was a second class one in dermatology.

As a medical student, Laing became fascinated with hypnosis. He formed an interest group with three other students and they met regularly over the course of three years to discuss theory and hypnotize each other.[96] Alongside his medical studies, Laing continued his exploration of religion, philosophy, literature, and music, as well as drinking and meeting women. He was friendly with George MacLeod who was the founder and leader of the Iona Community, a Christian project in which Laing participated.[97] The Community set out to rebuild the Abbey Monastery on Iona and it also trained young men to work in industrial areas of Scotland. MacLeod emphasized the role of the congregation, rather than relying on a single preacher. He described himself as 'an uncomfortable socialist and a reluctant pacifist'.[98] He went on to become Moderator of the General Assembly of the Church of Scotland in May 1957.

During his time at university, Laing set up the Socratic Club.[99] The purpose was to 'bring together people from all walks of life and persuasions to discuss issues which troubled him intellectually'.[100] Hugh MacDiarmid was invited and Bertrand Russell was asked to be President, a role which he accepted.[101] Isobel Hunter-Brown, who had

[93] Laing, *Wisdom, Madness and Folly*, p. 85.

[94] Ibid., pp. 85–7.

[95] MS Laing R34. University of Glasgow, Faculty of Medicine. Certificate on Laing.

[96] MS Laing A662.

[97] Laing, A., *A Biography*, p. 35.

[98] Ferguson, R. (1990). *George MacLeod: Founder of the Iona Community*. Collins, London. MacLeod, G. (1958). *Only One Way Left*. Iona Community, Glasgow, which gives information about MacLeod on front free end paper.

[99] Laing, A., *A Biography*, p. 37.

[100] Ibid., p. 38.

[101] Clay, *R.D. Laing*, p. 27.

enrolled as a medical student at Glasgow three years after Laing, was a member of the Socratic Club. She recalled, that at this stage of his career, Laing was courteous to the other participants and 'was even then a charismatic figure'.[102] According to Clay, Laing found time to attend some lectures on philosophy,[103] and he also possessed a book of lecture notes on philosophy for students by C.A. Campbell of the Glasgow University Philosophy Department. One of his friends, and fellow medical student at the time, James Hood, has left an affectionate memoir of Laing, whom he described as 'one of the three most talented and probably the most intelligent and entertaining of all the men I have ever met':[104]

> To his medical peer group in Glasgow Laing showed himself an extraordinarily gifted musician, scholar and discussant . . . He introduced us to psychoanalysis. In a population still heavily influenced by puritan values, and by highly respectable civic expectations, his behavioural example, and the range of his mind were exhilarating.[105]

Hood also remembers the young Laing as a 'combination of Groucho and Chico Marx', and that he was an 'outrageously outspoken, mischievous, and funny man'.[106] He also 'played piano like an angel' and was to be found in the Men's Student Union coffee room, playing classical music, as well as jazz, blues, and Boogie-Woogie to an admiring audience.[107] Hood writes:

> Laing's speaking voice, with his rich educated Glasgow accent, showed a remarkable range of pitch and timbre, bringing to mind, highly esteemed preachers of the Protestant faith . . . Laing's everyday self-presentation was modest, and he was neither shy nor unduly loquacious. He was always willing to listen to what the other person had to say. When engaged with a person or subject that interested him, he became animated, persistently thoughtful, and probing.[108]

Hood recalls that Laing had been drinking more heavily than his fellow students since at least the age of 18. Where they were reluctant to venture outside the university bars, Laing went to more working-class establishments. Interestingly, Laing was brought up in a fairly abstemious household. He recalled that, when he was a child, no alcohol was permitted in the house, although at New Year, his father had a glass of sweet sherry and his mother had a glass of elderberry wine.[109] Laing had told the young and obviously impressed Hood that he was sexually experienced, having seduced or been seduced by one of his music teachers when he was 16 years old.

---

[102] Hunter-Brown, *R.D. Laing*, p. 59.

[103] Clay, *R.D. Laing*, p. 31.

[104] Hood, J. (2001). 'The young R.D. Laing: a personal memoir and some hypotheses'. In Steiner, R. and Johns, J. (eds). *Within Time & Beyond Time: A Festschrift for Pearl King*. Karnac, London, pp. 39–53.

[105] Ibid., p. 40.

[106] Ibid., pp. 42–3.

[107] Ibid., p. 43.

[108] Ibid., p. 43.

[109] MS Laing K4. Autobiographical notes, c. 1970.

Laing was also a member of the university mountaineering club, which explored the West Highlands. His closest companion there was Douglas Hutchison, a fellow medical student. Hood remembers that Laing was 'devastated' some years later when Hutchison died in a mountaineering accident in January 1959. His wife was eight and half months pregnant with their first child.[110] Hutcheson was described by Hood as Laing's 'soul-mate, and primary male confidant'. He had exercised a restraining influence on Laing's more reckless behaviour and Hood believes that his death was to mark a turning point in Laing's life. He agrees with the remark of Adrian Laing, that when his father's friend died, 'something died in Ronald'.[111] Laing himself was to say, 'In Douglas's death I have lost my brother.'[112] Curiously, in *Wisdom, Madness and Folly*, Laing does not mention this major episode in his life. Was it too painful to recount? Or was Laing reluctant to admit that he relied on others?

The mountaineering expeditions provided Laing with the opportunity to bring along his non-student friends, such as John Duffy. Hood observes that Ronnie was amused to have his working-class acquaintances mix with what he felt was the 'puritanical bourgeoisie'.[113] However, they all got on well: singing sessions would ensue and Scottish ballads would feature heavily in the repertoire. Interestingly, Hood felt that Laing's Scottish background and culture were crucial elements in his later development:

> . . . lowland Scots historical traditions were an all-important source of Laing's intense emotionality and defiantly individual stance among his elders and his English-speaking and North American public. He spoke and sang in the Anglo-Scots and vernacular language and traditions, which found their paramount expression in the poetry and in the original and collected songs of Robert Burns. In a childhood and adolescent milieu characterized by strongly moral Presbyterian religion, Burns's celebratory alcoholic indulgence, anger at man's inhumanity to man, ambivalent conflicted attitude to women, preference for mocking satirical or bawdy humour, and hatred of prissy genteel and 'holier than thou' attitudes were exemplary.[114]

During his days as a medical student, Laing met Marcelle Vincent, an 18-year-old student from the Sorbonne, who was teaching French in Glasgow secondary schools as part of an exchange scheme.[115] Laing had met her one Saturday night at a concert by the Scottish National Orchestra in Saint Andrews Hall. She came from Grenoble and her father had fought in the Resistance. As he recalled: 'She was the first female of the species I had met who had read Kafka, and, indeed, Camus, let alone Rimbaud and Baudelaire.'[116] Laing fell in love with her and after two years they became lovers 'one marvellous April in Paris', when he was 19.[117] The surviving letters between the two

---

[110] MS Laing A505. Glasgow Past and Present. A Personal Memoir by R.D. Laing, p. 51.

[111] Laing, A., *A Biography*, p. 65.

[112] Ibid.

[113] Hood, *The Young R.D. Laing*, p. 45.

[114] Ibid., p. 47.

[115] Clay, *R.D. Laing*, pp. 31–2.

[116] MS Laing A522. Autobiographical sketches. November, 1977.

[117] MS Laing A522. Also Mullan, *R.D. Laing: Creative Destroyer*.

showed that they discussed a wide range of intellectual topics, such as the work of Camus and Sartre, poetry, music, and politics. Laing proposed to her on more than one occasion. Marcelle remained ambivalent and was unsure about settling permanently in Glasgow. She was also disconcerted by Laing's mercurial character and his tendency to nihilism and despair. She herself suffered from bouts of depression and was worried that they would bring each other down.[118] Laing was later to describe the failure of their relationship as 'absolutely heartbreaking',[119] but they remained friends for the rest of Laing's life. As with the loss of Douglas Hutchison, Laing placed little emphasis on his break-up with Marcelle in his published accounts of his life story.

Laing failed all his final examinations and commented later: 'I have never known why.'[120] Writing about the subject some two decades later, he rehearsed the argument he was to employ in *Wisdom, Madness and Folly*, that he had somehow upset the medical establishment. He wrote:

> My guess is that at our Final Year Dinner, I told some of my professors, including the Dean, what a fuck up medical education was, and had the amazing stupidity, being somewhat drunk, to outline my system for passing their exams, whilst knowing nothing about their subjects . . . Perhaps they decided to teach me a lesson.[121]

In his autobiography he gave a more temperate account:

> I've always wondered whether my failure might have had something to do with our Final Year Dinner, when, sitting with the professors at the top of the table, as an after dinner speaker, I drank too much whiskey, claret and port, and expressed far too candidly, what I felt about a few things in medicine.[122]

For someone as competitive as Laing, the exam failure must have been a terrible blow, and it is perhaps not surprising that he sought refuge in constructing a conspiracy theory to explain his downfall. It also lent an air of drama to his story. However, the reason for Laing's failure may have been more prosaic. As a result of all his extra-curricular activities, perhaps he simply did not expend enough time on his studies. Contemporaries of Laing who talked to Daniel Burston certainly favoured this explanation rather the conspiratorial one put forward by Laing and they pointed out that outspoken challenges to authority were not all that unusual at Glasgow University during the late 1940s.[123] They felt that Laing was trying to save face and shift the blame for his failure. Clay suggests a psychological explanation. Like his father, who became agitated when faced with the prospect of promotion, was Laing baulking at the last hurdle, fearful of success, or was he subconsciously taking revenge on his mother who was anxious he do well?[124]

---

[118] Burston, *The Wing of Madness*, p. 26.
[119] Mullan, *Mad to be Normal*, p. 76.
[120] MS Laing K1, p. 68.
[121] Ibid., pp. 68–9.
[122] Laing, *Wisdom, Madness and Folly*, pp. 87–8,
[123] Burston, *The Wing of Madness*, p. 27.
[124] Clay, *R.D. Laing*, p. 37.

Laing filled in the next six months while he waited to resit his exams, as a House Physician at the Psychiatric Unit at Stobhill Hospital. The Unit housed about eighty men and women whom Laing remembered as 'the largest surviving colony of devastated survivors of the 1927 epidemic of encephalitis lethargica'.[125] The drug Artane was being introduced and he recalled witnessing patients transformed by it.[126] Despite claims that Laing must have found the day-to-day experience unedifying and would only have been going through the motions in his clinical work,[127] contemporary reports paint a different picture. One of the consultants, Dr Ivy MacKenzie reported that Laing earned the confidence and appreciation of both patients and staff, and spoke highly of his abilities and his erudition.[128] Laing writes about this clinician in *The Facts of Life* in his story of Dr MacKenzie prescribing intra-muscular turpentine injections to men suffering from involuntial melancholia in order to give them an experience of 'hell fire'.[129] Laing claimed that this unusual treatment had a 100% success rate, though one does wonder about the accuracy of the story. It was at Stobhill that he met his future colleague, Aaron Esterson, who was one of the many Jews with whom Laing would discuss his work.

Laing's failure in his final exams caused even greater consternation at home than his failure in second year. He decided to leave the family home. Two days before he was due to resit the final examinations, the family's doctor contacted him to say that his mother was ill. She had eaten very little for some time and was now very thin and weak. She weighed less than five stone. Laing went to see her and found her very pale but 'still very beautiful'.[130] She told him that she loved him more than anything in the world. She wanted him to pass his exam and she had vowed that she would not eat again until she had heard that he had. Laing passed his finals on 13 January 1951 at the age of 23.[131] He observed: 'Never had it been so hard not to fail an exam.'[132] When he was 40, Laing recalled: 'I have been failing examinations for more than the last 17 years in my dreams.'[133]

Beginning as a doctor

In January 1951, Laing began work at the Glasgow and West of Scotland neurosurgical unit at Killearn, near Loch Lomond. At this stage, Laing recalled that his neurological outlook had been formed by the tradition of Hughlings Jackson and Sherrington.

[125] MS Laing K45. Reflections on medical training and the Psychiatric Unit, Stobhill Hospital, Glasgow, c. 1970.

[126] Mullan, *Mad to be Normal*, p. 115. Also MS Laing K45.

[127] Burston, *The Wing of Madness*, p. 28.

[128] Letter to the Secretary, Western Regional Health Board about Laing from Ivy Mackenzie, 6 October 1953.

[129] Laing, *The Facts of Life*, pp. 85–6.

[130] MS Laing K1, p. 69.

[131] MS Laing R34. University of Glasgow, Faculty of Medicine. Certificate on Laing. Laing dates his graduation as 14 February 1951.

[132] MS Laing K1, p. 70.

[133] Ibid., p. 70.

He knew of the theories of Pavlov and he was aware of the work of Lashley and Penfield, which was appearing when he was a medical student. It fascinated and puzzled him.[134] In a notebook entry he remembers:

> Despite being physically on the stretch all the time, and the fact that a neurosurgical unit is no place for armchair speculation about mind and matter, I was in frequently bodily and mental agony at the baffling theoretical problems that were continually being exposed by my day to day, night to night practical work.[135]

Laing's tasks were to perform neurological examinations, put up drips, take blood, do lumbar punctures, and put in canulae through cranial burr holes. In *Wisdom, Madness and Folly*, he describes the case of a 10-year-old boy with hydrocephalus caused by an inoperable brain tumour. He was in terrible pain and Laing's task was to drain fluid from his skull with a long needle twice a day. The boy knew he was dying and asked God to let him finish *The Pickwick Papers* before he died. He died before it was half-finished.[136] In the same book Laing described the case of a 19-year-old circus-horse rider.[137] She and the horse had fallen, and the animal had rolled over her head. She was unconscious for several days, and when she regained consciousness, 'she *was* a horse'. She looked and behaved like a horse, even grazing on grass, naked and on all fours, outside the ward. After a few weeks she became herself again. With Laing, it is difficult to be sure that this is an entirely accurate account of events and how much faulty memory or literary embellishment distorted the picture. Of the circus-horse rider, Laing comments: 'I wanted *desperately* to *understand* this sort of thing.'[138] He goes on to quote Thomas Traherne, the seventeenth-century English mystic and poet, who is credited with being the first person to use the word 'self'.[139] These two examples from his time at Killearn show that, from an early stage, Laing was bringing a literary and religious perspective to his clinical work.

There were three neurosurgical chiefs at the unit in Killearn: Paterson, Robertson, and Schorstein. Laing remembered that there was a 'lobotomy controversy'[140] raging at the time, and, of the three, only Robertson performed the operation, and then only occasionally.[141] One of the neurosurgeons, J. Eric Paterson, wrote a reference for Laing after he left. He said that he had formed a high opinion of him and he described Laing as a 'clever fellow, keenly interested in his work, especially in its psychological aspects, with a brilliant, rather original type of mind'.[142] Burston has suggested that Paterson

[134] MS Laing K45.

[135] Ibid., no page number.

[136] Laing, *Bird of Paradise*, pp. 145–6.

[137] Laing, *Wisdom, Madness and Folly*, p. 94.

[138] Laing, *Wisdom, Madness and Folly*, p. 94.

[139] In 1674 Traherne wrote: 'A secret self I had enclos'd within ,/That was not bounded with my clothes or skin'. As discussed in Hacker PMS (2007). *Human Nature: the Categorical Framework*. Blackwell, Oxford, pp. 237–84.

[140] Laing, *Wisdom, Madness and Folly*, p. 90.

[141] Ibid.

[142] Letter to The Secretary Western Regional Hospital Board from J. Eric Paterson on Laing, 30 September 1953.

had 'scorned Laing's metaphysical vapours', but his comments about Laing do not bear this out.[143] Laing, for his part, remembered Paterson as a good clinician, who also advised him against a career in neurosurgery:

> ... Paterson assured me that I had no instinct for brain surgery though he fully encouraged me in my neurological ambitions. Of course he was right, and I had never seriously entertained the prospect of being a brain surgeon (a carpenter) ... [144]

Joe Schorstein

Joe Schorstein was a leading neurosurgeon, whom Laing was later to describe as 'my spiritual father' and as 'a spiritual intellectual gift from heaven'.[145] Schorstein, the son of a Viennese rabbi, was immersed in European philosophy and helped to further Laing's knowledge of continental thinkers. As Kenneth Collins[146] has shown, Schorstein was crucial to Laing's development. Burston[147] feels he was secondary only to Gregory Bateson in his influence on Laing. According to Adrian Laing, Ronald was closer to Schorstein than he was to his own father.[148] Joseph Schorstein was born in 1909 in Moravia and was the son of a Hassidic Rabbi.[149] He graduated in medicine from the University of Vienna in 1931 and moved to England the following year before the Nazis seized power in Germany. He trained in neurosurgery in Manchester and served as a neurosurgeon in the Royal Army Medical Corps (RAMC) with the British Army during the Second World War. The strain of wartime surgery with its very long hours and dangerous working conditions took its toll on Schorstein and, after the war, he spent time as an inpatient in the Crichton Royal Hospital under the care of Dr Mayer-Gross. Schorstein subsequently took up a post as a neurosurgeon at the West of Scotland Neurosurgical Unit at Killearn. Schorstein was sceptical about scientific and medical advances, describing patients as 'prisoners of progress'.[150] He was concerned that the preoccupation with technological advances meant that the patient as an individual was in danger of being overlooked.

Laing writes of a memorable meeting he had with Schorstein:

> At three o' clock in the morning in the changing room after one operating session that had been going for hours, Joe Schorstein decided to check me out. He proceeded to grill me from Heraclitus and, in between, Kant, Hegel, Nietzsche, Husserl, Heidegger, in very specific detail. The interrogation went on for over two hours before Joe was 'convinced'.

---

[143] Burston, *The Wing of Madness*, p. 29.

[144] MS Laing K4.

[145] MS Laing A531/2. Joe Schorstein.

[146] Collins, K. (2008). 'Joseph Schorstein: R.D. Laing's "rabbi"'. *History of Psychiatry*, **19**(2), 185–201.

[147] Burston, D. (2000). *The Crucible of Experience: R.D. Laing and the Crisis of Psychotherapy.* Harvard University Press, Cambridge, Massachusetts, p. 4.

[148] Laing, A., *A Biography*, p. 45.

[149] Background information on Schorstein is taken from Collins, *Schorstein*.

[150] Collins, *Schorstein*.

Then began a real argument that went on for another two hours. No one, before or since, has put me through such a grinder.[151]

Some[152] have found this account rather melodramatic, and it could certainly be viewed as our Hero, like Hercules, facing up to his first task and emerging triumphant. It could also be seen as the young Laing being selected by a master of arcane philosophy, surviving the initiation rite, and being rewarded with the gift of secret knowledge. As we have seen, Laing was keen to undergo a 'personal apprenticeship' and Schorstein fulfilled the role of 'master philosopher'. Schorstein brought with him a knowledge of and a link to the 'rich Jewish cultural milieu of Central Europe'.[153] He had been acquainted with Buber and Heidegger and kept in touch with Karl Jaspers after he fled from Nazi Europe.[154] Laing described Schorstein as having a desperate religious fight with nihilism, which he saw all around him.[155] He had an impassioned objection to the prevailing epistemological presuppositions of Western science. He did not think that science could solve all the problems of humanity and wrote that to believe that 'a profound knowledge of electronics and neuro-anatomy suffices to give the scientist a superior insight into the meaning and aim of human existence, which is Job's concern, is both arrogant and confused'.[156] Schorstein was worried that science was leading to the manipulation and control of man,[157] and to the denial of his freedom.

Schorstein had come to the conviction that science would eventually wipe out humanity.[158] Such convictions were not uncommon in the post-war period following Hiroshima and Nagasaki, and Laing shared them. We can get an idea of Schorstein's thinking from a paper he wrote, entitled 'The Metaphysics of the Atom Bomb'.[159] It was a meditation on man's alienation from the world. He referred to Heidegger and quoted his statement: 'Since the dreadful has already happened for what awaits this helpless fear.' This was an observation with which Laing was greatly taken and he repeated it in his writing and his conversation.[160] Schorstein's paper also referred to Plato, Hegel, and Jaspers, and there were liberal quotations from poets, such as Holderlin, Rilke, T.S. Eliot, and Yeats. As Marcelle Vincent observed, Laing and

---

[151] Laing, *Wisdom, Madness and Folly*, pp. 91–2.

[152] Collins, *Schorstein*.

[153] Collins, *Schorstein*.

[154] Glasgow University Archive DC 81 295. The impact of existential philosophy on psychology by J. Schorstein. Some idea of Schorstein's acquaintance with the major European figures can be gleaned from his series of lectures on existential philosophy, in which he makes statements like 'Martin Heidegger once said to me' (lecture 1, p. 6).

[155] MS Laing A531/2.

[156] Schorstein, J. (1960). *The Present State of Consciousness*. Penguin Science Survey B, London. Quoted in Collins, *Schorstein*.

[157] During this period the term 'man' was used to describe all of humanity, both male and female. To avoid anachronism, this term will be used throughout the book when it is deemed appropriate to the historical context.

[158] MS Laing A531/2. Joe Schorstein, p. 5.

[159] Schorstein, J. (1964). 'The metaphysics of the atom bomb'. *The Philosophical Journal*, **1**, 33–46.

[160] For example in Laing, *The Politics of Experience*, p. 46.

Schorstein felt isolated from others as a result of their erudition.[161] There were further similarities. Both were musical, both liked drinking, and they were also prone to depression.

Karl Abenheimer

Another influence on Laing at this time was the Jewish émigré Karl Abenheimer. Abenheimer[162] was born in Mannheim in 1898 and graduated in law at Heidelberg. He had studied psychology under Karl Jaspers as early as 1919, and later worked with Frieda Fromm-Reichmann, and also with Jung in Zurich. By October 1936 he had fled to Glasgow where he was recruited to the post of analyst by the Superintendent of Gartavel Royal Mental Hospital, Dr Angus MacNiven. He developed a reputation as a therapist, writer, and lecturer, and was later to become friends with Schorstein. Abenheimer was described by Laing as an existential Jungian psychotherapist.[163] Laing's friendship with Abenheimer and Schorstein made him feel he had been admitted to the living stream of European thought. As Collins[164] has shown, Scotland was the beneficiary of an influx of many Jewish medical refugees from Central Europe during the 1930s and this was to have a major impact on Scottish medicine, especially in psychiatry and psychoanalysis. Émigré European doctors were required to take the final examinations of one of the Royal Colleges of Medicine and Surgery, and whereas the English colleges increased the length of study required to take their examinations, the Scottish ones permitted requalification after one year. Unsurprisingly, most continental doctors made their way to Scotland.

Laing was part of a philosophical discussion group that met regularly in Glasgow. It has sometimes been called the Schorstein or Abenheimer group after the two Jewish members who had settled in Glasgow, but Laing himself said it had no name.[165] He also claimed that he had been an instigator of the group. It had a strong existentialist and personalist tradition. Ronald Gregor Smith, an expert on Martin Buber and the English translator of *I and Thou*, was a member, as was the philosopher John Macquarrie. Macquarrie was a lecturer in theology during the 1950s[166] and was working on his thesis about the relationship between the theology of Rudolf Bultmann, a German existential thinker, and the philosophy of Martin Heidegger. This became his first book, *An Existentialist Theology*. He also co-translated Heidegger's *Sein und Zeit* [*Being and Time*] and went on to write a lucid guide to existentialism. Other members included Ian Henderson, Professor of Systematic Theology at Glasgow University, who was the pioneer of Bultmann studies in Britain. There was also Archie Craig, who

---

[161] Clay, *R.D. Laing*, p. 41.

[162] Calder, R. (1978–1979). 'Abenheimer and Laing—some notes'. *Edinburgh Review*, **32**, 108–16; and Collins, *Schorstein*.

[163] MS Laing A531/2. Joe Shorstein, p. 3.

[164] Collins, K. (1985). 'Angus MacNiven and the Austrian psychoanalysts'. *Glasgow Medicine*, **2**, 18–9; and Collins, K. (1998). *Go and Learn—the International Story of the Jews and Medicine in Scotland 1739–1945*. Aberdeen University Press, Aberdeen.

[165] Mullan, *Mad to be Normal*, pp. 146–7.

[166] Macquarrie, J. (1999). *On Being a Theologian*. SCM Press, London.

was then secretary of the World Council of Churches, and Laing's Gartnavel colleague, Ian Cameron.

One member, Jack Rillie, has left a short account of the group.[167] It met in members' homes and the evening would begin with someone reading a paper. Most of the members had an interest in existentialism, or more specifically existentialist theology. Barth was 'out', while Bultmann and Tillich were 'in'. Baillie, Macmurray, and Buber were repeatedly invoked. Rillie described Schorstein as erudite, highly intelligent, 'often obsessively serious, but somewhat unpredictable and undisciplined'. Abenheimer was described as a 'large, genial man, speaking good English in a ruinous German accent'. Rillie provides an interesting picture of Laing at this period:

> Laing I remember at only three of the early meetings. He read drafts of *The Divided Self*. He was still at that time working at the local hospital dealing practically with the problems he tries to understand in his book, and his mind had an exciting kind of turbulence about it. His papers had an immediacy and urgency which made our normal discussions seem pale. He was very soon in London after that. I did not really get to know him in these short meetings. But he was manifestly remarkable, intellectually insatiable, committed, courageous, and always—I felt—near to physical exhaustion. But I wondered too whether he wasn't something of a neophiliac . . . perhaps too eclectic. On a personal level, I must confess— unfairly on such a slight acquaintance—I did not much take to him. (The educated Glaswegian sometimes feels a strong obligation to be 'gallus'—I thought he had enough insight to know better.)

The term 'gallus' is a Glaswegian slang to describe someone who is self-confident, exuberant, and stylish. Quite whether Rillie meant the term in this way is hard to determine. However, he does seem to suggest that Laing was putting on something of an act, and one that belied his educated background. In later years, others were to see Laing in the context of the cliché of the Glaswegian: the hard-drinking proletarian, who exudes authenticity, has a tendency to brooding menace, and maintains a passionate belief in social justice. Showalter's picture of Laing conforms to this, as does Clancy Sigal's fictional representation in *Zone of the Interior*. To some extent, Laing played up to this image, and, indeed, like all clichés they hold some truth.

Rillie also remembers that Laing received great deal of help from Abenheimer. Laing had read papers by Abenheimer, including his commentary on Binswanger's studies of schizophrenia.[168] Some years after Laing moved to London, however, they had a decisive break and Abenheimer never discussed Laing again. During this period Laing attended a lecture by Martin Buber when he visited Glasgow to talk at a Jewish society.[169] He remembered Buber as a short man with unkempt hair and a long white beard like 'a reincarnation of some Old Testament Prophet'. In the talk, Buber raged against God because of the Extermination Camps and what had happened to the Jews. Paul Tillich also visited Glasgow and Laing met him several times.[170]

---

[167] Rillie, J. (1988). 'The Abenheimer/Schorstein Group'. *Edinburgh Review*, **78–9**, 104–7.
[168] MS Laing A230. A critique of Binswanger's 'Ellen West'.
[169] Laing, *Wisdom, Madness and Folly*, pp. 138–9.
[170] Ibid., pp. 155–6.

Laing's time in Glasgow was crucial to his later intellectual development, but this has often been ignored by commentators, who have been surprised that the early Laing was so well versed in Continental philosophy, coming as he did from that supposed outpost of civilization, the West of Scotland. For example, Kotowicz expressed surprise that Laing knew anything about existential philosophy and regarded the appearance of *The Divided Self* in the English-speaking world as 'absolutely unique, almost alien'.[171] In their book *The Eclipse of Scottish Culture*, Beveridge and Turnbull have emphasized that, during this period, there was, in fact, a thriving philosophical tradition at Glasgow to which Laing had been exposed.[172] Laing's first book, *The Divided Self*, makes specific mention of one of the leading Scottish personalist philosophers, John Macmurray, who argued that the techniques of natural science were inappropriate to the study of people. George Davie has observed that the Glasgow University philosophy department during this period was 'German-Hegelian' in its orientation. J.J. Russell was particularly concerned with phenomenology, and Davie has judged that Laing continued this work 'with striking success'.[173] Beveridge and Turnbull have pointed out that there was an interplay between native Scottish ideas and the European tradition:

> Laing is not, as has often been assumed, an isolated figure in recent Scottish intellectual history. An inclination to question the claims of science (without, however, lapsing into any kind of irrationalism); the concern with the threat posed to ethics by the spread of positivist modes of thought; the refusal to ignore or disesteem the dimensions of experience, reasoning and reality which are beyond the scope of natural scientific knowledge; an insistence on the phenomenon of *personhood,* and concern about its fate in modern cultural conditions—these attitudes and interests . . . link Laing to a number of other recent Scottish thinkers, such as the theologians John Baillie, Ronald Gregor Smith and John Macquarrie, and the philosophers John Macmurray (an acknowledged influence) and C.A. Campbell (whose classes at Glasgow Laing attended). This 'personalist' movement in Scotland reflected a strong interest in the work of German and Jewish thinkers, especially Martin Buber . . .[174]

The British Army

After his placement at Killearn, Laing planned to study with Karl Jaspers, the philosopher-psychiatrist, who was known personally to Schorstein. Laing had corresponded with Jaspers, who had agreed to take him on and had arranged for him to attend the Neuropsychiatric Department at Basel. Laing was given a scholarship through Glasgow University but the authorities decreed that he should serve in the British Army. The Korean War was being fought and Laing remembers that the prospect of military service threw him into one of the most extreme crises in his life.[175] He did not want to

---

[171] Kotowicz, Z. (1997). *R.D. Laing and the Paths of Anti-Psychiatry.* Routledge, London, p. 2.

[172] Beveridge, C. and Turnbull, R. (1989). *The Eclipse of Scottish Culture: Inferiorism and the Intellectuals.* Polygon, Edinburgh.

[173] Davie, G. (1986). *The Crisis of the Democratic Intellect.* Polygon, Edinburgh, p. 176.

[174] Beveridge, C. and Turnbull, R. (1998). Introduction to R.D. Laing, *Wisdom, Madness and Folly.* Canongate, Edinburgh (originally published in 1985) p. xii.

[175] MS Laing A662. Draft notes.

die and he worried as to whether he would be able to cope with the stress of warfare as he was already feeling under pressure and pushed to the limit in his post as a junior doctor at Killearn.

Laing was sent to the central British Army Psychiatric Unit at Netley in England in November 1951. The Royal Victoria Military Hospital had opened in Netley in 1863.[176] The lunatic asylum department had opened in 1870 and was set apart from the rest of the hospital.[177] During the First World War it treated countless cases of shell-shock including the poet, Wilfred Owens. Biographers have generally taken Laing's lead and described Netley as a grim place devoid of humanity or any kind of meaningful therapy. They have also accepted Laing's account that he was the only one who had qualms about the use of physical treatments. Philip Hoare, in his book on Netley, paints a particularly bleak picture of the psychiatric department of the hospital.[178] He largely sees the place through Laing's eyes and contrasts the seemingly repressive and cruel ethos of the institution with that of the sensitive young Glasgow doctor, trying to bring compassion to the inmates. Hoare makes much of the hospital's use of insulin coma therapy, and electroconvulsive therapy (ECT), which he compares to the Nazi medical experiments.

Despite Laing's criticisms of the unit, there seems to have been more to it than just physical treatments. In his CV of 23 September 1953, Laing outlined the other treatment options available: group therapy, psychodrama, and art therapy.[179] In *Wisdom, Madness and Folly*,[180] Laing had made the claim that staff in the psychosis unit were under strict orders not to talk to the patients and to discourage patients from talking to each other. This especially applied to patients suffering from schizophrenia as it was felt that it aggravated the psychotic process. Both Burston[181] and Hoare[182] somewhat misleadingly give the impression that this policy, if indeed it was in force, applied to all psychiatric patients, but it was not the approach of the Psychoneurotic Wing where Laing worked. He did individual analytical work with patients and asked them to tell them about their dreams.

We get some idea of Laing at Netley from a referee's report about him completed by his senior colleague, J.F.D. Murphy.[183] He noted that Laing had already read extensively before he took up the post at Netley and that he continued to read. His interest was directed mainly towards 'the psychoneurotic' and he was employed in the 200-bedded Psychoneurotic Wing. 'His bent was obviously analytic', observed Murphy. Laing worked hard and was very thorough. He was described as having a good approach and manner with patients. He was regarded as a sociable fellow, was 'a good group member',

[176] Hoare, P. (2002). *Spike Island: The Memory of a Military Hospital.* Fourth Estate, London.

[177] Jones, E. and Wessely, S. (2005) *Shell Shock to PTSD. Military Psychiatry from 1900 to the Gulf War.* Psychology Press, Hove and New York.

[178] Hoare, *Spike Island*, pp. 310–28.

[179] Application by Laing for post of registrar at the Royal Mental Hospital, Glasgow, 23 September 1953.

[180] Laing, *Wisdom, Madness and Folly*, p. 100.

[181] Burston, *The Wing of Madness*, pp. 32–3.

[182] Hoare, *Spike Island*, pp. 310–28.

[183] Letter to The Secretary of the Western Regional Health Board on Laing by JFD Murphy, 29 September 1953.

and was popular with colleagues. Murphy went on to say: 'Perhaps of a somewhat mercurial temperament and at times carried away with enthusiasms—and perhaps all the more likeable for that.' Years later, Murphy remembered Laing as 'a loner, steeped in psychoanalysis, intellectual pursuits, very positive ideas, different'.[184] Murphy's initial verdict was given in the context of providing a reference, which may have constrained what he wrote. However, the second verdict was given some years after Laing's death and may have been shaped by his posthumous reputation.

In the account of his Army days that he gave to Peter Mezan,[185] Laing complained that there was no one he could talk to. He claimed that the only person with whom he could have an ordinary conversation was a young psychotic man he encountered in a padded cell. This seems part of Laing's mythologizing of his past. In his version, he is the lone hero who prefers the company of the mad to that of his colleagues. Of course, in Laing's defence, it could be argued that he was able to maintain the sociable front with his colleagues that Murphy observed, but that, behind the front, he felt estranged. Certainly his Army diaries and letters exude discontent and dissatisfaction with his lot. One entry reads:

> Durer's melancholy—nothing to work for—no enthusiasm—not ultimately concerned (Tillich) even the torture of doubt, of a paradoxical faith which is always in question is to be preferred to this depression without tears, or sadness or retardation. A painted ship upon a painted ocean.[186]

At times he questioned his own sanity: 'I am not sure that I am not going insane. The psychiatrist and the disease. Who is the cat and who is the mouse?'[187] Another entry reads:

> alcoholism, madness, suicide.
> Only if I don't run away from myself can I ever hope not to marry and despair: and however 'happy' I may be, despair will remain the worm at the heart. I must have my cake and eat it.[188]

The reference to alcoholism is significant in view of Laing's later problems. In his notebooks he commented about his drinking; for example, he wrote: 'The essence of what it is that I seek to achieve by drunkenness is still unrevealed to me.'[189] He was concerned about the harmful effects of alcohol: 'Will my brain tolerate two years of pickling? What irreversible brain changes will develop.'[190] In the same entry he observes:

> A subtle change has overtaken me. I am very drunk as I write this and yet here I am coherent, articulate, coordinated, fluent: and not very garrulous. It must be a simple thing to gain

[184] Interview of Dr Desmond Murphy by Edgar Jones on 26 November 1998.

[185] Mezan, P. (1972). 'After Freud and Jung, now comes R.D. Laing'. *Esquire*, **77**, 92–7, 160–78.

[186] MS Laing K14. Notebook and diary covering Laing's stay at the military hospitals at Netley and Catterick, January 1952 to June 1953.

[187] Ibid.

[188] Ibid., p. 3.

[189] Ibid., 2 February 1952.

[190] Ibid., Thursday, February 1952.

self-mastery. but why? why should one? why not just get drunk: why not commit suicide? Suicide is the end of pleasure as well as of pain.[191]

Later he advised himself:

Don't drink to run away from suffering but to bear it easier: but to tolerate it better. To make it more tolerable is not to run away. Even this is not permissible. But by what, or whose, rules is it not permissible? That one should be so intelligent and so informed, and lacking in wisdom.[192]

In *The Varieties of Religious Experience*, William James suggested a possible reason why people like Laing were attracted to alcohol:

The sway of alcohol over mankind is unquestionably due to its power to stimulate the mystical faculties of human nature, usually crushed to earth by the cold facts and dry criticisms of the sober hour. Sobriety diminishes, discriminates, and says no; drunkenness expands, unites, and says yes.[193]

It is clear that Laing's reservations about the use of physical treatments in mental illness were increased by his experience in the Army. He had already been exposed to Joe Schorstein's impassioned rejection of psychosurgery during his time at Killearn. In his autobiography Laing claimed that he first began to have doubts about psychiatric treatment during his time in the Army:

I was just beginning to suspect that insulin and electric shocks did more harm than good. In fact, I had begun to have to call into question my own sanity, because I was beginning to suspect that insulin and electric shocks, not to mention lobotomy and the whole environment of a psychiatric unit, were ways of destroying people and driving people crazy if they were not so before, and crazier if they were. But I had to put it to myself—maybe I was completely mistaken. How could the whole of psychiatry be doing the opposite of what I assumed psychiatry was about—treating, curing if possible, arresting the course of mental illness. Was Artaud right?[194]

He ends the passage by referring to Antonin Artaud, the French playwright and former psychiatric patient who had written a vehement critique of psychiatry, entitled 'Van Gogh, The Man Suicided by Society',[195] which Laing had read and which we will consider in Chapter 6. Laing comments further on his experience of Army psychiatry: 'It was only in retrospect that I realized the full extent to which I did not accept psychiatric theory and practice and I began to realize that, with such an attitude, I was going to have a very strange professional career.'[196]

At Netley, Laing met his first wife, Anne Hearne, who was working as a sister in the hospital. She became pregnant and they married on 11 October 1952 in the Richmond

---

[191] Ibid.

[192] Ibid.

[193] James, W. (1902). *The Varieties of Religious Experience*. Longmans, Green, and Co, London, p. 387.

[194] Laing, *Wisdom, Madness and Folly*, p. 106.

[195] Clay, *R.D. Laing*, p. 30. Hirschman, J. (1965). *Antonin Artaud Anthology*. City Lights Books, San Francisco, pp. 135–63.

[196] Laing, *Wisdom, Madness and Folly*, p. 108.

Registry Office. He wrote a farewell letter to Marcelle.[197] After a year at Netley, Laing was transferred to Northern Command at Catterick in Yorkshire in September 1952. Laing became a captain in charge of the psychiatric and detention wards of Catterick Military Hospital. Along with Murray Brookes, an ear, nose and throat (ENT) specialist at the unit, he wrote a paper about determining whether soldiers were genuinely deaf or malingering. Brookes was one of the few colleagues at Catterick that Laing liked and whom he considered was not part of 'the herd'. In a letter to his friend John Duffy on the 22 November 1952, he expanded on this and reveals how he saw himself and others during this period:

> My last few weeks here have been enlivened by the companionship of a doctor [Murray Brookes] here who has now been posted. He was one of the 'Initiates'. We spoke the same language . . . I've met quite a few people now in the Army yet the past year I think I've met only four people who could be called 'initiates' . . . In what way are they different? The average run of doctors, is not essentially different from the average run of shipyard worker or ship's engineer. Certainly I find I have nothing in common with them. Looking for a phrase for them I can think of nothing more dignified than 'small-minded cunts'.[198]

Laing went on to try and define the attributes of an 'initiate', and concluded that they encompassed being unconventional, living a life of alcoholic and sexual excess, being reckless, and knowing 'what it is all about'. Here we see Laing expressing his belief in his superiority to the common run of humanity. In one of his frequent stock-taking exercises, Laing recorded in his notebook on 18 May 1953.

> Almost finished N.S.[National Service] 4 months to go.
> What have I achieved?
> Fuck all.
> Yet I have now a baby girl, I am married, I own a flat.
> A great deal of piss has been knocked out of me.
> I have retained my friends.
> I have done perhaps inestimable harm to one person.
> I have become more reconciled with my parents.
> I have been forced to my knees: forced back to the Bible, Plato, Kant.
> I can hardly say I have furthered my career.[199]

The line 'inestimable harm to one person' probably refers to Marcelle who had been upset to learn of Laing's relationship with and subsequent marriage to Anne. After leaving the Army, Laing and his wife Anne and daughter Fiona set up home in Glasgow, eventually finding a flat at 104 Novar Drive in the West End of the city. When he returned to his parents' home to collect his belongings, he discovered that his mother had thrown out his writing desk, which contained numerous bits of writing he had composed in the previous years. According to Laing, this included a journal in the

---

[197] Laing, A., *A Biography*, p. 53.
[198] Mullan, *Creative Destroyer*. Letter from Laing to John Duffy, 22 November 1952, pp. 109–10.
[199] MS Laing K14.

manner of Gogol's *Diary of a Madman*.[200] Laing confided despairingly in his diary: 'The loss of everything I have written before the age of 24! These writings were my past, my memory, myself. In their loss or destruction, I've lost part of myself. There it is.'[201] Such comments suggest that Laing saw his autobiographical writing as central to his self-construction.

Gartnavel Royal Mental Hospital

Laing's first civilian posting began in October 1953 at Glasgow's Gartnavel Royal Mental Hospital, whose superintendent was the humane if eccentric Angus MacNiven, whom Laing had encountered as a medical student. MacNiven took a sceptical view of the newly emerging physical treatments, and staff at Gartnavel during this period, were open to alternative social and psychodynamic methods of therapy. Laing was allocated a female 'refractory' ward. In a poetic account of the place, Laing wrote:

> A refractory ward in a mental hospital is a strange place to be reminded of Homer. But these women in the refractory ward brought back to me Homer's description of the ghosts in Hades, separated on their side from the living by the widths of the Ocean, and, on the part of the living, by the Rivers of Fear. Ulysses goes to the land of the dead to meet his mother. Although he can see her, he is dismayed to find he cannot embrace her. She explains to him that she has no sinews, no bones, no body keeping the bones and flesh together. Once the life force has gone from her white bones, all is consumed by the fierce heat of a blazing fear, and the soul slips away like a dream and flutters in the air.
>
> From what experience of life had that description come? It seemed to be so far and yet so near.
>
> How can we entice these ghosts to life, across *their* oceanic abyss, across *our* rivers of fear.[202]

Dr MacNiven formed a high opinion of Laing.[203] He thought he had an exceptional knowledge of psychiatric literature, particularly in the psychoanalytic field. He was very impressed with Laing's contributions to staff discussions of clinical problems. He thought he established a very good relationship with his patients. In addition to the routine work of the hospital, which he did with great energy and enthusiasm, he treated certain patients by psychotherapy 'with considerable success'. MacNiven felt that Laing was 'a very intelligent young man' who had 'a great capacity for hard work and study'. He observed that he had a stimulating influence on his colleagues, and was well liked. MacNiven considered that Laing was a man of 'outstanding ability'. He wrote that Laing had: 'a very keen, critical, analytic mind. He showed a great capacity for grasping the essential points in a case . . . he was prepared to have them subjected to rigorous criticism'.[204] Further, and somewhat ironically in view of Laing's later difficulties,

---

[200] Mullan, *Mad to be Normal*, p. 55. Also in Clay, *R.D. Laing*, p. 53.

[201] MS Laing K14.

[202] Laing, *Wisdom, Madness and Folly*, p. 121.

[203] Letter to Secretary of the Paddington Group Hospital Management Committee about Laing from Angus MacNiven, 12 June 1956.

[204] Letter to Dr Max M Levin, Foundations' Fund for Research in Psychiatry, New Haven, Connecticut from Dr MacNiven, 30 March 1960.

MacNiven stated that he was not 'a man who is likely to arouse antagonism or obstruction in the pursuit of his scientific work'. Of course MacNiven was giving his opinion in 1960 before Laing became a counter-culture guru. The admiring observations of the young Laing by MacNiven and others during this period raise questions. Did fame have a catastrophic effect on his further development? Were there signs early on which might have predicted his later fall from grace? Certainly his contemporaries underline how seriously Laing took his work at this stage and there are counter retrospective assessments that he was a charlatan and had been so from the beginning. Laing for his part thought highly of the Gartnavel superintendent. When MacNiven retired in 1965, Laing wrote to him, apologizing for being unable to make the dinner, and adding: 'I am sure you are aware how much I have always respected your work and how much inspiration I have drawn from your personal example of dedication to the service of the patients at Gartnavel.'[205]

On 20 January 1954, Laing confided to his diary:

> What to do now? There are various practical things I *must* do.
> 1. German.
> 2. Either MD and/or MRCPE. Wait until news of Senior Registrar's job before starting on 2 . . .[206]

He also determined to join a library and to write a critical survey of the Kleinian system.

The Southern General Hospital

In December 1954 Laing gained the Diploma in Psychological Medicine, and on 19 February 1955 he left Gartnavel to take a National Health Service job as a senior registrar with Professor Ferguson Rodger at the Southern General Hospital, where the Department of Psychological Medicine of Glasgow University was located. Rodger had supported his application for the post. Laing later told a colleague that it was Rodger's example that made him determined to make use of the copious clinical material and notes that he had been collecting since he had qualified.[207] In his autobiography, Laing was less charitable and his only reference to Rodger was to mention that the professor told him 'not to get too close to' patients.[208] In his autobiography, Laing joked that his new place of work was nicknamed the 'Department of Psycho-Semites' because five of its senior members were Jews.[209] Laing emphasized that he had several Jewish friends and seemed proud to relate that he was invited by them to a lecture at the Jewish Society, where he was the only Gentile present. Once again we see Laing continuing to involve himself in Jewish culture, and there is also the implication that he had been especially chosen by the Jewish community.

---

[205] Unarchived letter from Laing to MacNiven, 18 May 1965.
[206] MS Laing K16. Notebook, July 1953 to August 1962.
[207] Hood, *The Young R.D. Laing*, p. 40.
[208] Laing, *Wisdom, Madness and Folly*, p. 154.
[209] Ibid., pp. 138–9.

Laing resumed his working relationship with Joe Schorstein and they set up a headache clinic together.[210] Both men felt that the interpersonal process was crucial to recovery. An example of their work was 'The case of Nan', which Schorstein[211] wrote up in a paper and to which Laing referred in his autobiography. Schorstein wrote: 'We were so fascinated by our technical abilities, so keen to create new records of survival, that in the dramatic recoveries which we witnessed we were forgetting the main actor—the patient.'[212]

Laing later claimed that when he first started working in psychiatric hospitals in Glasgow, he 'was absolutely shocked with the inhumanity and the disgrace of what was going on in psychiatry . . . There was fury and indignation and outrage working in me'.[213] However, Laing's time in Glasgow was to prove crucial to his career, both clinically and intellectually. The majority of patients he discusses in *The Divided Self* are from Gartnavel Hospital, and in later books Laing frequently returns to consider patients from this institution. Intellectually, Laing had participated in philosophical discussion groups, most notably with Schorstein and Abenheimer.

London

As Laing informed Dr Angus MacNiven, he had been keen to move to London for some time before he actually went there in October 1956.[214] He took advantage of a new scheme which had been set up to allow promising young psychiatrists from outside London to come to the Tavistock Clinic and the Institute of Psychoanalysis to study and undergo a free analysis. Professor Ferguson Rodger was a friend of Dr Jock Sutherland who was the Director of the Tavistock Clinic, and he recommended Laing to Sutherland. Angus MacNiven observed that Laing could have continued as a National Health psychiatrist and would have been rapidly promoted.[215] This would have greatly improved his financial situation. At this stage he had a wife and a young family to support. MacNiven felt that Laing's decision to go to London would have further stretched his financial resources as his salary was not increased. He saw this as a sign of Laing's strength of character and his determination to pursue his work without regard to personal comfort or material security. Laing later commented that neither he nor his first wife, Anne, were particularly interested in material possessions.[216] MacNiven did not feel that Laing was being egotistical or ruthless in pursuing his goals, or that he was neglecting the needs of his family. On the contrary, he stated that Laing was 'a most devoted husband and father'.

[210] Collins, *Schorstein.*
[211] Schorstein, J. (1961). 'The story of Nan: a case of severe head injury'. *Physiotherapy,* **47,** 335–6.
[212] Schorstein, *Nan.* Also quoted in Collins, *Schorstein.*
[213] Mullan, *Mad to be Normal,* p. 75.
[214] Letter from Laing to Dr MacNiven, 11 June 1956.
[215] Letter to Dr Max M Levin from Dr MacNiven about Laing, 30 March 1960.
[216] Mullan, *Mad to be Normal,* p. 76.

Looking back at the move, Laing wrote:

> When I left Glasgow to go to London to work at the Tavistock Clinic and undergo a training at the British Institute of Psychoanalysis I was clear about what I wanted to address myself to, for the foreseeable future in theory and practice.
>
> I wanted to see further and more clearly what person to person communication was all about. I wanted to find out how far such an understanding of communication could contribute to understanding mis-communication, non-communication and excommunication. Maybe this approach could be a helpful contribution to the problems of Western Psychiatry and its patients.[217]

As Daniel Burston[218] has noted, the Institute of Psychoanalysis was bitterly divided by a dispute between two rival factions, who followed either Anna Freud or Melanie Klein. Those who were repelled by the dogmatisms of the Freudians and the Kleinians joined the so-called 'Middle Group', which included Michael Balint, Jock Sutherland, John Bowlby, D.W. Winnicott, Charles Rycroft, and Marion Milner. During Laing's time there, Ernest Jones, Wilfred Bion, Melanie Klein, and Donald Winnicott all gave lectures or seminars at the Institute. Laing also met Ronald Fairbairn and Harry Guntrip.[219] Laing recalls being unpleasantly surprised to find that the Tavistock was an outpatient organization. Furthermore:

> These were ordinary people who lived in Hampstead and all very white and very middle-class, and none of them seemed to be anymore disturbed than I was or anyone else. I had a lot of sympathy with the Maudsley argument that they dealt with the really ill, and serious cases, and that the Tavistock was a sort of dilettante outpost of an organization that dealt with normal people.[220]

In another notebook, Laing struck a more personal note and admitted there were problems with the move. He remembered:

> I sorely missed the intellectual companionship of Glasgow, Joe Schorstein, Karl Abenheimer, Penry Jones, Ian Cameron, John McQuarrie, Ian Henderson, Archie Craig, as well as my professional colleagues and my drinking pals.
>
> At the Tavistock and the Institute of Psychoanalysis there was no one, and there was at first no one else in London I knew, who were interested in, or had even heard in [sic] Kierkegaard, Tillich, et al.[221]

James Hood, a fellow Glasgow graduate, had also moved to London to train in psychoanalysis. He remembered that Laing still had a strong sense of his Glasgow connection, and, at this stage, spoke warmly about his psychiatric colleagues, especially Professor Ferguson Rodger.[222] Laing tried to interest his new colleagues in existential philosophy and phenomenology, but no one saw the relevance of it. Laing remembers Winnicott making several, unsuccessful attempts to pronounce the word 'phenomenology' in

---

[217] MS Laing A713. Drafts.

[218] Burston, *The Wing of Madness*, pp. 47–9.

[219] Mullan, *Mad to be Normal*, p. 155.

[220] Ibid., pp. 147–8.

[221] MS Laing A685. Travels, London from Glasgow, p. 1.

[222] Hood, *The Young R.D. Laing*, p. 40.

front of him.[223] Whether or not Winnicott was deliberately trying to be provocative and was assuming the air of the self-satisfied Englishman who views anything foreign or intellectual as beneath his contempt, we do not know. Certainly this is how Laing viewed the situation. But it was not just the English who were unreceptive to European philosophy. Laing suggested to Dr Jock Sutherland, who was Scottish and was the Director of the Clinic, that Kierkegaard's *The Sickness unto Death* was well worth reading. Sutherland judged that it was 'a very good example of early nineteenth century psychopathology'.[224] Laing felt that the culture of the Tavistock was devoid of any sort of camaraderie or rapport with the people who were patients.[225] However, Laing did eventually find a group of like-minded individuals and they started meeting for discussion evenings in each other's houses, in much the same way that he had been used to in Glasgow. The circle included Jan Resnick, David Cooper, John Heaton, and Paul Senft, who helped Laing understand the ideas of Husserl.[226]

On 29 December 1956, Laing, who was then living in Harlow with his wife and children, wrote in his diary:

> The end of another year
> 3 children
> Fiona, Susan, Karen
> Another due to come out in this world which his/her father has never quite got used to. But for me, I will not say it has been a bad world. That I do not dwell in Jerusalem is not the fault of Harlow Development Corporation or of God, but it is because I still yet hanker after a cauldron of illicit loves in Carthage or Babylon, or more subtly ... I still do not see Samarkand as a mirage. It is all a question of whether Heaven is 'enjoyment', 'torment' and insanity.[227]

Laing reveals that he used the end of the working day in London to write, and this seems entirely convincing, given what we know about his very driven behaviour and his output during this period.[228] He was involved with a group working on a project, seemingly inspired by Laing, to publish a series of French and German 'classics' of psychiatric literature. It was under the aegis of Tavistock Publications, and Michel Foucault's *Madness and Civilisation* was one of the books published. A colleague, Robert Gosling, recalls asking Laing how he had the stamina to begin his literary work at the end of the day. Laing replied: 'Well, Freud did, didn't he?'[229]

The training analyst chosen for Laing was Charles Rycroft. For the next four years Laing saw him five times a week for an hour.[230] Laing did not think there was much the matter with himself apart from some wheezing, but he did look forward to the experience to see what illumination it would throw on his life.[231] Rycroft was to

[223] MS Laing A685, p. 1.

[224] Ibid., p. 2.

[225] Mullan, *Mad to be Normal*, p. 164.

[226] Ibid., p. 291.

[227] MS Laing K16.

[228] Research Fellowship Application by Laing to Foundations' Fund for Research in Psychiatry, 21 March 1960, pp. 5–6.

[229] Clay, *R.D. Laing*, p. 65.

[230] Laing, A., *A Biography*, p. 62.

[231] Mullan, *Mad to be Normal*, pp. 162–3.

comment that Laing had 'an extremely effective schizoid defence mechanism against exhibiting signs of depression'.[232] He was an only child and, in Rycroft's opinion, this led to a tendency to self-dramatize. Only children became the author, actor, and audience of their own internalized world. Laing was to develop a high regard for Rycroft. Reviewing one of his books in later years, he described it as 'breath of fresh air'.[233] He stated that Rycroft had come to believe that the main problem for psycho-analysts was to emancipate themselves from the 'humanly emaciating doctrine of psychoanalysis'.

Laing's supervisors for his work with patients were Donald Winnicott and Marion Milner. He remembers supervision sessions at 5 o'clock with Winnicott, who would produce a bottle of wine. Because of his poor attendance at seminars and lectures there was a dispute about whether Laing should be allowed to qualify as a psychoanalyst. Milner, Winnicott, Rycroft, Bowlby, and Sutherland were in favour. Wride and Hellman were against and, in a letter to Rycroft, they expressed their concerns:

> 24 October 1960
> Dear Dr Rycroft,
>   With reference to the correspondence about Dr Laing, the Training Committee has asked us to write to you . . .
>   They were worried, however, by the fact that Dr Laing is apparently a very disturbed and ill person and wondered what the effect of this obvious disturbance would be on patients he would have to interview . . . It is also felt as unsatisfactory that the Training Committee should be put into the position of qualifying candidates in an obviously disturbed condition.
> Yours sincerely,
> Fanny Wride (Chairman)
> Ilse Hellmann (Secretary), Training Committee.[234]

We learn from Adrian Laing's biography that his father was seriously ill at the time and nearly died.[235] Hood speculates that this illness might have been a reaction to the death of Douglas Hutchison, who had died the year before. Milner wrote in Laing's defence, pointing out that to delay his qualification would reflect badly on the psycho-analytic society and demonstrate it was not flexible enough to meet the needs of a 'specially brilliant student'.[236] She added: 'I found him a pleasure to work with because I never feel he is distorting the material to make it fit into a preconceived theory or formula, he never gives ready made or cliché interpretations.' Both Rycroft and Winnicott wrote letters supporting Laing. Rycroft contrasted Laing's originality and drive with the usual type of Institute student, who was passive and unimaginative.[237] Winnicott felt that a continuation of the teacher–student relationship would be

---

[232] Laing, A., *A Biography*, p. 63.
[233] MS Laing 511/2. Drafts of a review for the New Scientist of 'Psychoanalysis and beyond' by Charles Rycroft, 1985.
[234] Laing, A., *A Biography*, pp. 66–7.
[235] Ibid., p. 67.
[236] Clay, *R.D. Laing*, p. 68.
[237] Quoted in Burston, *The Wing of Madness*, pp. 52–3.

harmful to Laing's future personal development.[238] The training committee relented and granted Laing his qualification.

Looking back at his move to the Tavistock, Laing judged, 'that's where I felt that I went down the drain in my career'.[239] At first sight, this seems an extraordinary statement. However, Laing was plainly more at home with the severely disturbed patients of the Glasgow hospitals than with the clientele of the Tavistock, whom he considered to be relatively normal. Nevertheless, the move to London had also involved study at the Institute of Psychoanalysis and this exposed Laing to many of the leading figures in the field. Although he was later to be rather coy as to the influence of these London-based analysts, he sought their opinions of his draft manuscript of *The Divided Self* and the book clearly owes a debt to object relations theory and, in particular, to Donald Winnicott.

When he completed the manuscript of *The Divided Self*, Laing, in an undated entry in his notebook, imagined what the frontispiece of his book would look like. At this stage the subtitle was: 'A Phenomenological Study of Schizoid and Schizophrenic States'. He noted:

> Well, it's written—a book, but not the one I thought I was going to write on G.M.H.
> [Gerard Manley Hopkins] The ice has been broken—at any rate, as far as I am concerned.
> Now for publishers (?Maschler) and the public.
>   MONEY.[240]

In the same entry he planned his next book which was to be titled *The New Man: An Existential Analysis/Study of William Blake*. In 1960, *The Divided Self*, the book which Laing had been working on since his days in Glasgow was finally published. In November of that year, Laing had another stock-taking exercise, which he recorded in his diaries. He congratulated himself that *The Divided Self* had been published and that *The Self and Others* would be published 'even if I die'.[241] He planned to write on Husserl, Bleuler, Jaspers, Minkowski, and Boss. He chided himself: 'None of this really done yet. Do it first!!!' He also advised himself that he should try to meet such eminent people as Jung, Sartre, and Ionesco. He added: 'Do so this year. It is time'. He concluded: 'I am now of course an Assoc. Member of Inst. Of Psych-Analysis. A fantastic anti-climax to 10 years or 14 years ago'.[242]

At the time of the publication of *The Divided Self*, Laing was living with his wife and three children in Harlow. After qualifying as an analyst, Laing had set up practice in Wimpole Street. A print of 'The Death of Icarus' by Breughel hung on the wall. Icarus, according to the myth, flew too near to the sun, melting the wax by which his wings were attached and he plummeted to his death. The parallels with Laing's subsequent glittering ascendancy on the world stage and his dramatic fall from favour are obvious.

---

[238] Ibid., p. 53.

[239] Mullan, *Mad to be Normal*, p. 149.

[240] MS Laing K16.

[241] Ibid.

[242] Ibid.

Chapter 2

Portrait of the psychiatrist as an intellectual: Laing's early notebooks, personal library, essays, papers, and talks

Towards the end of his life when he sat to have his portrait painted, Laing told the artist, Victoria Crowe, that he would like the picture to make him look like a 'mid-European intellectual'.[1] In fact, from a young age Laing was determined to be an intellectual. His early writings, both private and personal, chart his scholarly questing and provide a detailed map of the cultural terrains over which he travelled. He filled notebooks with extracts of verse by Keats, Blake, and T.S. Eliot. He copied out quotations by such thinkers as Nietzsche, Marx, and Freud, and he made lists of books he had read and those he had yet to read. There is no doubt that he was a serious young man, fired by a mission to become a leading intellectual. The sheer range of his reading and the dedication to his self-appointed task of mastering the work of the Greats is undeniably impressive. In *Wisdom, Madness and Folly* (1985), Laing recounted his intellectual wakening:

> I had started eating [sic] my way through the library from A to Z . . . This way I first came across Freud, Kierkegaard, Marx and Nietzsche. Somewhere among what they were going on about lay my obsessions. I was so grateful for books, for libraries, for the endowers and organizers of public libraries. I wanted to be a writer. Or rather, I was convinced I *was* a writer, like them, and that it was my duty, my necessity to become the writer I was. I gave myself the age of thirty as an absolute deadline for the publication of my first book . . .
>
> I was sure I could write, but I was not sure when I would have anything I felt justified to write about.
>
> I knew what I wanted to write about. I wanted to ferret out some truth about what was going on in the human world . . .
>
> I could read books and write them anyway. I did not need, I felt, to learn anything at university as to what and how to read or what or how to write. No one was ever going to make me sit another examination on that.[2]

The title of Laing's autobiography, *Wisdom, Madness and Folly* is significant. It is taken from the Bible, Ecclesiastes, 1:17: 'And I gave my heart to know wisdom and to know madness and folly: I perceived that this is also vexation of spirit. For in much

---

[1] Mullan, B. (1997). *R.D. Laing. Creative Destroyer.* Cassel, London, p. 120.

[2] Laing, R.D. (1985). *Wisdom, Madness and Folly. The Making of a Psychiatrist 1927–57.* (1998 reprint). Canongate, Edinburgh, pp. 71–2.

wisdom is much vexation; and he that increases knowledge increases sorrow.' The extract highlights the limitations of knowledge and the thin line between wisdom and madness.[3] As a young man, Laing had also read *In Praise of Folly* by Erasmus, in which the Renaissance wit catalogued the widespread craziness of his fellow humans, a theme that Laing was to expand upon in his later writing.[4]

The quest to be an intellectual: the notebooks

Laing's notebooks allow us to see how he organized his campaign to become an intellectual. They reveal the boldness of his plans and the enormous body of work he set himself to master. They show his recurrent doubts about his ability to fulfil his ambition: he wonders whether he is too lazy, too melancholic, too dissipated, or whether he has anything important to say. Alongside his doubts, Laing also expresses his self-belief: he feels entitled to compare himself to the major figures in European culture and anticipates becoming one of their number.

In his notebooks, Laing repeatedly planned and discussed the course of his intellectual journey, which he envisaged would take him through the classics of world literature and philosophy. As he surveyed the path before him, he was both exhilarated and daunted. He counselled himself on the best way of attaining his ambition: sleep less, drink less, and read more. Laing felt that until the age of 14 he had been under the dominance of Christian teaching and had missed out on contemporary culture. He observed that it took him the next three years 'to catch up, in a scrappy way, intellectually, with the 20th C'.[5] He recounted:

> Even at this time, I was amazed, how in two months of my time (aged 16–17) I traversed 25 years of historical time. I realised also that this was not 'progress', but simply the acquisition of a contemporary sensibility. At school I read Homer, Sophocles, Virgil and Catullus. At home I moved from the dead end of English literature, from Hardy to Lawrence, Joyce, Pound. In philosophy, I discovered Wittgenstein. In psychology, Freud, in politics, Marx. By 1946, a year after World War II ended, I had got as far as the threshold of World War I.[6]

From the outset Laing was desperate to compete with his intellectual heroes and compared his progress with theirs. As he wrote:

> When I was nineteen I had read somewhere in Havelock Ellis, that at the age of nineteen he had determined to have his first book published by the age of thirty—which he did— his study on criminology. I formed the same resolve. And this remained a background strategic priority. Whatever else I did, I would nail this one to the wall anyway before thirty. But the book would be only an external token, that I had not wasted my time entirely.[7]

---

[3] Collins, K. (2008). 'Joseph Schorstein: RD Laing's "rabbi"'. *History of Psychiatry*, **19**(2), 185–201.

[4] Mullan, B. (1995) *Mad to be Normal. Conversations with R.D. Laing*. Free Association Press, London, p. 76.

[5] MS Laing K1, Elements for an Autobiography. p. 52.

[6] Ibid., p. 54.

[7] MS Laing K4. Autobiographical notes. c. 1970.

In another notebook he observed that Christ began his ministry when he was 30 and that Freud had published *The Interpretation of Dreams* when he was 40.[8] Publishing his first book by the age of 30 was clearly important to Laing. Although *The Divided Self* was published in 1960 when Laing was 33, he was to claim in the 1965 Preface to the Pelican edition that he was 28 when he wrote it.[9] In an autobiographical account, written when he was 40, Laing outlined his intellectual aspirations:

> By 19 I had worked out my plan. I would consolidate Greek and Latin. Learn French, German, Italian, and possibly Spanish. Acquire a touch of Hebrew, Aramaic, Arabic and Sanskrit. Read through in the original language, with a crib if necessary, a list of somewhat over 100 key books from the world's literature. Ignore the commentators, and second level thinkers. Age 27, I would begin to put down on paper for publication, my first definitive views on what it was all about, with a view to its publication in my 30th year.[10]

Laing stated that he had worked out his 'programme' alongside a detailed comparison of the dates of eminent European men who had lived over the last hundred years— men 'whom I considered worthy to compare myself'. His girlfriend of the time, Marcelle Vincent, remembered that from an early age Laing saw himself as 'a man of talent'.[11] But when Laing looked at the example of his intellectual heroes, he felt anxious: 'I realised I was in for it. Freud had said that Meynert had said to him that you could not expect to get anywhere in medicine with over five hours sleep a night'.[12] He also noticed that some of the teachers he admired at medical school, such as Dr Harrison in the embryology department or Professor Hamilton did not sleep for more than four hours. The sheer volume of knowledge to master was daunting. He despaired:

> ... every subject was accumulating faster than anyone could keep up with. How was I ever going to catch up anywhere and really get to the growing point where alone one could begin to be in a position to make what was called a 'worthwhile contribution'.[13]

In addition, there were temptations from elsewhere, primarily drinking and women. Laing, as we know, enjoyed partying whilst at University, and he worried that he was wasting valuable time in such hedonistic pursuits. He admonished himself to follow what he called 'a burning categorical imperative'. He reflected:

> I must do the right thing if there was a right thing to be done. I was thoroughly imbued with Kierkegaard, Nietzsche, Marx, Lenin, Freud, aspects of Kant, Jaspers, Camus, on top of my upbringing as a Scottish Presbyterian in the tradition from Calvin to T.H. Huxley, Herbert Spencer, H.G. Wells, Julian Huxley and religious atheism or atheistic religiosity, difficult to tell when it came to Albert Schweitzer and Paul Tillich.[14]

---

[8] MS Freud K1, p. 56. Laing was wrong as Freud was actually in his early forties.

[9] Laing, R.D. (1965). 'Preface'. In *The Divided Self*. Pelican, London.

[10] MS Laing K1, p. 55.

[11] Mullan, *Creative Destroyer*, p. 67.

[12] MS Laing K4. Theodor Meynert (1833–1892) was an Austrian professor of psychiatry who was interested in the biology of the brain. See Shorter, E. (2005). *A Historical Dictionary of Psychiatry*. Oxford University Press, New York.

[13] MS Laing K4.

[14] Ibid.

In this we see Laing's great aspirations and the range of his interests. There is also something of an intellectual swagger about this passage and possibly a degree of boastfulness about his acquaintance with the great philosophers. He was fond of reeling off lists of intellectual heavyweights and these lists appear throughout his notebooks. In one entry Laing wrote that he was trying 'to give body to the homeless and drifting souls of my thoughts and so to end their death'.[15] Although it is not clear whether it was a quotation or an original observation, it serves as a suitable description of what Laing was attempting in his diaries. From an early stage, Laing carried out his intellectual conversations with dead authors, or authors he was unlikely to meet: in other words he used books as a means of creating a dialogue about ideas with the great thinkers of the world, past and present.[16]

For example, Laing described reading Nietzsche with a pencil in hand, awarding the philosopher marks out of 100 for his aphorisms.[17] He was both the pupil and the examiner. He read Sartre in French, and claimed he had learnt German by reading Heidegger's *Sein und Zeit* in the original language. He sat with a dictionary and looked up every word until he made sense of it. Characteristically, Laing averred that Heidegger was very simple if you were not German, but that it was very difficult for native Germans to read.[18] He maintained that he first read Jaspers' *General Psychopathology* in a French translation. Laing observed that Darwin had the habit of noting down any facts that seemed to run against his theories.[19] Laing felt he, too, should cultivate the same habit. From the age of 13 he had also made a point of never forgetting anything that was painful.[20]

In his notebooks, Laing wrote down copious extracts from books and countless poems. The notebooks also contain numerous entries where Laing lays down commands to himself. For example: 'Finish: Hegel "Phenomenology of Mind", Hume "Treatise on Human Nature", Husserl "Ideas". Start German'.[21] Another entry reads:

To be done:-
Brush up French
German} linguaphone.
Italian
German
Binswanger
Dilthey
Goethe's Colour Theory and other 'scientific' works. (nature)
Italian
++Dante

[15] MS Laing K15. Notebook begun on 12 March 1953.
[16] Mullan, *Mad to be Normal*, p. 160.
[17] Ibid., p. 98.
[18] Ibid., p. 110.
[19] Letter from Laing to Marcelle Vincent, undated. Quoted in Mullan, *Creative Destroyer*, p. 71.
[20] Evans, R.I. (1976). *R.D. Laing. The Man and his Ideas*. New York, E.P. Dutton & Co., p. lxxii.
[21] MS Laing K14. Notebook and diary covering Laing's stay at the military hospitals at Netley and Catterick, January 1952 to June 1953.

Basic Reading
Racine
Revise Aeschylus, Sophocles, etc.
+++Heraclitus
Dante
Goethe
Read Leonardo's Notebooks properly.
++Boehme.[22]

In one entry he tells himself: 'Return to Hamilton–Reid, Hulme [sic], Dugald Stewart, *my own heritage.*'[23] Laing was trying to articulate his own personal philosophy and, in his notebooks, he often berated his approach: 'The weakness in my reading of philosophy is the lack of an explicit, articulate, self-aware standpoint, or point of view of my own.'[24] He asked himself: 'What is man? What can I hope? What ought I to do? What can I know?'[25] In an entry which anticipated his later poems, he wrote:

> I can attempt the impossible.
> Therefore it is not meaningless to do so.
> I cannot achieve the impossible. I *can* attempt to achieve the impossible.
> Therefore it may be that I ought.
> What ought I to do?[26]

In a notebook entry which echoes Kierkegaard's contention that philosophy had to be personally meaningful, Laing outlined the requirements of the type of philosophy he required:

> It must be relevant to, and indeed be an articulation of, my own needs. It will have general application in so far as my needs are apprehended essentially and hence in their essential identity with the needs of every other human being. It must start from me, and my situation, my time and place, the present day etc . . . It must be an explicit statement of a philosophical faith. Otherwise best to say nothing.[27]

Laing frequently chided himself for personal failings:

> There is an abominable staleness in my life—a lack of grip. Sloth and laziness—of action and thought. So far I have been far too happy to rest on my own estimate of my potentialities. Whenever I felt I had mastered something, that I could if I wanted,—as soon as [I] got sufficiently near [the] summit to satisfy myself that I could reach it, that was all I required. That extra effort was superfluous. I had already won my point . . . But I realise

---

[22] MS Laing K16. Notebook, July 1953 to August 1962.

[23] MS Laing K14.

[24] MS Laing K14.

[25] Ibid.

[26] Ibid.

[27] Ibid.

that this is not enough. Neither for myself nor other people. Henceforth my life must consist in actually doing what I know, or imagine I know I can do.[28]

And again: 'My trouble is that I'm too lazy and in too great a hurry. To act you must be able to forget. Nietzsche.'[29] Laing wondered whether a life of excess was compatible with his philosophical ambitions:

> There have been drunken and dissipated poets, musicians, doctors, and men of action, learned men, and even men of great goodness and love. But as far as I know there is no philosopher of distinction who has produced any systematic work and who has also been a drinker and fornicator. The practice of philosophy demands a considerable element of not-doing—esp. anything Dionysian. Philosophy demands sobriety, reflection, clarity, a fine precision of utterance. So of course does the work of any artist but it would seem that there are some things radically forbidden to the philosopher which are not denied the artist so absolutely.[30]

At times he wondered if he had anything to say:

> After K[ierkegaard] N[ietzshe] Dost[oyevsky] and later Freud, Sartre, Camus, Heidegger, Jaspers, what I often feel, [what is there] now to say. Merely interpretate [sic], to pick this from here, and that from there, add a little salt, and to a reasonable consistency.[31]

Laing also had religious doubts about his intellectual quest. As he wrote:

> Intelligire! That has been my desire for so long. But in itself I realise its 'vanity'—ie. its total impertinence as regards God and Grace and Salvation. But I don't believe in God or Grace and Salvation—so I tell myself and others—most of the time at least.[32]

He asked himself why he shouldn't give up philosophy and replied: 'I have gone so far. I am in mid stream. Too late to turn back—if I give up I drown . . . I can't stop thinking anymore than a spider can stop itself spinning its web'.[33] Laing linked his intellectual ambitions to his desire to be famous: put simply he wanted 'the fame of the wise man'.[34] In a letter to Marcelle Vincent, Laing wrote:

> I think of myself as a man of talent. I don't doubt that the raw material, the sheer pre potentiality that I have, is sufficient for me to be able to fulfil the worldly requirements of any position that lie in the line of the career I have chosen to pursue. In that sense I have confidence in myself. I certainly am afraid of 'coming to nothing' in a worldly sense—for all manner of reasons, my own folly, bad luck, lack of influence or the wrong sort of influence etc., but in this sense I am as well placed as anyone could wish to be for my age.[35]

---

[28] Ibid.

[29] Ibid.

[30] Ibid.

[31] Ibid.

[32] Ibid.

[33] Ibid.

[34] Evans, R.I. (1976). *R.D. Laing: The Man and his Ideas.* Dutton, New York, p. lxxi.

[35] Quoted in Clay, *R.D. Laing*, p. 45.

Laing also contrasted his intellectual ambitions with what he saw as the trap of domesticity:

> What a task I have: but unless I can do something, for myself, even though others are not helped, I shall be crippled in all purposeful activity. I shall take to a hearth or home, put my slippered feet up . . . warm bed . . . wife . . . children—fundamentally, a hideous failure.[36]

Laing worried that he would follow the path of his paternal grandfather who lost his 'brilliant career as a naval architect' when he was forty and had taken to drink. He thought that if he could achieve something intellectually he might avoid the 'involutional depression which I have been afraid of since 17 or 18'.[37] In middle age he looked back at this period and again observed that his hope had been to ward off melancholia by making a real contribution to the world of ideas.[38]

Leaving medical school: what path to follow?

When Laing left medical school he had to decide which career path to follow. He was attracted towards psychiatry, psychoanalysis, and neurology, but what sort of doctor should he be? Should he become an academic and do research? If so, should he embrace the natural scientific model which explained mental disorder in terms of biological malfunction? Or was this approach profoundly misguided? What role did social factors play in mental illness? Was mental disturbance really the outward manifestation of a spiritual crisis? Alongside these questions Laing was also trying to find a niche that would accommodate his deep interest in philosophy, religion, and literature. In a notebook entry, Laing looked back on his frame of mind at the time of his graduation from medical school.

> When I graduated in medicine from Glasgow University in January 1951, aged twenty four, I had my eyes firmly set on a medical career, steering a course somewhere through neurology, psychoanalysis, and neuropsychiatry. However I had already become completely committed to 'la vie intellectuelle' in an unlimited extensive sense, and so medicine and neurology in particular offered a focus upon which my many sided interests could converge their different styles of attention.
>
> I was at times . . . literally burning with the fever of the sense of urgency and crisis in my life. Everything was basically alright. I kept reminding myself that my problems were occasioned by a glut of possibility. Nevertheless I could feel more intensely intolerably alive and more suicidal at the same moment than ever before or since . . . I had regarded my student days, as student days. But now, it was now or never.[39]

On leaving medical school, Laing's sense of urgency intensified as he struggled to reconcile the theoretical with the practical. In *Wisdom, Madness and Folly*, he gives a description of his intellectual pre-occupations at this time:

> . . . my mind was in a theoretical ferment: historical materialism, nihilism, theology, philosophy, psychology, neurology, the discovery of phenomenology; Heidegger, Sartre,

---

[36] MS Laing K14, p. 4.
[37] MS Laing K1, p. 56.
[38] MS Laing A685. Drafts on travels.
[39] MS Laing K4.

Merleau-Ponty, Husserl; the discovery of the distinctions between understanding and explanation; the translation of the hermeneutics of the text to the hermeneutics of interpersonal relations; the twin figures, for me, of Kierkegaard and Nietzsche, Christ and Anti-Christ, the knight of faith, the destiny of nihilism; Nietzsche's critique of 'convictions' and his disposal of ego, free will, and the problems of psychiatry and psychopathology; Heidegger and the question of being, what is it to be? Wittgenstein: the destruction of that question. Nietzsche and Wittgenstein: history. The socio-economic material reality of society . . .[40]

The natural scientific method

In the end, of course, Laing chose psychiatry. He immersed himself in reading about the subject and began working out his response to what he witnessed in the wards and clinics. Initially he felt he might be able to make a 'real scientific contribution'. During his period as an Army psychiatrist, Laing reflected:

> There are numerous things I observe in the Insulin Unit. There are innumerable casual observations that could be pushed thro' to a conclusion. Kraep[elin] wrote his first paper as a medical student . . . Why did I not act like Kraep[elin]?[41]

Here we see Laing envying Emil Kraepelin for having published a scientific paper so early in his career, but he also wondered whether he felt comfortable with the natural scientific model, to which the German professor and many other researchers, subscribed. In his notebooks he confessed:

> I would 'like' to be positivistic, [and do] research; but I can't impress myself sufficiently by the 'importance' of any possible research which I can imagine, to embark upon it . . . The terrible secret is that I don't believe in natural science. And yet I do, I do.[42]

He continued:

> I was interested to read Schilder's brilliant book on 'The Body Image' but I know I will never write a book of that kind because I don't believe in the value (for me) of doing so. Ultimately what is its value? It has value as being interesting, fascinating, full of clever observations and some brilliant theorising. For what end? For whose good? I don't ask this rhetorically? In K[ierkegaard]'s terms I can bring to such reading and such work no ethical or religious meaning.[43]

Here Laing is referring to work of the Austrian psychiatrist, Paul Ferdinand Schilder, whose book, *The Image and Appearance of the Human Body,* was published in 1936. Laing wondered why he was responding in such a way:

> I am not incurious. Is my ambivalence to scientific observation to be accounted in p[sycho]. analytic terms? Undoubtedly so. But what does a p[sycho]. a[nalytical] 'explanation' explain?

---

[40] Laing, *Wisdom, Madness and Folly,* p. 96.
[41] MS Laing K14, no page number.
[42] Ibid., pp. 2–3.
[43] Ibid., p. 3.

O for the naivete of the young Maudsley! Or the dogmatism of Sargant—no more meta-physics! The denial of metaphysics is the denial of one's own being.[44]

Laing mentions Henry Maudsley, the eminent Victorian alienist who held uncom-promisingly materialist views about the nature of insanity. William Sargant, a twentieth century London psychiatrist, was dismissive of psychoanalysis and was a zealous proponent of physical treatments such as ECT and psychosurgery. Laing went on to consider clinical research:

> . . . the ideal of modern clinical research—I can regard only as a form of self-punishment for self-indulgence in 'speculation' . . . I can hardly believe that I shall even become engaged in this type of work. I am not esp. concerned to demonstrate to myself or others what changes take place in the blood cells or chemistry during or after insulin coma, what changes there are in C.S.F., reflexes etc.—I am prepared to believe that changes take place . . . I am interested to read about it, I shall remember it for a little while and then forget it . . . So what. What does it tell me about this man who is in an insulin coma because he persisted in wandering around his Unit 'in search of God' as he told people—perhaps his brain does not utilise glutamic acid the way my brain does or perhaps it does and mine doesn't—I can't remember and I don't care very much . . . what is glutamic acid to me, or me to glutamic acid?[45]

For Laing, a knowledge of biochemistry did not contribute to an understanding of human distress. Typically, he used an example with a religious theme to support his argument. And typically, he referred to Kierkegaard to expose the limitations of the scientific method:

> Curiosity, looking down a microscope or thro a telescope is a 'joke'—as K[ierkegaard] puts it. But a joke only in terms of the paradoxical—of the irony of trying/hoping to find what cannot be found by such a method . . . As K[ierkegaard] says—that a man should simply or profoundly say that he can't explain consciousness is fine but that he should look down a mic[roscope] for years and years and say that he still can't explain consc[iousness] is ridiculous![46]

Having looked at Laing's campaign to become a man of intellectual substance, we will now examine what he was actually reading during this formative period.

Laing's library

Laing's personal library, which is now housed at Glasgow University, offers an illumi-nating insight into his intellectual background and the works he was devouring in these early years.[47] Even confining the survey to books published before 1960, one is struck by how wide-ranging his reading was. Laing often tried to read authors in their original tongue and he took a keen interest in learning languages. His collection includes books on French, German, Greek, and Italian. In literature, he read Greek

---

[44] Ibid., p. 3.

[45] Ibid., no page number.

[46] Ibid.

[47] Glasgow University Library Special Collections. Laing's personal library.

drama, French poetry, mediaeval Latin lyrics, Chinese poems, as well as Shakespeare, Dickens, Orwell, Gogol, Tolstoy, Dostoyevsky, Goethe, Kafka, Thomas Mann, Rilke, Cervantes, Strindberg, Mallarme, Baudelaire, Genet, Diderot, Camus, Sartre, Flaubert, James Joyce, Samuel Beckett, Herman Melville, and Hemingway. There are several Scottish works, such as the poems of Hugh MacDiarmid, William Dunbar, and William McGonagall, Border ballads, *The Golden Treasury of Scottish Poetry, Modern Scottish Poetry*, Eric Linklater's *Poet's Pub*, Compton MacKenzie's *Carnival*, Walter Scott's *The Existence of Evil Spirits Proved, and their Agency Particularly in Relation to the Human Race*, and Thomas Carlyle's *Sartor Resartus*. In a notebook, Laing had remarked that Carlyle's world was one of work and duty.[48] At an early stage Laing was interested in his native culture, but, initially he made little reference to it in his published work.

Laing read widely on religion, taking in Christian work such as *St Theresa of Avila by Herself, The Confessions of Saint Augustine, The Life and Words of Christ* by Cunningham Geikie, *The Life of Jesus* by Ernest Renan, as well as the Bible and hymn books. He had two works by his friend George Macleod, leader of the Iona Community. These were *Bombs and Bishops* and *Only One Way Left*. In the latter Laing had marked the passage which read: '. . . Christian man went wild. He forgot the word "companion" which means the sharer of the loaf'.[49] In his autobiography, *Wisdom, Madness and Folly*,[50] Laing was to discuss the concept of companionship, a quality he felt was lacking in psychiatric hospitals. Laing had written on the back of his copy of MacLeod's book: 'Whether we have this faith to despair . . . for life begins in the far side of despair'.[51] Laing read mystical writers such as Jacob Boehme, Pseudo-Dionysius the Aeopagite, Master Eckhart, and books on theosophy, the Qabalah, and *The Tibetan Book of the Great Liberation*. He also read the *Upanishads, Religion and Thought in Ancient Egypt, The Life of the Buddha*, and Norman Cohn's *The Pursuit of the Millennium*.

He had a large collection of philosophy books by such thinkers as Plato, Aristotle, Descartes, Voltaire, Hegel, Schopenhauer, Nietzsche, Marx, Husserl, Heidegger, Jaspers, Locke, Berkeley, Popper, Russell, Wittgenstein, Merleau-Ponty, and Sartre. He also had Strawson's *Individuals*, Koestler's *The Yogi and the Commissar*, and Hannah Arendt's *The Human Condition*, as well as books on Indian philosophy, the Neo-Platonists, early Greek philosophy, and the Scholastics. He read Scottish works such as John Macmurray's *The Self as Agent*, Thomas Brown's *Lectures on Philosophy of the Human Mind*, Alexander Bain's *Mental and Moral Science*, David Hume's *A Treatise of Human Nature*, and William Hamilton's *Lectures on Metaphysics*. He made extensive notes on *The Scottish Philosophy from Hutcheson to Hamilton* by James McCosh.[52] He had a copy of *Philosophical Lecture-Notes: for the use of students in the Logic Ordinary Class of Glasgow University* by C.A. Campbell. Following his

---

[48] MS Laing K12. Notebook, 1951–1952, p. 96.
[49] Glasgow University Library Special Collection. Laing's personal library 646. Macleod, G. (1958). *Only One Way Left*. Glasgow, Iona Community, p. 6.
[50] Laing, *Wisdom, Madness and Folly*, p. 126.
[51] Macleod, *Only One Way Left*, back flyleaf of book.
[52] MS Laing A689. Handwritten extracts.

commands to himself in his notebooks, Laing made great efforts to familiarize himself with the philosophical tradition of his own country.

Laing was very interested in biographies and compared his progress with that of the Great Men in world culture. He had the lives of Pope, Shelley, Kafka, Baudelaire, Dostoyevsky, and two on William Blake. He also had the curiously titled *The Life of Professor John Stuart Blackie, the most distinguished Scotsman of the day*. He read *The Confessions* of Rousseau, as well as the autobiographies of Benjamin Franklin, Charles Darwin, John Stuart Mill, and Igor Stravinsky. Laing also read James Joyce's fictional autobiography *The Portrait of the Artist as a Young Man*.[53] In one diary entry he wrote: 'There are certain "lives" I must know about more specifically e.g. Yeats, Coleridge, Beethoven, Goethe. Study the *method* of biography'.[54] He also made notes on an autobiography of Arthur Koestler.[55] He wondered why we read biography. Was it to idealize or to denigrate the person? When he came to construct his own autobiographical narrative Laing would draw on this reading.

He had books on film and history and books on Beethoven and Bach. He also possessed Ernst Kris's *Psychoanalytic Explorations in Art* and many books on artists, such as Hieronymus Bosch, Breughel, Matisse, Modigliani, Picasso, Klee, and Chagall. He had the notebooks of Leonardo Da Vinci, the journal of Delacroix, and Herbert Read's *Education through Art*. In one of his notebooks, Laing commented on the genius of Leonardo, using the terminology of Kierkegaard:

> Instead of applying the categories of morbidity to Leonardo, the neurotic must be estimated in terms of Leonardo. Yet it is not an aesthetic, or even ethical (in K[ierkegaard]'s terms) superiority which the great man has.[56]

As may be expected, he had a large collection of books on psychiatry and psychology. As well as books by William James, Bleuler, Jung, Ernest Jones, Medard Boss, Binswanger, Pierre Janet, and Henry Ey, he had Havelock Ellis's *Sex in Relation to Society*, Ian Suttie's *The Origins of Love and Hate*, and Ida Macalpine's *Schizophrenia 1677*. He also possessed *The Psychology of Insanity* by Bernard Hart, who worked at the National Hospital, Queen's Square in London.

It is interesting to see what subjects did *not* interest Laing. There are comparatively few books on science compared with those on the arts. There are hardly any books on politics, though there is a biography of Trotsky and a book by Lenin. Given the Left's adoption of Laing in the 1960s this might seem surprising, but he was actually more interested in change from within than without. One of his books, Arthur Koestler's *The Yogi and the Commissar* explored this dichotomy. For Koestler, the commissar represented the political approach which sought to change the structure of society. The yogi represented the religious approach which attended to the inner world. It seems clear that Laing, in Koestler's classification, was a yogi. When Laing came to discuss politics in his notebooks, his focus was on the individual and their relation

---

[53] Glasgow University Library Special Collections. Laing's personal library 351. Joyce, J. (1942). *Portrait of the Artist as a Young Man*. Jonathan Cape, London.

[54] MS Laing K16.

[55] MS Laing K14.

[56] Ibid.

to society. He was much less interested in providing a sustained political critique than in examining the difficulties that conformity posed for the individual. There are occasional references to Marx, but in his discussions with his girlfriend, Marcelle Vincent, he argued against Marxism.[57] In later interviews Laing stated that he had never been attracted to Marx, at least in its narrow economic focus.[58] Curiously, he maintained that his first literary project was to be a biography of John Maclean, the Glasgow communist, who became the first overseas Bolshevik consulate in the early part of the twentieth century.[59] As a student, Laing had read Tom Johnston's *A History of the Working Class of Scotland* and began to feel that Scotland was a colony which was owned by English capitalists.[60] It is evident, though, that Laing was more interested in thinkers such as Nietzsche and Kierkegaard, who focused on the individual.

In addition to books, Laing also read magazines, such as *Les Temps Moderne*, which was edited by Sartre and Merleau-Ponty and which could be purchased in Glasgow. He read *Horizon*,[61] an 'avant-garde intellectual journal of the 1940s',[62] edited by Cyril Connolly. The last editorial reviewed the previous ten years of the journal and observed:

> We became a display window for Sartre and Camus and the French writers . . . and were in danger of becoming an advertisement for international fashions of the mind . . . One can perceive the inner trend of the Forties as maintaining this desperate struggle of the modern movement, between man, *betrayed by science, bereft of religion,* deserted by the pleasant imaginings of humanism.[63]

Laing recalled this magazine in *The Bird of Paradise*, which he wrote in 1967:

> Bookshop, Glasgow. Usual copy of *Horizon*. The last number!
> 'It is closing time in the Gardens of the West. From now on a writer will be judged by the resonances of his silence and the quality of his despair.'[64]

Laing retorted to this passage in the magazine with a passionate outburst that may have reflected his feelings at the time:

> All right—you did not have a circulation of more than eighty thousand. You ran out of money. But you bastard, speak for yourself. Write *Horizon* off and wish yourself off. Don't write me off. I'll be judged by my music not by my silence and by the quality of whatever pathetic shreds of faith, hope and charity still cling to me.[65]

---

[57] Clay, *RD Laing,* pp. 31–2.
[58] For example, Charlesworth, M. (1976). *The Existentialists and Jean-Paul Sartre.* George Prior, London, pp. 49–50.
[59] Mullan, *Mad to be Normal,* p. 89.
[60] Mullan, *Mad to be Normal,* p. 89.
[61] Laing, *The Politics of Experience and the Bird of Paradise,* p.144.
[62] Howarth-Williams, M. (1977). *R.D. Laing. His Work and its Relevance for Sociology.* Routledge and Kegan Paul, London, p. 4.
[63] Quoted in Harcourt-Williams, *Laing,* p. 4.
[64] Laing, *The Politics of Experience and the Bird of Paradise,* p. 144.
[65] Ibid., p. 144.

Medical school: first public pronouncements and early writings

A medical institution is not the place to find freedom of thought and speech. I learned at school and at university to voice my thoughts and feelings with the greatest precaution and circumspection to teachers, tutors or professors.[66]

During his time as a medical student, Laing gave talks and wrote essays. We first encounter the public Laing in January 1947 as a second year medical student, addressing his colleagues at the Medico-Chirurgical Society.[67] He sounds assured and intellectually precocious. He discusses what he perceives as the three types of students and their reaction to the knowledge they are receiving. The first type refuses to accept it. He observes: 'I'm sure Professor Hamilton's hair would stand on end had he the faintest idea of the number of students in Second Year Medicine who, as they put it "don't believe in evolution".' The second type keep their medical knowledge separate from what else they know. 'Thus any difficult problems which ought to be arising in their minds simply do not arise.' He then outlines the characteristics of the last group, to which he clearly feels he belongs:

> Thirdly there are the students who attempt as far as they can to bring what they learn in their studies here into line with ideas derived from other sources. They seek to apply their new-found knowledge to more general problems. This is quite a difficult thing to do if it is done honestly . . . Students of this type tend to separate themselves into two well-defined camps. Some see in everything a purpose, a meaning, 'a directiveness of organic activities', a design and hence a Designer. Their studies confirm & strengthen what religious convictions they already have. Others again see equally clearly that there is no purpose or aim behind organic processes, that the forces at work are blind.[68]

Here we see Laing emphasizing the inter-relatedness of different fields of knowledge. In this he exemplified what George Davie[69] has described as 'the democratic intellect', which he held to be a characteristic feature of the Scottish approach to education. Davie maintained that the Scots were interested in generalization rather than specialization; the latter approach he identified with the English educational system. In this talk, we also see Laing suggesting that medical knowledge should be applied to wider problems. Later he will use his psychiatric skills to diagnose society at large. In this passage Laing speaks of those who believe in a Designer and those who believe that

---

[66] MS Laing A685, p. 17.

[67] MS Laing A519. Impressions of a Second Year Med. Student. A paper delivered to The G.U. Medico-Chirurgical Society.

[68] MS Laing A519.

[69] Davie, G.E. (1961). *The Democratic Intellect. Scotland and her Universities in the Nineteenth Century.* Edinburgh University Press, Edinburgh. Davie's thesis has attracted its critics, for example, Robert Anderson (1983). *Education and Opportunity in Victorian Scotland.* Edinburgh University Press, Edinburgh. Anderson stresses the practical, socializing function of Scottish education.

there is no purpose to existence. Laing, himself, swung between these two poles, from belief to unbelief. He went on to describe his own outlook:

> Speaking for myself, I have become much more critical and sceptical since I came to the varsity and this is largely [owing] to the nature of my studies . . . I simply mean a refusal to accept things at their face value or merely on authority . . . If my studies have made me critical my fellow students have made me more tolerant.[70]

Health and happiness

Whilst he was a medical student Laing managed to have two articles published and win an essay prize. These and the associated draft versions give a good indication of his intellectual pre-occupations at the time. Laing's first literary success was a composition, entitled 'Health and happiness',[71] which won the Students Essay Prize in 1948 in a competition held by the International Psychoanalytic Society for British undergraduates. An ambitious essay which shows signs of precocity in the range of intellectual references cited, it is also something of an exercise in showing-off. At its core is an orthodox Freudian perspective on the state of humanity. At this stage Laing has mastered the basics of psychoanalytic theory and appears to use it in a very accepting and uncritical way to discuss the attainment of happiness. However, as he quite reasonably commented later, because he was entering a competition set by psychoanalysts, he emphasized the Freudian perspective. To this basic brew of psychoanalytic theory, he stirs in references to Rabelais, Swift, Camus, Rilke, Lewis Carroll, Havelock Ellis, Andre Breton, Max Ernst, Auden, T.S. Eliot, Donne, Dostoyevsky, Bergson, Jean-Paul Sartre, Robert Louis Stevenson, Thomas Mann, Maxim Gorky, Mayakovsky, Martin Buber, and Ian Suttie. There are also quotations in Latin.

Certain themes in this early essay, though crudely and somewhat artlessly expressed, anticipate Laing's later, more mature work. First, there is the theme that madness and sanity are on a spectrum and are not distinct conditions. As he writes: 'We cannot look upon the insane as a race apart anymore.'[72] Laing observes that Freud had demonstrated that the minds of the mad and the 'normal' are 'exactly the same'.[73] This contention very much foreshadowed Laing's later pleas for treating the mentally ill with humanity. A second theme in the essay is the oppressive influence of parental upbringing and education. The child's curiosity about the world, particularly sexuality, is 'brought to an abrupt end by energetic repression'. Education serves to distort and constrain the personality. It blocks the child's spontaneity. Laing was to amplify this claim in his 1967 counter-culture best-seller, *The Politics of Experience*, in which he writes:

> From the moment of birth, when the stone-age baby confronts the twentieth century mother, the baby is subjected to . . . forces of violence called love, as its mother and father

---

[70] MS Laing A519.

[71] MS Laing A64. 'Health and happiness', 1948.

[72] Ibid., p. 1.

[73] Although Hunter-Brown (*R.D. Laing*, p. 70) observed that Angus MacNiven held similar ideas, it was a commonplace of Freudian thinking, and Laing was not claiming to be original.

have been, and their parents, and their parents before them. These forces are mainly concerned with destroying most of its potentialities. This enterprise is on the whole successful. By the time the new human being is fifteen or so, we are left with a being like ourselves. A half-crazed creature, more or less adjusted to a mad world. This is normality in our present age.[74]

The third and most recurring theme in the essay is the contrast between the creative individual and the ignorant and unimaginative masses. Laing holds that most of the masses are happy because they uncritically accepted life's 'illusions'. Those individuals with more 'insight and knowledge', whom Laing deems 'our brightest people', are 'frustrated and unhappy'. Thus a mark of one's sophistication and worth is the degree to which one is miserable. There are certain individuals, he observes, who are prepared to face 'greater mental distress in the interests of truth than the "normal" man'. It seems clear that Laing includes himself in this category of the despairing but knowing. To achieve knowledge, one has to follow Freud in his in-depth exploration of the unconscious. Anything less is 'pseudo-self-knowledge', and people who settle for this 'tend to be proud of the superficial schools of psychology such as Adler's'. Laing adds contemptuously, '[they] are very common amongst psychiatrists'. This certainly could be viewed as arrogance, and it does seem to anticipate Laing's later, negative views about his psychiatric colleagues.

Of the general population, Laing writes: 'The enlightened individual comes to despise the mass: and the mass, when it does not ignore or ridicule him, attempts to control him.' Once again, Laing appears to be writing about himself, and he sets up a dichotomy between the superiority of the gifted individual and the dull, uncomprehending mass. Much of Laing's later writing repeated and amplified this theme. He evinces an antagonism if not contempt for 'normal' society, and his heroes are the outsiders—the artists, the thinkers, and the mad. They are in perpetual battle with the forces of conformism, which try to grind them down or lock them up. Laing concludes his essay with the thesis that it is more important to change man from within than to change his external circumstances. He observes:

> The discoveries of Freud will have a much greater influence for good in the world than those of Marx. They are no less revolutionary but in a much truer and more profound sense. The Marxist imagines that a revolution in the Politico-economico structure of society will revolutionise man's mind. But it may well be that a change of mind can revolutionise society.[75]

Despite his later association with radical left-wing politics, Laing continued to maintain that it was more important to attend to the inner man than to the outer society. He ends the essay by hoping that if enough people are able to change from within—along the lines stipulated by Freud—it will 'save society from destroying its best individuals through its own ignorance and incompetence'. The essay also displays Laing's knowledge and interest in literature. Creative and unusual people emerge as

---

[74] Laing, R.D. (1967). *The Politics of Experience and the Bird of Paradise*. Penguin Books, London, p. 50.

[75] Laing, R.D., *Health and happiness*, p.16.

his heroes. Laing refers approvingly to a quotation from Dostoyevsky: 'The nobler type of people are all mentally ill nowadays. Only the mediocre and the untalented are heartily capable of enjoying life.'

At this stage Laing presents an orthodox Freudian outlook but it is filtered through his own perspective which champions the individual (if they are gifted) over the herd. There are other aspects of the essay which reveal Laing's pre-occupations. For example, in a passage which seems to acutely describe his own spiritual position, he writes, 'Many have lost their faith but have not lost the sense of sin nor attained the saving belief in redemption.' Years later, in his autobiography, Laing spoke of seeing love 'crucified' but could not see its 'resurrection'.[76]

Philosophy and medicine

His second essay was a short history of medical psychology and it appeared in the Glasgow University magazine, *Surgo*, in 1949 under the title, 'Philosophy and medicine'.[77] Laing was heavily influenced by Gregory Zilboorg's *A History of Medical Psychology*,[78] which had appeared in 1941, and from which he had made copious notes. The draft version of the paper is more extensive than the published *Surgo* version. It begins with the sixteenth-century Spanish clinician, Juan Luis Vives, whom Laing, following the opinion of Zilboorg, describes as 'one of the founders of modern psychiatry'. He quotes Vives as saying: 'What the soul (anima) is, is of no concern for us to know: what it is like, what its manifestations are, is of very great importance.' Laing remarks that the writings of philosophers and theologians about the soul have made a great contribution to the development of medical psychology. He applauds Plato's contention that it is an error to have physicians for the body and physicians for the soul, as mind and body are one and indivisible.

Typically, Laing is interested in Plato's view that madness and genius are related. As Laing notes, Plato claimed that there were two types of insanity, one which is the result of disease and the other which is a gift from the gods. Laing observes:

> The rational, immortal soul of man may in a state of ecstasy, act so forcibly on the body as to cause a form of madness. This sort of thing may possess a poet or a philosopher in moments of inspiration.[79]

Laing concedes that not everyone accepts that there *is* a link between the genius and the mad man, but he asserts that in both cases 'unconscious material' is 'brought to the surface of the mind'. He observes that the Surrealists explored the unconscious for symbols and images. Andre Breton, Laing notes with admiration, probably mingled with a touch of envy, had started the Surrealist movement as a medical student. He quotes Breton as saying: 'It is only at the approach of the fantastic, at a point where human

---

[76] Laing, *Wisdom, Madness and Folly*, p. 96.

[77] MS Laing A408, Philosophy and Medical Psychology (1948). Laing, R.D. (1949). 'Philosophy and medicine', *Surgo*, June, 134–5.

[78] Zilboorg, G. (1941). *A History of Medical Psychology*. (in collaboration with Henry GW) WW Norton & Co., New York.

[79] MS Laing A408, no page numbers.

reason loses its control that the most profound emotion of the individual has the fullest opportunity to express itself.' In subsequent years, Laing was to exalt the positive aspects of insanity, hailing it as leading to emotional growth and authenticity, most emphatically and most notoriously in *The Politics of Experience and the Bird of Paradise*.

In the essay, Laing considers the mind–body problem and attempts to find a physical location for the workings of the mind. He dismisses these attempts in a phrase he lifted from Zilboorg's *A History of Medical Psychology*, as examples of 'brain mythology'. Laing declares that he does not think that the mind–body problem will ever be solved by trying to establish the primacy of mind over matter or *vice versa*. In a response he was to use again in his later work, for example, in his Schumacher lecture,[80] he states: 'What is mind? No matter: what is matter? Never mind!' Laing quotes the work of the English neurophysiologist, Sir Charles Sherrington who pointed to the lack of physical evidence for a materialist explanation of mind. He then goes on to consider the views of Schopenhauer, Nietzsche, Freud, and Spinoza, who, he maintains, all questioned the notion of the free will. He concludes:

> If there is any lesson we can learn from the history of philosophy and science it is that knowledge is indivisible. Despite the present departmentalism in our educational system and the specialization in research and all branches of medicine this fact remains true . . . The acquisition of learning and factual knowledge is of very limited value unless such learning and knowledge are related to the rest of human wisdom.[81]

Once again, Laing emphasizes the inter-relatedness of all branches of knowledge and stresses that facts, on their own, taken out of their human context, are of dubious worth. This was to become a major theme of his later work. In the published essay, Laing changes the ending. In this version, he concludes by praising the Greeks for combining the study of the arts with that of medicine. This was another recurring theme in his later work. In both the essay and draft, Laing's writing once again reflects his wide reading and his tendency to intellectually name-drop.

Health and society

A third article, entitled 'Health and society'[82] appeared in the 1950 Candlemas issue of *Surgo* and was based on his 'Winning Senior Address, Medico-Chirurgical Society Members' Night'. It opens with a sentiment that Laing was to repeatedly return to in later years: 'It is a mistake to regard the normal person as necessarily a healthy person.' He goes on to consider man in his social context and the role that society plays in ill-health. He states that orthodox medicine has been reluctant to look at this area, but since the end of the nineteenth century, it has been clear that Western civilization has been prone to conditions that do not afflict other societies. He quotes the American neurologist, George Beard, who described neurasthenia, and also the German sexologist, Kraft-Ebbing, who talked about the 'syphilisation and society'. He cites Freud,

---

[80] Laing, R.D. (1980). 'What is the matter with mind?'. In Kumar, S. (ed.) *The Schumacher Lectures*. Blond & Briggs, London, pp. 1–19.

[81] MS Laing A408, pp. 6–7.

[82] Laing, R.D. (1950). 'Health and society'. *Surgo*, Candlemas, 91–2.

who held that the rapid and vast changes in society had produced deleterious changes in the nervous systems of the people. Laing considers the interplay between the individual and society in the creation of illness. He refers approvingly to the Glasgow physician, J.L. Halliday, who had written about psychosocial medicine and who had concluded that it was not the patient but society that was sick.

Laing's reference to J.L. Halliday is interesting. Halliday was a Glasgow doctor, who like Laing, had a background in the arts and the classics.[83] Unusually for a physician, he had undergone analytic training and held a part-time appointment as a psychotherapist at the Lansdowne Clinic in Glasgow. He wrote *Mr Carlyle, My Patient*, a biography of the eminent Scotsman whose chronic dyspepsia he investigated along psychosomatic lines. In 1948, Halliday published his internationally celebrated book *Psychosocial Medicine*, in which he combined his experience in Public Health with Freudian theory to analyse health trends in society.[84] He claimed that statistics showed physical health was improving, but that psychological ill-health was rising. He outlined a picture of what he called the 'sick society'. The increasing application of science to the physical environment had brought about major changes in the structure of society. Halliday contended that before the Industrial Revolution children were allowed to develop emotionally at their own pace, but from the 1870s onwards they were subjected to an ordered regime of toilet-training and feeding by the clock, combined with the fussy over-protection of their parents. This and the decline of religious faith, which gave a sense of purpose to life, had led to the increase in mental problems among the population. Laing is clearly influenced by Halliday in this student essay, but he also drew on his ideas when he came to write his more mature work.

In the remainder of the essay, Laing considers what effect a sick society can have on its citizens. He warns: 'It is not immediately obvious that traits we regard as normal may by people in the future be regarded as grossly abnormal.'[85] He refers to the witch trials in eighteenth century New England and observes: 'today the "witches" would be in Crookston Old Folks' home [in Glasgow] and their executioners would be having a course of E.C.T. or leucotomy at Gartnavel'.[86] Laing goes on to speculate that even some of society's most admired individuals, for example, from politics or the business world, might be judged as insane in the future. He quotes Spinoza who suggested that greed and ambition were forms of insanity, and also Erich Fromm and Kierkegaard who had both questioned the validity of the distinction between sanity and insanity. Laing concludes that a healthy society is a necessary prerequisite for healthy citizens. The present society is unhealthy, resulting in an increased incidence of psychoses, neuroses, and psychosomatic disease. He ends provocatively:

> I suggest that it may be that the standard of normalcy accepted in our culture prevents some people from realizing their full potentialities as human beings and that many

83 ACM (1983). 'Obituary of JL Halliday'. *British Medical Journal*, **28**, 697.

84 Halliday, J.L. (1949). *Psychological Medicine. A Study of the Sick Society*. William Heinemann, London. For an account of Halliday, see Brown, J.A.C. (1964). *Freud and the Post-Freudians*. Penguin, Harmondsworth, pp. 97–100.

85 Laing, *Health and society,* p. 92.

86 Ibid., p. 92.

normal people in our present time are far from being healthy as judged by an objective standard.[87]

This passage reflects Laing's abiding preoccupation with the definition of 'normalcy'. He holds that society uses the category of 'abnormality' to repress the more imaginative of its citizens.

Laing's three student essays reveal him as precocious and eclectic in his reading. He sounds self-assured in his discussions of major intellectual issues, verging at times on arrogance. In a remarkable way these articles anticipate most of the major themes that would dominate his later work.

The individual and society

One theme from the student essays in particular—the relationship between the individual and society—continued to preoccupy Laing throughout his life. For example, in notebooks written during his time in the Army, he again ponders the issue. He asks himself what *he* can do about the 'established order' of society. He tells himself:

> Do as much as you can. But if that much is not enough to make any appreciable difference to the Est[ablished order]why bother? . . . One can do what one can, one should at least do that. That is all one can ever do. But we have all come to value our actions not by their subjective absoluteness, but by their objective effect. One can 'bear witness', 'testify' to what one believes. But what is the point of testifying to dumb ears (e.g. Nazi or Russian torture chamber).[88]

He comments: 'Anything which overthrows the established order or calls it in question, is profoundly suspect and will always be attacked. e.g. Socrates, Christ.'[89] He considers that there are five categories of deviance: cranks, heretics, great reformers, criminals, and the mad. The most threatening category to society is that of the mad. But how, Laing wonders, does society define madness? Is it a deviation from a statistical 'norm'? Against this notion, Laing argues: 'If a sufficient number of people were hallucinated, hallucinations would not be regarded as basically "morbid"'.[90] Further, he contends:

> To be sane is to share the world, lived in by the statistical majority, to share the experiences and make the same judgements about real and non-real etc. of the majority in our culture—or at least to act more or less as though one did so. It is to share the sensus communis . . . the 'common' sense of the community. A creative genius does not live in this world . . . [91]

Perhaps madness is defined by non-conformity? One has to adapt to the expectations of society, but one has to be careful not to be too intense about it. Laing writes:

> He is perhaps expected to bear the suffering 'common to mankind' but he is not called upon to take upon unnecessary suffering—if he does so he is a *masochist*. He is expected to be as enthusiastic and as hard working as the most [sic], but not to be too enthusiastic,

---

[87] Ibid., p. 92.
[88] MS Laing K15.
[89] Ibid.
[90] MS Laing K14.
[91] Ibid.

or too devoted to his work. If he is, he is *ipso facto*, an *hypomanic*. He is expected to strive after efficiency and perfection. If he has too an exacting ideal he is, ipso facto, a perfectionist for which a psychopathology will be found.[92]

In another extract, which anticipates Richard Bentall's[93] ironic proposal that happiness should be classified as a psychiatric disorder, Laing questions the diagnosis of depression:

He's got depression. What about saying 'He's got happiness'. And this is not merely a form of words. It's a way of thinking. Depression is reified, it is state, a condition, a syndrome, a disease.[94]

Laing's early discussions about how society defined madness anticipated his later work, such as *The Politics of Experience and the Bird of Paradise*. He would continue to believe that society exercised a repressive and malign effect on its citizens, and that the best and brightest suffered the most, at times being driven to insanity. He repeatedly questioned whether 'normality' necessarily equated with sanity. Burston contrasts Laing's questioning of the concept of normality with its unexamined acceptance by many psychiatrists, who, nevertheless, do not define what they mean by it.[95] Laing did not believe that the exceptional individual should cut themselves off from society; a life of splendid isolation also carried risks. Surely the creative person wanted to communicate with others, or why would they bother to make their work public. With Holderlin and Nietzsche in mind, and perhaps also himself, Laing wrote:

The *risk* of the genius—madness—despite himself—if his effort fails—if he remains too long without being able to establish contact, rapport—to share his world—the risk of madness.[96]

Early papers

Deception and the Ganser syndrome

During his period in the Army, Laing pursued his interest in the subject of lying, an interest, which we have seen, began in childhood when he first discovered that he could tell untruths to adults and not be found out. When he came to examine soldiers, Laing was fascinated by the problem of differentiating lies from *bona fide* mental or physical disorders. Along with his colleague, Murray Brookes, an Ear, Nose, and Throat specialist, Laing wrote a paper, entitled 'On the recognition of simulated and functional deafness'.[97] The authors state:

A malingerer is one who is lying; that is, he makes a statement which he himself believes to be false. He deliberately simulates a disease for the sake of personal gain. He lies and

---

[92] MS Laing K15.

[93] Bentall, R. (1992). 'A proposal to classify happiness as a psychiatric disorder'. *Journal of Medical Ethics*, **18**, 94–8.

[94] MS Laing K16.

[95] Burston, D. (2000). *The Crucible of Experience. R.D. Laing and the Crisis of Psychotherapy*. Harvard University Press, Cambridge, Massachusetts.

[96] MS Laing K14.

[97] MS Laing A518. Lieutenant Murray Brookes and Captain Ronald D Laing, 'On the recognition of simulated and functional deafness'. Unpublished manuscript.

knows he is lying. In contra-distinction the hysteric is deceiving himself, and believes himself to be suffering from his disability, as in fact he is. The liar is deceiving only other people and has constantly to be on his guard.[98]

In the paper, the authors make reference to *The Road to En-dor*. This was a book by Elias Henry Jones, a Welsh officer in the Indian Army who, along with a fellow-soldier, tried to escape from the Yozgad prisoner of war camp in Turkey during the First World War by faking madness. Laing continued to be interested in the area of deception throughout his life. In an eloquent passage in a 1960 paper on existential analysis, he wrote:

Between . . . 'truth' and a lie there is room for the most curious and subtle ambiguities and complexities in the person's disclosure/concealment of himself. For instance, one may say with confidence, 'His smile gave him away', or, 'That expression is just put on', 'Or that rings true', and so on. But what has been revealed, what concealed, and to whom, in the Gioconda smile, in the 'twixt earnest and joke' of Blake's angel, in the infinite pathos—or is it apathy—of a Harlequin of Picasso? [99]

Later still, in his book, *Knots*, Laing examined human communication and how people lied to each other and themselves.

In 1953, Laing, or rather Lieutenant Ronald D. Laing, published his first professional article,[100] which was concerned with the Ganser syndrome, a type of hysterical condition. He describes the case of a young soldier and draws on psychodynamic and object relations theory. He also makes reference to Henderson and Gillespie's *Textbook of Psychiatry*, the well-respected Glasgow primer he had used as a medical student. He concludes his article by stating: 'This Ganser-like reaction may be understood as a massive, desperate and temporary defence to a situation fraught with both internal and external danger to the ego.' We will consider this article in more detail when we look at Laing's clinical work as an Army psychiatrist.

Papers on Paul Tillich and human-relatedness

While he was a registrar at the Glasgow Royal Mental Hospital, Laing wrote a draft paper, entitled, 'An examination of Tillich's theory of anxiety and neurosis',[101] which he sent to *The British Journal of Medical Psychology*. It arrived on 19 February 1954. The draft was an attempt to introduce the work of the philosopher, Paul Tillich to a general audience and to relate his writing on anxiety to psychoanalysis. Tillich was a German philosopher and theologian whose writing was in the tradition of Christian existentialism. In the mid-twentieth century his work struck a chord with the general public as it dealt with the widespread post-war anxiety about the apparent meaninglessness

---

[98] Ibid., p. 2.

[99] MS Laing A116–7. Laing, R.D. (1960). 'The development of existential analysis. A paper submitted to RMPA, December 1960', p. 20.

[100] Laing, R.D. (1953). 'An instance of the Ganser Syndrome'. *Journal of the Royal Army Medical Corps*, **99**, 169–72.

[101] MS Laing A112. (1954). R.D. Laing, 'An examination of Tillich's theory of anxiety and neurosis'.

of life.[102] Tillich had fled Nazi Germany in 1933 for America, where he went on to pursue a highly successful university career, eventually becoming a professor at Harvard. He was greatly respected in the academic world of theology and philosophy but, with the publication of *The Courage to Be* in 1952, his work burst upon the wider American cultural scene and he became an intellectual celebrity. According to Gomes, Tillich's book became a classic, was on every college reading list, and its very title—*The Courage to Be*—entered the language of campus debate.[103] There are, of course, parallels with Laing's period of popular acclaim in the mid-1960s when *his* work was widely read and quoted by American students, and by many others. Tillich would have been another example to Laing of the intellectual as a lauded public figure who imparts his wisdom to an eager audience. As we have noted, Laing actually met Tillich several times in 1955 and 1956 when the latter gave lectures in Glasgow.[104] Interestingly, in view of Laing's subsequent public performances, he remembers that Tillich 'went pretty far over the edge for some'.

Laing's original draft paper on Tillich is a rather cumbersome and opaque piece, but it does reflect some of his pre-occupations in these early years. First, he states that relying on medical psychology to explain anxiety is too limiting, and that other perspectives, particularly that of philosophy, should be considered. He acknowledges that some readers might be dismayed at the discussion of philosophical matters in a 'scientific' journal, but he argues that notions of the soul and of being cannot be dismissed as 'irrelevant'. As in his student essay on the history of medical psychology, Laing uses the same quotation from Vives, the sixteenth century Spanish clinician, but this time he is critical of the idea that, 'What the soul (anima) is, is of no concern for us to know.' In a colourful passage, Laing maintains that Vives' words are no longer appropriate:

> They were, I imagine, bitter words. They were the assertion of the right of a young science to go its own way, unfettered by the sterile and restrictive authority of the traditional philosophy and theology of the day. That day has passed. Theology is a queen without a crown, and like some royal émigrés, she has been pathetically reduced, at times, to soliciting casual favours from the new lords of the sun. But surely the time is gone when scientists of fact need any longer strike a pose of defiance and contemptuous indifference to scientists of essence.[105]

Laing contends that a science of man which does not take account of his being becomes—and here he quoted Jaspers—a 'demonology'.[106] Laing argues that ontology precedes the empirical sciences. He goes on to consider Tillich's theory of anxiety. Individuals are prone to anxiety about three major topics: death; guilt and condemnation; and doubt and meaninglessness. Laing states that it is central to Tillich's thesis

---

[102] Gomes, P.J. (2000). 'Introduction to Tillich P' (1952). *The Courage to Be* (second edition). Yale University Press, New Haven and London, pp. xi–xxxiii.

[103] Ibid., p. xii.

[104] Laing, *Wisdom, Madness and Folly*, pp. 155–6.

[105] MS Laing A112, p. 3.

[106] Ibid., p. 4. Laing quotes Jaspers (1950). *The Perennial Scope of Philosophy*. Routledge Kegan, London, pp. 117–28.

that a person can be full of anxiety without being aware of it. The effort to prevent the anxiety becoming manifest might lead to neurosis and psychosis. However, Laing observes that Tillich did not relate his theory of anxiety to interpersonal relations: he did not consider how other people make us feel anxious. At this point, Laing brings in Plato to express one of his own key concerns:

> Plato clearly states the problem, which remains the central one, philosophically and psychologically. We are separate beings, and yet we are not entirely isolated, or else interpersonal relationships would not be possible. It is necessary to give due weight both to our separateness and our relatedness.[107]

This central problem was to be addressed by Laing repeatedly throughout his later work, for example, in *The Self and Others*. As part of this problem, Laing considers the subject of love, which he defines as being able to fully recognize oneself as one *is*, and the other person as he or she *is*. Laing sees this as a test of maturity in the psychoanalytical sense, but also of 'authenticity' in the existentialist sense. In parallel, Laing sees the role of the psychotherapist as helping the patient 'to accept our separateness, and to actualize our potential relatedness'. He also claims that Jesus teaches this as well—that we should love not only our friend, but also 'our neighbour who is indifferent to us' and 'our enemy who hates us'. Laing was pre-occupied with the subject of love, and the observations in this early paper anticipate his later thoughts. Several diary entries find Laing pondering the Christian dictum to love thy neighbour and concluding it is an impossible task. Freud had also considered the subject, and like Laing, had decided that it was unreasonable to expect people to love their neighbours.[108]

Another Laingian preoccupation discussed in the paper is that of conformity. He writes:

> There is . . . the man who is above all anxious at the possibility of being in any way different from the statistical norm, whose whole life's project appears to be to achieve the maximum anonymity, to be absolutely 'one like many'; absolutely like everyone else.[109]

Borrowing from Tillich, Laing states that such a man is 'avoiding non-being by avoiding being': he deals with his anxiety about death by not engaging with life in an authentic manner. He may, for example, lose himself in his work and thereby fail to be true to himself. To the outside world, however, he may appear to be perfectly normal. This is an early examination by Laing of the issue of conformity, and one that reveals his critical approach to those who conform.

Laing's first draft received a mixed reception from the referees of *The British Journal of Medical Psychology*. On 15 July 1954, the editor, Jock Sutherland wrote to Laing to say that the referees were divided in their opinion of the paper but he was prepared to accept it if Laing amended it in the light of critical comments.[110] He enclosed one of the reports. The anonymous referees' comments make interesting reading because,

---

[107] Ibid., footnote to p. 9.

[108] Freud, S. (2002). *Civilization and its Discontents* (trans. McLintock D). Penguin Books, London (originally published in 1930), pp. 46–8.

[109] MS Laing A112, p.12.

[110] MS Laing A112. Letter from JD Sutherland to Laing, 15 July 1954.

although they make valid criticisms of the rather unstructured line of argument, they reveal the lack of familiarity and sympathy with European existential thought prevalent in British psychiatric and psychological circles at the time. The referee complained that the paper was 'full of jargon' and that certain statements were incomprehensible. The report continued:

> One paragraph consists of a single sentence: 'To love is to recognize the existence of the other person.' This is either bad poetry or jargon. One can recognize the existence of another person in Woolworth's, but that does not constitute loving them.

The statement was actually a direct quotation from Simone Weil, the French philosopher and religious thinker.

This last comment obviously stung Laing because he incorporated the 'Woolworth's' remark in *The Divided Self*.[111] Laing eventually sent a revised manuscript back to the journal some two and half years later and it was published in 1957. It was a much more concise paper and made great efforts to make Tillich's existential approach understandable and meaningful to the journal's readership.[112] The exercise must have been helpful to Laing. He was compelled to clarify his thoughts about European philosophy and to present them in a clear and accessible manner.

In the published version, Laing outlines Tillich's view that we all carry around with us various preconceptions about the nature of man, but that they usually remain unexamined. However, it is important that we examine them in order to clarify our thinking about the human condition. Laing explains that Tillich holds that man is faced with three existential threats: the feeling that life is utter meaninglessness; the tendency to complete self-condemnation; and death. To deny these possibilities is to live a life based on illusions; a state of mind which leads to anxiety.

In a companion paper entitled, 'Reflections on the ontology of human relations', which was also written in 1954, Laing considers human-relatedness and the nature of love.[113] It contains ideas that he was to develop more fully in *The Divided Self*, and he refers once again to Tillich, but also to Kierkegaard, Heidegger, Buber, and Sartre. In defining what he means by ontology, Laing quotes Kierkegaard's dictum that 'every human being must be assumed to be in essential possession of what essentially belongs to being a man'.[114] Laing considers that this dictum is often ignored and gives as an example a person whose opinion is dismissed because he is mad. Laing writes that no one 'has the right to "include out" any human being whose action he finds unaccountable even though his behaviour may seem more strange to him than the birds in his garden'.[115] In this statement, Laing is expressing what is probably the key idea of his clinical outlook: the mentally ill have as much right as anyone else to be heard. He also makes an allusion to Eugen Bleuler's admission that his schizophrenic patients

---

[111] Laing, *The Divided Self*, p. 104.

[112] Laing, R.D. (1957). 'An examination of Tillich's theory of anxiety and neurosis'. *The British Journal of Medical Psychology*, **30**, 88–91.

[113] MS Laing A113. R.D. Laing (1954). 'Reflections on the ontology of human relations'.

[114] Ibid., p. 2.

[115] Ibid., p. 3.

were as strange to him as the birds in his garden. It was a remark that Laing was to quote in *The Divided Self*. [116] The paper was never published but it gave Laing an opportunity to clarify his thoughts on existential philosophy.

Lecture in Dublin

In 1955, Laing was invited to give a lecture to theology students at Trinity College in Dublin.[117] The talk is interesting for several reasons. Laing discusses John Bowlby, demonstrating he was familiar with his work before he went to London. Secondly, and characteristically, he voices his concerns about the applicability of scientific models to human emotion. Thirdly, instead of providing answers to the questions he poses, he asks the audience for their thoughts. This was a strategy that Laing was to employ both in psychotherapy and in his writing. He begins his lecture with an observation which anticipates his remark on the last page of *Wisdom, Madness and Folly*, that: 'Psychiatry tries to be as scientific, impersonal and objective as possible about what is most personal and subjective.'[118] In the Dublin talk, Laing says:

> Psychiatry, in some ways, involves us all the most personally and intimately of all the sciences. Because psychiatry is now more than a branch of medicine—it is a body of facts and theory which has as its specific object of study, you and me as people. It studies our loves, and hates, and fears . . . It also however, constitutes a body of theory—which is an attempt to interpret these facts.[119]

Laing goes on to consider the theories of John Bowlby, and in particular his notion that children need a loving mother if they are to develop along healthy and sociable lines. Laing outlines Bowlby's nostrum that if children do not receive a mother's love, of a certain kind, at a certain time, then they are unlikely to be able to love or be loved in later life. As adults, they will tend to be cold, detached, uncaring, and prone to crime. Laing asks if this is a specific and unvarying formula. Is it like the formation of bone which depended on receiving the right amount of vitamin D and calcium? Are some people 'condemned' to elude love because of the 'accident' of their upbringing? If Bowlby is right, what is the use of commanding such people to behave differently? Or, has Bowlby led us to approach the problem in a false way? Having posed these questions, Laing ends his talk by stating he does not know the answer to them. He says to his audience: 'I would like you to tell me.' Of course, by asking such questions, Laing is slyly suggesting that Bowlby's theory is untenable.

Analytic groups

When he was a senior registrar at the Southern General Hospital, Laing wrote a paper with Aaron Esterson on 'The collusive function of pairing in analytic groups',

---

[116] Laing, *The Divided Self*, p. 28.
[117] MS Laing A154. Notes for a lecture at Trinity, Dublin, 1955.
[118] Laing, *Wisdom, Madness and Folly*, p. 158.
[119] MS Laing A154, pp. 2–3.

which appeared in the *British Journal of Medical Psychology* in 1958.[120] He returned to the subject of the group in *The Self and Others*.[121] In the original paper, Laing and Esterson state that their group is run on the principles described by Sutherland and Ezriel. The paper demonstrates that Laing had experience of analytic groups before he went to London, although the final and revised version of the paper was written after he had moved south. It shows that Laing was aware of Wilfred Bion's writing on the subject. Ferguson Rodger, the Professor of Psychiatry at the Southern General, was interested in Bion and had copies of his papers in his personal collection.[122] Laing and Esterson were also acquainted with the work of Sartre. They discussed his play, *Huis Clos* and quoted the famous line: 'L'enfer, c'est les autres' (Hell is other people). Perhaps the most interesting aspect of their paper was the description of one of the patients, called 'Richards'. His story was later incorporated into *The Divided Self* as the case of 'James'.[123] According to the paper:

> He was an extremely schizoid individual. Once, recently, he had left his books to have a walk in the park. It was a beautiful evening in early autumn. As he sat watching the lovers together, and the sun setting, he began to feel 'at one' with the whole scene, with the whole of nature, with the cosmos. He got up and ran home in panic. It was a relief when he 'came to himself' again. Identity for Richards could be sustained only in isolation. Any relationship threatened him with loss of identity—being engulfed, fusing, merging, losing his separate distinctiveness. He could only *be*, by himself.

Here we see Laing employing the term 'engulfing' for the first time. This would be a key schizoid mechanism in *The Divided Self*. In the book he would relate this passage to Gerard Manley Hopkins and his view that mortal beauty was dangerous. Laing was to repeat this passage in *The Self and Others*, but somewhat confusingly the patient was now called 'Richard'.[124] In this book, Laing gave an account of the group which was based on the 'The collusive functioning of pairing in analytic groups'. In *The Self and Others*, Laing ended his account of the group by comparing the role of the therapist to that of a Zen Master. Both had to point out that suffering was not the result of being deprived of 'the answer', but that it was the state of desire that assumed that there was an answer, coupled with the frustration of never getting it.

This chapter has looked at Laing's early notebooks, the contents of his library, his essays, papers, and talks to build up a picture of his intellectual world. It has revealed how wide-ranging he was, and how, from the outset, he was determined, to borrow Freud's description of himself, to become an intellectual 'conquistador'.[125]

---

[120] Laing, R.D., Esterson, A. (1958). 'The collusive function of pairing in analytic groups'. *British Journal of Medical Psychology*, **31**, 117–23.

[121] Laing, R.D. (1961). *The Self and Others*. Tavistock, London, pp. 109–15.

[122] Glasgow University Archive. DC81. Ferguson Rodger 450–2. WR Bion: Experiences in Groups Parts 1–3.

[123] Laing, *The Divided Self*, pp. 91–2.

[124] Laing, *The Self and Others*, p. 109.

[125] Quoted in Sulloway, F.J. (1980). *Freud. Biologist of the Mind. Beyond the Psychoanalytic Legend*. Fontana, London, p. 477.

Chapter 3

Laing and psychiatric theory

History of psychiatry

In working out his theoretical and clinical stance towards madness, Laing was, in fact, participating in a long tradition of debate about the nature of mental disturbance.[1] In their account of the historical development of ideas about insanity, Fulford, Thornton, and Graham[2] have described how these ideas have veered between the twin poles of the 'medical' and the 'moral': between the belief that madness is the result of brain disease and the belief that it is a psychological or spiritual problem. This conflict was apparent at least two thousand years ago, when Hippocrates espoused a humeral theory of madness in contrast to Plato, who believed that insanity reflected a disturbance of the soul.

A key stage in the development of ideas about insanity occurred in the eighteenth century with the dawn of the European Enlightenment, out of which evolved the modern-day medical discipline of psychiatry. Enlightenment thinkers held that reason rather than prejudice, superstition, imposed belief, or tradition would be the guide to the problems of humanity. In the field of madness, and partly in response to the excesses of the witch trials of the previous centuries, medical rather than religious explanations of insanity were favoured. There was a reassertion of the theory that madness was the result of natural causes. Laing was troubled as to which position he should adopt in this debate. Should he see himself as a secular medical scientist in the tradition of the Enlightenment? Or was the Enlightenment project to promote human reason over the divine a misguided one? Was the legacy of the Enlightenment a modern-day psychiatry which was unable to deal with the spiritual dimension of the human condition?

In fact it is simplistic to portray eighteenth and early nineteenth century clinicians as in thrall to a materialist model of madness. Many if not most adhered to the Christian faith and, as Laing knew from his reading of the classic medical texts of the period, there was also a healthy scepticism about the benefits of physical treatments. The late eighteenth century saw the emergence of 'moral therapy', a type of treatment introduced by the Quaker William Tuke at the York Retreat, which advocated a psychological rather than a somatic approach to patients. In place of physical restraints and medications, moral therapy stressed the value of treating the patient with kindness and respect. Laing was to see himself as part of this tradition. When he was a

---

[1] Fulford, K.W.M., Thornton, T. and Graham, G. (2006). *Oxford Textbook of Philosophy and Psychiatry*. Oxford University Press, Oxford, pp. 140–59. For a discussion of the philosophical background to the history of ideas about madness.

[2] Ibid.

young doctor at Gartnavel Royal Hospital in the 1950s and chlorpromazine was being introduced, he was sceptical about the benefits of a drug that would come to be seen by many as the first effective anti-psychotic medication.

Alternative histories of psychiatry

Fulford and his colleagues' account of the development of ideas about madness is of course not the only one. In contrast to their dialectical narrative in which psychiatric theory zigzags between physical and psychological explanations of insanity, there are narratives in which there is linear progress. Edward Shorter's *A History of Psychiatry* charts what he sees as the triumph of biological psychiatry.[3] A book which Laing knew well told a similar story of triumph, but this time it was psychological rather than physical therapy which emerged as the victor. The book was Gregory Zilboorg's (1941) *A History of Medical Psychology*, which Laing had read as a medical student and from which he had made extensive notes.[4] In Zilboorg's account, psychiatry was seen as evolving out of the darkness of previous times towards the golden age of Freud and psychodynamic theory. Past clinicians and thinkers were examined in the light of Freud and judged as to how closely they approximated or anticipated him. Physical approaches were generally viewed as leading to a therapeutic dead end, while psychological ones were hailed as the forerunners of psychoanalysis. The book took a Whiggish perspective that saw the history of psychiatry as one of progress. Laing seems to have found the book's championing of psychological over physical approaches to mental illness congenial to his own outlook. In a notebook entry he declared, 'Away from Galen, Maudsley, Cabanis, Sargant!'[5] Such names represented the physicalist approach to human suffering, and from Laing's point of view they were the villains of the story.

Both Shorter and Zilboorg told a story of the progress of psychiatry, though they disagreed as to what elements led to its success. In contrast, Michel Foucault, in his ground-breaking 1961 book, *Madness and Civilisation*, challenged the very idea that the history of psychiatry was a narrative of progress.[6] Foucault contended that the new discipline of psychiatry, as it emerged at the time of the Enlightenment, had actually introduced more sophisticated forms of control. Instead of the chains of pre-Enlightenment times, the more subtle methods of moral therapy, were developed to restrain the mad: patients were induced to construct their own 'chains', but these were mental in origin and served to constrict self-expression or any deviance from bourgeois ideas of decorum— they were, to quote the words of William Blake, 'mind-forg'd manacles'. By these

[3] Shorter, E. (1997). *A History of Psychiatry. From the Era of the Asylum to the Age of Prozac.* John Wiley and Sons, New York.

[4] MS Laing K13. R.D. Laing: Notebook, 1951–1960, un-numbered; Zilboorg, G. (1941). *A History of Medical Psychology* (in collaboration with Henry GW). W.W. Norton & Co., New York.

[5] MS Laing K14. R.D. Laing: Notebook and partial diary covering Laing's stay at the military hospitals at Netley and Catterick, January 1952 to June 1953.

[6] Foucault, M. (1967). *Madness and Civilisation. A History of Insanity in the Age of Reason* (trans. R. Howard). Tavistock, London (originally published in French in 1961).

means, Foucault argued, 'the voice of unreason' was silenced.[7] Interestingly, he suggested that the voice of unreason could still be heard in those creative people who had gone over the edge of sanity: Friedrich Holderlin, Friedrich Nietzsche, Gerard de Nerval, Vincent Van Gogh, and Antonin Artaud. The names of these individuals were all very familiar to Laing, and, like Foucault, he was fascinated by what their experiences revealed about madness. Like Foucault, Laing felt that psychiatry often served to suppress the voice of the mad. In his discussion of *Madness and Civilization*, Laing observed:

> It is not the account of the supposed madmen of the 17th century to the 19th century that is particularly terrifying about this book . . . What we do hear through these pages is how the men of reason experienced and treated the men of unreason. Victory belonged to those who could control the power structures of society . . . The madness of Europe is revealed not in the persons of the madmen of Europe, but in the action of the self-validated sane ones who wrote the books, sanctified, and authorised by State, Church, and the representatives of bourgeois morality.[8]

In the conflict between the forces of reason and unreason, Laing tended to identify with the latter, and this was to cause him much disquiet in his chosen career as a psychiatrist. As we have seen, Laing played a part in ensuring that Foucault's *Madness and Civilization* was published in English.[9] He was a reader for Tavistock and wrote that Foucault's work presented a 'thesis that thoroughly' shook 'the assumptions of traditional psychiatry'.[10]

Classic texts

Laing was very interested in history and wrote that it had been his first love.[11] He took a particular interest in the history of his own discipline, psychiatry. He read classic early works in the field of psychiatry, such as William Battie's *A Treatise on Madness* (1758). A classical scholar, Battie was physician to St Luke's Hospital in London, which he helped to found, and he was also the first teacher of psychiatry in England.[12] One of his patients was the poet Christopher Smart. Implicit in Battie's approach was

---

[7] Hacking has observed that 'unreason' and 'madness' are not used synonymously by Foucault and the former term disappears like Alice's Cheshire cat in subsequent editions of *Madness and Civilisation*. See Hacking, I. (2006). 'Foreword'. In Foucault, M. *History of Madness*, pp. ix–xii (trans. Murphy, J. and Khalfa, J.). Routledge, London.

[8] Laing, R.D. (1996). 'The invention of madness'. In Smart, B. (ed.) *Michel Foucault. Critical Assessments*. Volume IV. Routledge, London, pp. 76–9. Originally published in *New Statesman*, 1987, 16 June, p. 843.

[9] Mullan, B. (1995). *Mad to be Normal. Conversations with R.D. Laing*. Free Association Books, London, p. 204. Laing claimed he was a series editor for Tavistock.

[10] Laing's original reader's report dated 29 April 1965 for Tavistock is reproduced on the first page of Foucault, M. (2006). *History of Madness* (trans. Murphy, J. and Khalfa, J.). Routledge, London.

[11] Research Fellowship Application for Foundations' Fund for Research in Psychiatry, p. 5.

[12] Hunter, R. and Macalpine, I. (1963). *Three Hundred Years of Psychiatry 1535–1860*. Oxford University Press, London, pp. 402–10.

a shift from seeing madness as a uniform entity to the observation and management of individual patients. Battie had also discovered that patients sometimes recovered spontaneously without treatment. In fact some recovered after the treatment was *stopped*. Battie declared: 'tho' it may seem almost haeretical to impeach their antimaniacal virtues, many a Lunatic, who by repetition of vomits and other convulsive stimuli would have been strained into downright Idiotism, has when given over as incurable recovered his understanding'. Battie's approach has been seen as anticipating the 'moral treatment' of the nineteenth century.[13] Moral treatment which emphasized treating patients with kindness and respecting their autonomy struck a chord with Laing.

Laing also read William Pargeter's *Observations on Maniacal Disorder* (1792). Following in the wake of Battie, who held that humane treatment or 'management' did more for the patient than medicines, Pargeter was the first physician to show how much could be achieved by 'management' and the influence of the doctor.[14] The doctor by his manner could help to calm the patient and even halt incipient madness. Pargeter sought to make immediate contact with patients and gain their 'good opinion'. Pargeter did not think diagnosis was very important. Once again we can see how such views anticipated and most probably influenced those of Laing.

Another book Laing read was Thomas Arnold's *Observations on the Management of the Insane; and Particularly on the Agency and Importance of Humane and Kind Treatment in Effecting their Cure* (1809), whose title stressed the need for a humanitarian approach.

Laing was particularly interested in John Conolly, who maintained that there was more similarity between the sane and insane than was often thought. Conolly wrote:

> They [medical men] have sought for, and imagined, a strong and definable boundary between sanity and insanity, which has not only been imaginary, and arbitrarily placed, but, by being supposed to separate all of whom were of unsound mind from the rest of men, has unfortunately been considered a justification of certain measures against the portion condemned, which, in the case of the majority, were unnecessary and afflicting.[15]

This statement, albeit couched in nineteenth century language, expresses a core belief of Laing's. The sane and the insane were on a spectrum and any denial of this led to the risk of perceiving the mad as somehow less than fully human. Once this step was taken, it paved the way for inhumane treatment. Conolly also advocated non-restraint in the treatment of the mentally ill. Although Laing was often critical of Henry Maudsley, the eminent Victorian alienist and contemporary of Conolly, he supported Maudsley's contention that chemical restraint of the brain cells was equivalent to physical restraint of the body. Laing interpreted this to include medication and physical methods of treatment.

---

[13] Ibid.

[14] Ibid., pp. 538–42.

[15] Ibid., p. 806.

One of Laing's heroes was Sir William Osler, who was Professor of Medicine at Harvard University in the early part of the twentieth century and who emphasized the importance of the bedside manner.[16] He brought a humanitarian perspective to clinical work and advocated treating the patient as person who had a disease, rather than just focusing on the disease process. He felt that medicines should be used sparingly.

Laing also read classic works by patients, such as Daniel Schreber's *Memoirs of My Nervous Illness*, which he referred to in *The Divided Self*. Schreber's *Memoirs* had been translated into English by Ida Macalpine and Richard Hunter and published in 1955.[17] Schreber was a senior German judge who developed paranoid schizophrenia and in his memoirs he gave a very detailed account of his experience of psychosis. Macalpine and Hunter provided a useful introduction to the case of Schreber and how he had been viewed by psychiatrists and psychoanalysts. Laing would have read that it was Eugen Bleuler who introduced Schreber to a psychiatric audience by writing about him in his *Dementia Praecox: or the Group of Schizophrenias*. This attracted the notice of Freud who analysed Schreber's text in his 1911 paper, 'Psychoanalytic notes upon an autobiographical account of a case of paranoia (Dementia Paranoides)'. Freud's essay was one of the first attempts to apply psychoanalysis to a psychotic patient. He considered that Schreber's delusions were a manifestation of his unconscious homosexual longings. Laing would have been interested in Macalpine and Hunter's account of the reception of Freud's attempt to analyse a psychotic patient. Freud's thesis that paranoid delusions were linked to unconscious homosexual feelings was readily accepted by the psychoanalytic community. Macalpine and Hunter offered a more sceptical view, although they were, at this stage in their careers, broadly sympathetic to psychological approaches to psychosis.

They provided a blistering attack on physical approaches to schizophrenia. Laing would have read:

> Psychoses . . . diseases of the mind or soul as opposed to brain, are still often considered to originate from yet undiscovered brain pathology, the mental symptoms being merely incidental and without significance. The mirage created by general paralysis of the insane continues to spur on a psychiatry without psychology to find physical pathology for mental diseases . . . psychoses are at present widely treated by coma hypoglycaemia, electrically-induced convulsions, and surgical destruction of the brain . . . [18]

The authors observed ruefully that if Schreber were a patient in the 1950s he would have been subjected to such physical procedures and as a result would never have written his memoirs nor made such a good recovery. Laing would, of course, have been receptive to such views. Laing also read Clifford Beers' *A Mind that Found Itself*. Beers was an American businessman who developed a manic-depressive illness and spent time in mental institutions. After his recovery he set up the Mental Hygiene movement whose aim was to improve the treatment of the mentally ill.

---

[16] Mullan, *Mad to be Normal*, p.114.

[17] Macalpine, I. and Hunter, R.A. (1955) *Daniel Paul Schreber. Memoirs of My Nervous Illness.* Dawson & Sons, London.

[18] Ibid., pp. 17–18.

Psychiatric theories

Laing read widely in the field of psychiatric theory. He read textbooks, journals, and monographs, and made extensive notes. As a young psychiatrist in the 1950s, Laing confronted the many diverse approaches to mental illness which were current at the time. There was the approach exemplified by Emil Kraepelin which sought to delineate psychiatric syndromes on the basis of a careful description of signs and symptoms, and on the long-term course of the illness. There was the psychoanalytical approach which was less interested in diagnosis and which sought to relate symptoms to underlying unconscious forces. There were existential approaches which held that the patient's presentation was a meaningful and conscious response to the predicament in which they found themselves. Social psychiatrists examined how the environment influenced a patient's mental condition, while psychologists held that a person's behaviour was moulded by rewards and punishments. In his notebooks and clinical practice, Laing grappled with these different ideas as he tried to forge an approach of his own.

Sigmund Freud

> It seems to me, Freud represents a landmark in our contemporary human consciousness. Freud opened for us the world of childhood.[19]

So wrote Laing in one of his diaries. It is apparent that he was greatly influenced by Freud. As we have seen, his student essay, 'Health and happiness', revealed that he was acquainted with the work of Freud from an early age and that it informed his views on madness and society. As a trainee doctor Laing was not only exposed to senior clinicians who adopted a Freudian approach to patients, but he also read widely in the field of psychoanalytic literature. He recalled that he was more interested in the Freud of *The Psychopathology of Everyday Life*, with its concentration on specific clinical detail and the analysis of dreams, rather than his later, more speculative works.[20] Laing subsequently trained as a psychoanalyst in London, though he was to claim that he kept his philosophical objections in abeyance.[21]

As we have seen in the Introduction, accounts of Freud, both by himself and his followers, have taken the form of the Hero Myth, in which he is the lonely but fearless pioneer creating work of absolute originality in the face of hostility and ridicule from his scientific peers. Ellenberger and, later, Sulloway have done much to dispel the mythology surrounding Freud and place him in his historical and cultural context.[22] The basic outline of his career is well known: Sigmund Freud was born in Freiburg,

---

[19] MS Laing A343. Diary, page B.

[20] Mullan, *Mad to be Normal,* p. 145.

[21] Ibid., p. 145.

[22] Ellenberger, F.H. (1970). *The Discovery of the Unconscious. The History and Evolution of Dynamic Psychiatry*. Basic Books, New York; Sulloway, F.J. (1979). *Freud, Biologist of Mind. Beyond the Psychoanalytic Legend*. Basic Books, New York.

Austria-Hungary in 1856 and studied medicine in Vienna.[23] In 1886, he spent several months in Paris attending lectures on hypnotism and hysteria by Jean Martin-Charcot, the eminent neurologist and director of the Salpetriere. Returning to private practice in Vienna, Freud published, along with his colleague Josef Breuer, *Studies on Hysteria* in 1895. The authors maintained that hysterics suffered from painful, unpleasant, traumatic memories, which were repressed by the unconscious. These repressed memories were converted into the physical symptoms of hysteria.

Drawing on these early experiences with hysterical patients, Freud developed a method of therapy that, in 1896, he was to call 'psychoanalysis'. Rather than being hypnotized, as Charcot had advocated, the patient was asked to say whatever came into their head or to 'free associate'. By doing so, they would reveal clues about their neurosis which were considered to lie hidden and 'repressed' deep in their unconscious. In 1899 Freud published his *magnum opus, The Interpretation of Dreams*, in which he claimed that dreams represented the unconscious fulfilment of wishes which were often disturbing and sexual in nature; as a result, they had to be disguised. Freud called such disguises the 'manifest content' of the dream. This material was then 'interpreted' or translated by the psychoanalyst into the 'latent content', i.e. what the dream 'really' meant. The concept of 'interpretation' was to occupy a key place in the theory of psychoanalysis. In *The Psychopathology of Everyday Life*, which appeared the following year, Freud extended his method of interpretation to human behaviour generally. He claimed that supposedly accidental phenomena, such as slips of the tongue and forgetting words, were actually meaningful and that they revealed the speaker's unconscious wishes and desires.

In *The Interpretation of Dreams*, Freud had also examined Oedipus, whose story was related in *Oedipus Rex*, the Greek tragedy by Sophocles, which Laing knew well. Freud maintained that Oedipus acted out a wish that was universal in childhood: the son falls in love with his mother and wants rid of his father. Freud would later call this experience the 'Oedipus Complex'. In his 1905 work, *Three Essays on the Theory of Sexuality*, Freud outlined the stages of psycho-sexual development. He claimed that the infant progressed from an initial 'oral' stage through an 'anal' to a 'phallic' stage. This process was completed by around the age of five. The child then developed the Oedipus Complex, which, if male, led him to desire his mother and hate his father, whom he feared would castrate him; if the child was female, she would desire her father and conclude that she had *already* been castrated. At about the age of six, the Oedipus Complex was eventually repressed and the child's sex drive disappeared, only to re-emerge at puberty. If the infant failed to negotiate these stages and became arrested or 'fixated' at a particular stage, then neurotic symptoms would arise in later life. Neurosis in adulthood represented a return or a 'regression' to this early fixated level. In 1923, Freud proposed a new tripartite model of mind, which encompassed the Ego, the Id, and the Super-ego. The Id represented the primitive, unconscious basis of the psyche and was dominated by basic urges. The Ego was the guide to reality and acted

---

[23] For accounts of Freud, see Roazen, P. (1976). *Freud and his Followers*. Allen Lane, London; Clark, R.W. (1982). *Freud. The Man and the Cause*. Granada, Frogmore, St Albans; Gay, P. (1988). *Freud. A Life for Our Time*. Dent, Cambridge.

as an inhibiting agency. The Super-ego represented parental authority which had been internalized.

Increasingly in his later years, Freud commented on the wider society and the history of humanity. In 1920 he published *Beyond the Pleasure Principle*, in which he contended that human beings had a tendency to be drawn towards the 'pleasure principle', but that the 'reality principle' served to delay pleasure if there were risks involved. Humans strove to avoid unpleasure rather than actively pursue pleasure. In the same book Freud considered a phenomenon he called 'Repetition–Compulsion'. This was the tendency of the unconscious to repeat unpleasurable experiences. In *The Future of an Illusion* of 1928, he attacked religion as a 'universal obsessional neurosis'. In his 1930 book, *Civilization and its Discontents*, Freud observed that there was always an irreconcilable tension between the individual who sought instinctual freedom and society which demanded conformity and the repression of desire. As a result, Freud maintained, individuals were doomed to feelings of discontent. As we have seen, this was a theme that Laing warmed to in his student essays.

In his first book, *The Divided Self*, Laing paid homage to Freud as the pioneering explorer of the unconscious. Yet he also held highly critical opinions about Freud and psychoanalytical theory. In this Laing is not alone. Freud's legacy remains contested and there is now a vast literature, much of it critical, of the founder of psychoanalysis.[24] For Laing's part, he objected to the psychic determinism which he saw as lying at the heart of Freudian theory. This manifest itself in several ways: first, its mechanistic model of mind; secondly its contention that all mental life and behaviour were meaningful; thirdly its lack of an ethical dimension; and fourthly its neglect of the interpersonal and social context. In addition, such an approach to the human condition meant, in Laing's view, that Freudian theory could not account for such vital aspects of existence as spirituality and creativity.

Commenting on Freud's mechanistic model of the human mind, Laing wrote in his diary:

> Freud is still the great man but more and more 'the imbecile of genius' to me. Those ghostly hydraulics of the psyche! Mechanism. 19th [century] materialism translated into 'mental' terms.[25]

Laing borrowed the phrase 'the imbecile genius' from the French writer, Andre Gide. Laing was critical of the Freudian model because it implied that human beings were the passive playthings of mental mechanisms. Further, Freud's model was out-of-date, based, as it was, on the closed, deterministic world-view of nineteenth century physics.

---

[24] Fisher, S. and Greenberg, R. (1985). *The Scientific Credibility of Freud's Theories and Therapies.* Columbia University Press, Columbia; Gellner, E. (1992). *The Psychoanalytic Movement. The Cunning of Unreason* (second edition). Fontana, London; Torrey, E.F. (1992). *Freudian Fraud. The Malignant Effect of Freud's Theory on American Culture and Thought.* Harper-Collins, New York; Webster, R. (1996). *Why Freud was Wrong. Sin, Science and Psychoanalysis.* Fontana, London; Shorter, E. (1997). *A History of Psychiatry. From the Era of the Asylum to the Age of Prozac.* John Wiley and Sons, New York; Crews, F.C. (ed.) (1998). *Unauthorized Freud. Doubters Confront a Legend.* Viking Books, New York.

[25] MS Laing K14.

The deterministic orientation of Freudian theory meant that it held that all aspects of mental life were potentially meaningful, i.e. they could be understood. Slips of the tongue, dreams, jokes: all had an underlying meaning which could be discovered by means of Freudian analysis. As Laing wrote in one of his notebooks:

> One of the basic faiths of modern psychoanalysis (reminds me of Newton's faith that Nature must be rational, conform to laws) is that every form of expression can be given a 'meaning'.[26]

Freud's contention that psychic experience could be decoded had implications for the field of psychiatry. It meant that symptoms of mental illness, not just the neuroses but also the psychoses, could be understood. Laing was sympathetic to such a notion, and a central credo of *The Divided Self* was that madness was more comprehensible than many thought. However, Laing felt that the psychoanalytical approach was often misguided in its attempts to 'explain' mental symptoms. He wrote:

> In some ways psychoanalytic systems of 'interpretation', which try to make sense out of psychotic symptomatology, in making out that the patient means something totally different—if he or she means anything—from what he or she seems to mean, only widen the gulf.[27]

Laing felt that psychoanalytic theory denied the patient a voice; instead of attending to what the patient *actually* said, psychoanalysts 'translated' it into their own language.

For Laing, another consequence of Freud's psychic determinism was that it left no room for individual responsibility. If the behaviour of human beings was entirely the result of mental mechanisms, then they were not free to make ethical choices. They might think that they were making ethical decisions but this was an illusion; they were merely carrying out what had already been determined by the 'ghostly hydraulics' of the mind. As Laing wrote:

> Freud criticises the Modern Western Man. His system is, in a way, primarily a destructive analysis of the possible feelings, thoughts, beliefs or lack of beliefs . . . a man can have . . . For Freudian man, a genuinely 'moral action' (i.e. moral as to motive), is essentially impossible. He may believe in god. Subjectively it *can* be no more than an illusion, though by a happy chance, which is not improbable but possible, he *could* be right.[28]

Laing asked rhetorically: 'Who would place any validity in the dictates of conscience when he believes that it originates as the introjected penis of his father?'[29]

In another notebook, Laing argued that Freud had laid down two principles according to which all men, at all times, in every circumstance, always act.[30] These were the Pleasure–Reality Principle and the Repetition–Compulsive Principle. Laing wrote that

---

[26] Ibid.

[27] Ibid., pp. 7–8.

[28] MS Laing K14.

[29] Ibid.

[30] MS Laing K15. Notebook, begun 12 March 1953.

the first principle involved the seeking of pleasure and the avoidance of pain, although pleasure could be foregone in order to avoid disproportionately greater future pains. The second also involved the mastery of past pain by the compulsive repetition of painful past experiences. Laing felt that such a model implied that this was the *only* way that man *could* behave. If this were so it meant:

> A moral action, in Kant's sense, is thus impossible—for though a man may act according to the moral law, or even 'because' it is his duty . . . by doing his duty he will spare himself the more dangerous pains of the pangs of conscience . . . It follows, that a man who acts according to these two principles, acts as though his will was . . . 'determined'.[31]

He also reflected:

> . . . in general men seek pleasure and avoid pain . . . Freud's psychology is empirically correct. When all that is said, what has that [to] do with the ethical—what men ought to do.[32]

In his criticisms of what he saw as the ethical shortcomings of Freudian theory, Laing held to the view that individuals were free to choose how they conducted their life. For Laing, this also applied to mental illness: individuals made existential choices as to how they reacted to adversity and this could include the 'choice' of whether to go mad. Laing was also critical of what he called the 'mono-self psychology' of Freud, which he contrasted unfavourably with the interpersonal approach of others like Martin Buber.[33] Laing was to claim that he simply didn't meet people who had Freudian disorders, such as repressed homosexual fantasies.[34] This has parallels with his claim in *The Divided Self* that he didn't see patients who resembled the textbook descriptions of schizophrenia.[35] What unites these two observations is Laing's belief that a patient could not be seen in isolation, the presence of the psychiatrist with his or her particular preconceptions influenced how the patient behaved and this, in turn, affected how they were perceived by the psychiatrist. Laing felt that psychoanalytic theory could be depersonalizing and reifying in its discussion of people.[36] Just as somatic theories of mental illness were prone, in Laing's eyes, to turn people into objects, so psychoanalytic approaches could be equally guilty. Picturing the patient as a malfunctioning brain or as the victim of unconscious processes ran the risk of over-looking that the patient was a person.

Laing criticized Freud's account of religion. Freud held that belief in God was an illusion, and that only scientific knowledge was free from illusion. Laing argued that science could say nothing about the *object* of belief. The belief could be 'explained'

---

[31] Ibid.

[32] MS Laing K14.

[33] Ibid.

[34] Mullan, *Mad to be Normal*, p. 116.

[35] Laing, *The Divided Self*, p. 28.

[36] Laing in conversation with Charlesworth. In Charlesworth, M. (1976). *The Existentialists and Jean-Paul Sartre*. George Prior, London, pp. 46–55.

without having to consider whether the object existed or not. Freud's approach to the arts was also unsatisfactory. Laing observed of psychoanalysis:

> There is something—an essential something—profoundly opposed to the heart of the artistic attention in this method. This method admits that the artist may reveal truth but more or less unwittingly. It may come through in his work. But the expression of it, in so far as it is peculiarly 'artistic', is in a form which requires to be 'interpretated' [sic] in order to reveal in direct manner its latent content.[37]

Laing thus had a mixed response to Freud's work. As arguably the world's most influential and important psychological theorist, Freud represented a great intellectual magnet to the young Laing. He could not help but be impressed by his pre-eminence. But Laing would not have been Laing if he did not also see himself in competition with the Viennese analyst. In a letter to Marcelle Vincent when he was still a medical student, Laing had written about Freud and his notion of the unconscious:

> Freud, quite early, found a notion to exploit for the whole of his life. He found it in von Hartmann and Schopenhauer—he fully acknowledged his debt to them—the unconscious mind. Freud must have had a tremendously intense energy to carry through such a speculation in the face of its evident absurdity.[38]

In this passage Laing appears envious that Freud had managed to acquire a notion—one that wasn't even his own—and make a career out of it. Laing was of course correct in stating that Freud did not 'discover' the unconscious, although in popular culture he is often credited with doing so. Nevertheless, Laing was impressed by Freud's drive and by the fact that he had found a way to make money out of his interests.[39] Whether or not he agreed with all the tenets of psychoanalytic theory, Laing certainly took note of the way Freud had made a success of his career.

Emil Kraepelin

A major figure in the evolution of psychiatry is Emil Kraepelin; indeed he has been judged the most important psychiatrist who ever lived.[40] He was also an important figure for Laing, who, though he was totally out of sympathy with his clinical philosophy, had a grudging respect, as he invariably did, for anyone who gained professional success. He noted that Kraepelin had his first paper published when he was a medical student and Laing was always impressed, if not somewhat envious, of those who showed signs of intellectual precocity. Kraepelin represented the type of positivist psychiatry with its notion of the detached clinical gaze that Laing abhorred. Kraepelin's example, however, provided a useful model for Laing to measure his own ideas against, and he had great entertainment exposing what he saw as the flaws of Kraepelin's clinical approach in *The Divided Self.*

---

[37] MS Laing A410. R.D. Laing: Analytical notes on the poetry of Gerard Manley Hopkins. 21.5.54.
[38] Quoted in Clay, *R.D. Laing*, p. 35.
[39] Mullan, *Mad to be Normal*, p. 103.
[40] Fish, F. (1964). *Outline of Psychiatry*. Wright, Bristol.

Emil Kraepelin was born in 1856 in Neustrelitz in north Germany.[41] He attended the universities of Wurzburg, Munich, and Leipzig, where he came under the influence of the eminent psychologist, Wilhelm Wundt. In 1885 he was appointed Professor of Psychiatry at Dorpat in Estonia. Exposed to Estonian patients whose language he did not understand, Kraepelin paid little attention to doctor–patient communication or clinical investigation and instead concentrated on experimental laboratory research. In 1891 he moved to Heidelberg where he embarked on the clinical work which would ultimately lead to his ground-breaking distinction between manic-depressive psychosis and dementia praecox, now renamed schizophrenia.[42] Kraepelin announced this great division of the insanities to the world in his 1896 textbook. Later he moved to be director of the university psychiatric clinic at Munich, where he concerned himself with theories of degeneration, alcoholism, mental hygiene, and the threat, as he saw it, of homosexuality. Kraepelin increasingly focused on socio-political issues which he conceived of in biological and Darwinist terms. For him, the remedy lay in the eugenicist engineering of the population.

Kraepelin saw psychiatry as a clinical science and held that the experimental method was the best approach to study mental disease.[43] He had learnt about the experimental method from Wilhelm Wundt, with whom he had worked in the 'world's first laboratory for psychological research'.[44] As Kraepelin wrote:

> The methods developed by experimental psychology provide us with the means to define a more precise concept of the alterations of mental life, as nature produces them by its harmful influences.[45]

Kraepelin was less interested in those elements that could not be studied by the experimental method, such as subjective reports and the contribution of an individual's life experiences to their illness. Kraepelin believed that man was but a part of nature and could ultimately be understood by methods derived from the physical sciences. He felt that psychiatric illnesses represented natural entities which existed in the world completely independently of the researcher. The task of the medical scientist was to describe what he found—the idea that the scientist's preconceptions or theoretical position influenced what was found and how it was described was hardly considered. For Kraepelin, dementia praecox was an organic defect that led to the destruction of cortical neurones. The patient's personality might contribute to the development of the psychotic process but it was not a central factor.[46]

---

[41] Engstrom, E.J. and Weber, M.W. (1999). 'Emil Kraepelin (1856–1926)'. In Freeman, H. (ed.), *A Century of Psychiatry*. Mosby, London, pp. 49–51.

[42] See Berrios, G.E. (1987). 'Historical aspects of psychoses: 19th century issues'. *British Medical Bulletin*, **43**, 484–98; Berrios, G.E. (2000). 'Schizophrenia: a conceptual history'. In, Gelder, M.G., Lopez-Ibor, J.J. and Andreasen, N. (eds), *New Oxford Textbook of Psychiatry*. Volume 1. Oxford University Press, Oxford, pp. 567–71.

[43] Hoff, P. (1995). 'Kraepelin'. In Berrios, G. and Porter, R. (eds), *A History of Clinical Psychiatry*. Athlone, London, pp. 261–79.

[44] Ibid., p. 264.

[45] Ibid., pp. 267–8. The text was also translated by Hoff.

[46] Ibid., p. 272.

Hoff[47] considers that Kraepelin's work was successful because he offered a pragmatic and clinically based diagnostic system which was based on quantitative and naturalistic research methods and which avoided speculative theories as much as possible. This, however, had the weakness that it paid little attention to the patient's inner world and it made unexamined philosophical assumptions about the nature of psychiatric disease. Engstrom and Weber[48] have judged that Kraepelin's legacy is a mixed one. His division of the psychoses was very influential in the early part of the twentieth century and has shaped the diagnostic systems of the present day. However, his theories did not lead to any meaningful therapy. He had an uncritical faith in the impartiality of clinical observation and ignored the part played by interpersonal factors. These criticisms were the very ones that Laing made in *The Divided Self*.

Laing would have learnt from Gregory Zilboorg's *A History of Medical Psychology*[49] that Kraepelin's system suffered from artificiality in that it was forced to sacrifice too much of the rawness of human reality to maintain its diagnostic structure. In Zilboorg's view, the very clarity of Kraepelin's system was its weakness, because it left no room for the human personality; further, 'the mentally sick person' became merely 'a collection of symptoms'.[50] Such critical views of Kraepelin were common amongst psychoanalytically orientated psychiatrists in 1940s America, and Laing would have been familiar with them.

In his notebooks, Laing commented on the approach of the German clinician:

> Let us look at the behaviour of a young girl of 24 and an elderly man.
>
> The girl is emaciated, but she is in continual movement. She gets a few steps forward and then back again. She plaits her hair only to unloose it the next minute. The man looks at her carefully and from time to time addresses a number of other men who are looking at the girl with great curiosity and interest, and are listening to what the man says. As she moves about he steps in front of her and spreads out his arms. She tries to push him aside, but he won't move, so she slips thro' under his arms. Now he takes a firm hold of her. She starts to cry but she stops when he lets go. He sees that she has a crushed piece of bread in her left hand. He tries hard to force it from her but she absolutely won't let go. He comments to the audience that this demonstrates a senseless resistance against every outward influence, and remarks at the persistent obstinacy of the girl. . . . Even when he pricks her forehead with a pin she scarcely winces. He notes that she wanders back & forward like a beast of prey, after he has stuck this pin into her forehead and left it sticking in. He asks her some questions but she does not say anything to him. But she wails at times. O dear God, O dear God, O dear mother, O dear mother.[51]

---

[47] Ibid., p. 273.

[48] Engstrom, E.J. and Weber, M.W. (1999). 'Emil Kraepelin (1856–1926)'. In Freeman, H. (ed.), *A Century of Psychiatry*, Mosby, London, pp. 49–51.

[49] Zilboorg, *History*, pp. 450–64.

[50] Ibid., p. 452.

[51] MS Laing A260. Notes on depression and mania, c. 1960.

Laing had taken this case history from Emil Kraepelin's lecture on 'Katatonic Stupor' which has appeared in his *Lectures on Clinical Psychiatry*.[52] He felt that the text betrayed an essential inhumanity in the approach to the patient. Laing comments:

> The scene is a lecture room where Emil Kraepelin one of the greatest if not the greatest of psychiatrists is demonstrating a patient.
>
> It would require the genius of a Kierkegaard to convey the full comical/tragic pathos of the situation. The scene is like an ambiguous figure. Like all ambiguous figures, the other way of seeing it has to come from the reader. I simply ask you, who is more alienated from real life, the girl or the man: the girl distracted and in despair, so shut up in herself that a pin stuck in her forehead is almost disregarded: who evidently wants nothing more than to be alone, and as far as she can ignore the man who asks her questions, issues orders, stands in her way to prevent her turning, pins her arms to see what she will do, and tries to force a crumbled piece of bread from her, which incidentally means a great deal to her.[53]

Laing was to use this example from Kraepelin in *The Politics of Experience*.[54] He had of course used another extract from Kraepelin's *Lectures* in *The Divided Self* to bring out the flaws in the interview style of the German professor. Laing chose to engage in his battles with orthodox psychiatry on the subject of schizophrenia. It is natural that he saw Kraepelin as a prime adversary. He devoted much of his time to debunking the approach of the German professor.

Eugen Bleuler

Laing was more sympathetic to the work of Eugen Bleuler, the Swiss psychiatrist who had taken Kraepelin's term 'dementia praecox' and renamed it 'schizophrenia'.

In 1911 Bleuler published his classic book, *Dementia Praecox: or the Group of Schizophrenias,* in which he tried to employ Freudian theory to make sense of schizophrenia. In his notebooks, Laing judged that it was: 'A great book. A classic. The end of Kraepelin'.[55] Bleuler's appeal to many clinicians was his optimistic notion that schizophrenia could be stopped or reversed at any stage of its development.[56] This was achieved by a kind of 'moral treatment'. Bleuler used psychological and social interventions, which sometimes produced dramatic recoveries in his patients.

Bleuler has been the subject of historical myth-making, and has been regarded, like Pinel before him, as ushering in a new tradition: As German Berrios[57] has observed: 'He is

[52] Kraepelin, E. (1913). *Lectures on Clinical Psychiatry*. Bailliere, Tindall and Cox, London. Lecture IV, pp. 30–8.

[53] MS Laing A260.

[54] Laing, R.D. (1967) *The Politics of Experience and the Bird of Paradise*. Penguin Books, London. pp. 88–9.

[55] MS Laing K14.

[56] Ellenberger, H.F. (1970). *The Discovery of the Unconscious. The History and Evolution of Dynamic Psychiatry*. Basic Books, New York, p. 288.

[57] Berrios, G. (1987). '1911. Eugen Bleuler. The fundamental symptoms in dementia praecox or the group of schizophrenias'. In Thompson, C. (ed.), *The Origins of Modern Psychiatry*. Chichester, John Wiley & Sons, pp. 165–210.

seen as a humanitarian psychiatrist who broke away from the bad old days, psychologised madness and slayed the organicist dragon.' In fact, Bleuler's work was the culmination of a long tradition which had sought to introduce psychological concepts into an understanding of psychosis.

Bleuler was born of peasant stock in Zollikon near Zurich in 1857. As a school boy, he became aware that the first professors of psychiatry in Zurich had been imported from Germany and did not understand the local dialect of the patients. The lack of native clinicians apparently inspired Bleuler to become a psychiatrist.[58] Training in Waldau, Paris, and Munich, he took up the post of Director of the Burgholzli Mental Hospital in 1898, where he remained until his retirement in 1927.

In his book, *Dementia Praecox: or the Group of Schizophrenias*, Bleuler did not see himself as opposing Kraepelin's views; rather, he wanted to expand on his ideas, not disprove them.[59] However, Bleuler did introduce his own ideas about schizophrenia. Where Kraepelin's approach tried to be purely observational and empirical, Bleuler advanced a theory about the origin of symptoms. He postulated that there was an underlying cerebral process which caused what he termed the 'fundamental' symptoms. These included loosening of association of ideas and autistic features. The so-called 'accessory' symptoms, such as delusions and hallucinations were said to result from an individual's life experience. The second departure from Kraepelin was Bleuler's attempt to apply Freudian theory to his account of schizophrenia. Bleuler had close contact with Freud, and both Karl Abraham and Carl Jung had worked with him at the Burgholzli. Jung used psychoanalytic theory not only to make sense of the *content* of a patient's symptom but also to explain the *form* of the symptom and even the existence of the entire illness.

According to Berrios,[60] Bleuler allowed himself to become 'trapped in the Freudian web of total comprehensibility'. In other words Bleuler believed that the symptoms of schizophrenia were ultimately understandable. This was to be a key part of Laing's approach to schizophrenia and he judged other clinicians as to whether they thought that patients with schizophrenia were understandable or not. Laing had been struck by an observation by Gregory Zilboorg that Bleuler held that the schizophrenic patient should be approached as a person even in his most disturbed states.[61] The burden lay with the psychiatrist to understand the patient; it was not for the patient to learn the psychiatrist's reality. However, Laing observed that Bleuler, despite his sympathetic approach to people with schizophrenia, held the view that there was a chasm of understanding between himself and his patients. As Laing put it: 'Schizophrenia to Bleuler for all his understanding seem in point of strangeness to resemble "the birds he feeds"'.[62]

---

[58] Ellenberger, *The Discovery*, p. 286.

[59] Hoenig, J. (1995). 'Schizophrenia'. In Berrios, G. and Porter, R. (eds), *A History of Clinical Psychiatry*. Athlone, London. pp. 336–48.

[60] Berrios, *Eugen Bleuler*, p. 204.

[61] MS Laing A694. Laing comments on Zilboorg, 'The conceptual vicissitudes of the idea of schizophrenia'. No further reference details given by Laing.

[62] MS Laing K14.

Laing expressed other reservations in his notebooks:

> He is rather vague and at time seems to contradict himself as to what are the 'Fundamental' symptoms . . . 'explanation' is based on 'association' psychology. Seems to me to mingle 'description' with 'theory' and 'explanation'. Reminds me of the Golden Bough. Has that book's merits and defects. . . .'[63]

'Association' psychology, which had its origins in the writing of Locke, Hume, and David Hartley, held that, if simple elements such as ideas occurred together, or successively, or resembled each other, then they 'associated' to create more complex mental content and behaviour.[64] Association psychology offered a mechanistic picture of human beings, and one with which Laing would not have sympathized. The Scottish Common Sense philosophers, such as Thomas Reid and Thomas Brown, whom Laing had read, were opposed to the determinist approach of association psychology.

In this passage, Laing also referred to the writing of fellow Scotsman James G. Frazer and his monumental work, *The Golden Bough: A Study in Magic and Religion*. Frazer attempted to study classical mythology and religion in terms of the ancient and primitive mind and he aimed to illustrate 'the gradual evolution of human thought from savagery to civilisation'.[65] Although it appeared to offer insights into the evolution of human nature by examining primitive beliefs, Roger Smith has judged that Frazer's book 'fabricated general psychological explanation without reference to specific social context'.[66] Likewise, Laing was uneasy about Bleuler's attempts to provide a psychological explanation of the symptoms of schizophrenia. Laing added: 'Despite his championship of Fr[eud], a sense that Fr[eudian] concepts do not "fit" him comfortably (esp. chapter on Theory of Symptoms—delusions & stereotypes).'[67] Laing's criticisms seem fair and chime with what many other commentators have observed about Bleuler's book.

Carl Jung

Sonu Shamdasani has shown that Jung, like Freud, has been the subject of extensive mythologizing and that his ideas have often been misrepresented.[68] For Shamdasani, Jung played a pivotal role in the formation of the modern concept of schizophrenia, arguing it was psychological in origin and hence amenable to psychotherapy. During his collaboration with Freud, Jung was a principal architect of the psychoanalytic movement and he introduced the practice of the training analysis. He created the influential personality typology of 'introverts' and 'extraverts'. He emphasized the

---

[63] Ibid.

[64] Smith, R. (1997). *The Fontana History of the Human Sciences*. Fontana Press, London. pp. 250–9.

[65] Quoted in Smith, *History of the Human Sciences*, p. 763. Smith also provides a brief discussion of Frazer's work.

[66] Smith, *History of the Human Sciences*, p. 763.

[67] MS Laing K14.

[68] Shamdasani, S. (2003). *Jung and the Making of Modern Psychology. The Dream of a Science*. Cambridge University Press, Cambridge.

importance of myth in understanding how individuals and societies developed. His interest in Eastern thought anticipated the West's later exploration of this culture, and he sought to reconcile religion and science through psychology. Jung's interests and preoccupations were very similar to Laing's. However, Laing had reservations about the Swiss doctor. He thought his writing style was much inferior to that of Freud and that he borrowed heavily from Nietzsche, a philosopher that Jung freely acknowledged was a major influence on him. Laing commented rather dismissively that Jung 'seemed to be doing not much more than footnoting Nietzsche'.[69]

The son of a Protestant pastor, Carl Gustav Jung was born in 1875 in Kwessil, Switzerland.[70] His upbringing bears some similarities to that of Laing: both were only children; both had mothers who were mentally disturbed; and both had fathers who developed a depressive breakdown in mid-life. When Jung was in his teens, his father lost his faith, which precipitated a deep depression. He confided in Carl, who, like Laing, was to claim that his father was his first 'patient'.[71] In contrast to Laing's intervention, however, 'therapy' proved ineffective. After qualifying in medicine at the University of Basle, Jung worked as a psychiatrist in the Burgholzi mental hospital in Zurich, where he wrote his first book, a study of dementia praecox. In 1907, he met Freud and the two men enjoyed a close and productive working relationship until their fall out in 1912. Jung felt that Freud overestimated the extent to which human behaviour had a sexual basis and that he had unnecessarily restricted his theory to the early years of development, rather than considering a person's whole life. Jung went on to develop 'analytic psychology', which he later renamed 'complex psychology'. He put forward the theory of 'individuation', a process he saw as unfolding in certain gifted individuals during their middle years. He maintained that individuation was a journey to psychic wholeness and he used illustrations from alchemy, mythology, literature, and religion to sign-post the different stages a person would encounter on the way. Ellenberger has emphasized the fundamental difference in outlook between Freud and Jung.[72] Freud's psychoanalysis was the heir of positivism, scientism, and Darwinism, whereas Jung's analytic psychology rejected this tradition. Unlike Freud, Jung was sympathetic to spiritual accounts of existence and declared that man was naturally religious.

Laing, of course, had links with a therapist who had worked with Jung. This was Karl Abenheimer, the Jungian analyst, who was an early mentor of Laing. In one of his notebooks, Laing made an extensive critique of Jung's *The Psychology of Dementia Praecox*, which appeared in 1906.[73] Jung claimed it was the first monograph devoted

---

[69] Mullan, *Mad to be Normal*, p. 105.

[70] See Ellenberger, *The Discovery*, pp. 657–748; Storr, A. (1973). *Jung*. Fontana, Glasgow; Gregory, R. (ed.) (1987). 'Jung, Carl Gustav'. In *The Oxford Companion to Mind*. Oxford University Press, Oxford, pp. 403–05.

[71] Burston, D. and Frie, R. (2006). *Psychotherapy as a Human Science*. Duquesne University Press, Pittsburg, p. 110.

[72] Ellenberger, *The Discovery*, p. 657.

[73] MS Laing A580 (i). C.G. Jung (1906) *The Psychology of Dementia Praecox* (trans. A.A. Brill, 1936). Nervous and Mental Disease Publishing Company, USA.

to a 'depth-psychological' investigation of a psychotic patient.[74] He tried to show that a psychological approach to dementia praecox or schizophrenia could be productive. At this stage Jung was working with Eugen Bleuler, whom he described as his 'venerable chief', at the Burgholzli Clinic of Psychiatry in Zurich. Jung was influenced by Pierre Janet, a French clinician, whom Ellenberger[75] credits as being the first to found a new system of dynamic psychiatry. Jung was also influenced by Theodore Fluornoy, a Professor of Psychology at the University of Geneva, who was interested in the unconscious and parapsychology.[76] In his book Jung referred to the 'ingenious conceptions' of Freud, though he also expressed serious reservations. Jung's book was based on his experimental work with word association tests which he had administered to patients to test Freud's theories, particularly *The Interpretation of Dreams*. In a detailed study of one patient, a 60-year-old woman, Jung concluded that her seemingly incoherent utterances were an expression of wish fulfilment to compensate for a life of toil and deprivation. Laing felt it was a great advance for the time. However, he thought that Jung's theory did not allow the patient as an individual to emerge. In addition, he observed that Jung did not conceive of schizophrenia as an interpersonal problem and had no awareness that an individual's current social environment might contribute to their difficulties. Laing also felt that Jung's analysis of dreams was not radical enough.

In a review of Jung's *The Undiscovered Self* in 1959, Laing expressed further views on the Swiss doctor.[77] Laing was taken with Jung's view that there was a spiritual conflict between the individual and the organized 'Mass Man'. Laing saw Jung as sharing the same concerns as the existential tradition, in particular the focus on the individual. Laing maintained that the individual was faced with a crisis in which he or she could continue to develop, become engulfed by the masses, or go mad. Laing wrote that the crisis led to 'the appalling ordeal by solitude which is the present crucial test for the modern hero'. Further, Laing warned: 'We have already before us too much evidence of the devastation of the individual blinded and ravaged by solitude in "the time he calls his own".' Laing, who saw himself as a creative individual in conflict with the unappreciative masses, identified with the sentiments expressed in Jung's book.

Laing was also interested in *Symbols of Transformation*, in which Jung drew a parallel between a psychotic episode and a mythological journey or a transformation of the soul.[78] Jung had called this experience 'metanoia', a term Laing was to use later in his *The Politics of Experience and the Bird of Paradise*. Miller has argued that although Jung used the term, it is also to be found in the textual history of Christian scriptures.[79] 'Metanoia' is a Greek word, meaning 'change of mind', an inward shift of viewpoint. Miller contends that Laing was familiar with Christian hermeneutics and that this

---

[74] Ellenberger, *The Discovery*, p. 668.

[75] Ellenberger, *The Discovery*, p. 331.

[76] Ibid., p. 315.

[77] MS Laing A114. 'Review of *The Undiscovered Self* by C.G. Jung'. *Journal of Analytical Psychology* (1959) by Laing.

[78] Mullan, *Mad to be Normal*, p.104.

[79] Miller, G. (2009). 'How Scottish was R.D. Laing?' *History of Psychiatry*, **20**(2), 226–32.

would also have informed his use of the term. Laing read Jung's *Psychology of Religion*, but was disappointed that Jung had supported the view that Nietzsche had disintegrated mentally as a result of general paralysis of the insane. He was also disappointed that Jung had questioned the sanity of James Joyce and Picasso.

The Methodenstreit

As we have seen, Freud, Jung, Kraepelin, and Bleuler differed markedly in how they conceived of mental disturbance. Their differing perspectives should be seen in the context of a larger philosophical discussion about the 'science of man', in particular the *Methodenstreit* or Methodological Controversy, which took place during the late nineteenth and early twentieth century in Germany but which also referred to British and French thinkers. Essentially, this was a debate as to which was the most appropriate scientific technique to study human beings. At the core of the debate was the question: should all sciences model themselves on the natural sciences? On one side were positivist thinkers, such as John Stuart Mill, August Comte, and Emil Durkheim, who answered in the affirmative: humans were essentially no different from the rest of the natural world and thus the techniques of the physical sciences were appropriate for the study of people. On the other side were men such as Wilhelm Dilthey and Max Weber, who argued that the techniques of the natural sciences were *not* appropriate for studying human beings, who, they maintained, were distinct from the rest of nature as a result of possessing consciousness, free will, and the need to find meaning and value in their lives. The *human* sciences required specific techniques such as 'understanding' and 'interpretation'. Laing, who was aware of this debate, favoured the position of Dilthey and Weber, and much of his later work can be seen as an attempt to argue that human beings could not and should not be conceived of in terms of the natural sciences.

Laing made notes on Wilhelm Dilthey[80] and was to refer to him in *The Divided Self*.[81] Dilthey had made the distinction between 'explaining' and 'understanding', i.e. between rational grasping of causal relations and the intuitive feeling of one's way into another person's inner world. Dilthey[82] was writing in the context of hermeneutics or the art of interpretation, especially as it applied to historical texts. He maintained that we understood an author, artist, or historical actor by way of analogies to our own experiences, by imaginative sympathy. Dilthey believed that the human sciences expressed the spirit of their authors and we could only understand ('verstehen') them by grasping this spirit. Laing was taken by Dilthey's notion that the relationship between the expositor and the original author or historical actor was crucial in reaching an understanding. Laing felt that this notion particularly applied to the relationship between doctor and patient. However, where Dilthey had emphasized that expositor and author shared the same living experience, in *The Divided Self*, Laing

---

[80] MS Laing A258. Dilthey.
[81] Laing R.D. (1960). *The Divided Self*. Tavistock, London, pp. 32–4.
[82] See entries on Wilhelm Dilthey and on Hermeneutics in Honderich, T. (ed.) (1995). *The Oxford Companion to Philosophy*, Oxford University Press, Oxford, p. 201 and pp. 353–4.

noted that the sane and insane, by definition, did not share the same reality and, thus interpretation was problematic.

In draft notes[83] Laing pondered what he called the 'art' of understanding other people. Could such an art be given a 'scientific' basis? He stated that one could not understand anything in another person if one could not sense the potential for the same feeling in oneself. He went on to consider interpretation and pointed out that it was never a neutral activity. It always reflected the pre-suppositions of the person making the interpretation, whether it was Freud or Kraepelin. Laing compared the problem to language, suggesting that it was as though we said that English was the normal language and that German was a disorder of English. We would then be led to the conclusion that there were various disorders of vocabulary and syntax in the German speaker. The experience of the psychotic person was unlike our own. Laing observed: 'As long as we refer *his language* to *our* experience, it will be *senseless*. Rather we should allow his language to be a gateway, a means of access, a way of unveiling, of elucidating, of understanding *his* experience.'[84]

The debate about the natural sciences and whether they were appropriate to the study of human beings was not confined to the *Methodenstreit* of late nineteenth-century Germany, and many of the thinkers whom Laing admired, such as Kierkegaard, John Macmurray, and existential philosophers generally, opposed the notion that the physical sciences offered a valid way of understanding people. The *Methodenstreit* was to have a major influence on the German writer Karl Jaspers, 'psychiatry's first philosopher'[85] and author of *General Psychopathology*.

Karl Jaspers

Karl Jaspers was born in 1883 in Oldenburg, Northern Germany and between 1908 and 1915 he worked at the Heidelberg Clinic of Psychiatry, where he read widely in philosophy and psychiatry.[86] Jaspers described the state of psychiatry when he began his career:

> In the psychiatry of those days—about 1910—somatic medicine was still in control. Freud's influence was limited to small groups. Psychological efforts were considered subjective, futile, and unscientific . . . There seemed to be no common scientific psychiatry uniting all the workers in the field . . . One cause of this intellectual jumble seemed to me to lie in the nature of the case. For the subject matter of psychiatry was man, not just his body—or indeed his body least of all, but his soul, his personality, his self. I read not only Griesinger's somatic dogma—that mental diseases were diseases of the brain—but Schule's thesis that mental diseases were diseases of the personality.[87]

[83] MS Laing A708.

[84] Ibid.

[85] Fulford et al., *Oxford Textbook of Philosophy and Psychiatry*.

[86] Kirkbright, S. (2004). *Karl Jaspers. A Biography. Navigations in Truth*. Yale University Press, New Haven and London.

[87] Jaspers, J. (2000). 'Philosophical memoir'. In Ehrlich, E., Ehrlich, L.H. and Pepper, G.B. (eds), *Karl Jaspers: Basic Philosophical Writings*. Humanity Books, New York, p. 5.

Jaspers wanted a foot in both camps: to combine the techniques of the natural sciences, for example, examining brain tissue and function, with the approach of the human sciences, which focused on the experiences, aims, intentions, and subjective meanings of individual people. Jaspers argued that psychopathology was both a biological natural science seeking general explanations of mental disorders in terms of their neuropathological causes, but also a human science seeking to 'understand' the patient's individual experience. Fulford and his colleagues contend that Jaspers, who lived through psychiatry's first 'biological revolution', grappled with problems that we still face today: how to relate meaning to mechanism; and how to relate the patient's subjective experience to neuroscientific findings.[88]

Laing had mixed feelings about Jaspers. Early in his career, as we have seen, he had plans to go and study with him in Basle University where Jaspers held the chair of philosophy, though this fell through when Laing was conscripted to the British Army. Later Laing was to be critical of Jasper's thinking, especially with regard to his approach to people with schizophrenia and to artists who became mentally unbalanced.[89] Jaspers had condemned what he saw as attempts to extend understanding beyond its proper limits. He was particularly critical of Freud, but also of Bleuler and Jung, in their efforts to understand the symptoms of schizophrenia. Jaspers wrote:

> . . . attempts have been made to understand the contents of delusion as well as other psychotic symptoms in terms of the individual's wishes and longings. This approach has been extended to schizophrenia by the Zurich school (*Bleuler* and *Jung*). However they did not stop at the obviously meaningful contents but followed in Freud's footsteps and treated them as symbols. They have thus come to 'understand' almost all the contents of these psychoses by applying a procedure which as the results show only leads on into endlessness. In the most literal sense they have re-discovered the 'meaning of madness' or believe that they have.[90]
>
> The most profound distinction in psychic life seems to be that between what is meaningful and *allows empathy* and what in its particular way is *ununderstandable*, 'mad' in the literal sense, schizophrenic psychic life . . .[91]

Laing parted company with Jaspers on the question of whether schizophrenia was comprehensible or not. As Laing was to write:[92]

> Jaspers' use of process indicates that he fails to understand the dialectic of the person's life before the supposed alien, meaningless intrusion occurs. It is because he has lost track

[88] Fulford et al., *Oxford Textbook of Philosophy and Psychiatry*. See also Fulford, B., Morris, K., Sadler, J. and Stanghellini (eds) (2003). *Nature and Narrative. An Introduction to the New Philosophy of Psychiatry*. Oxford University Press, Oxford; and Thornton, T. (2007). *Essential Philosophy of Psychiatry*. Oxford University Press, Oxford.

[89] Kirsner, D. (1990). 'An abyss of difference: Laing, Sartre and Jaspers'. *Journal of the British Society for Phenomenology*, **21**, 209–15.

[90] Jaspers, K. (1963). *General Psychopathology* (trans. J. Hoenig and M. Hamilton). Manchester University Press, Manchester, p. 410.

[91] Ibid., p. 577.

[92] Laing, R.D. (1964). 'Review of Karl Jasper's General Psychopathology'. *International Journal of Psychoanalysis*, **45**, 590–3.

long before, that the person's experience finally loses all meaning to Jaspers, and process is then invented. I devoted a book, *The Divided Self*, largely to demonstrating that the way from apparent sanity to apparent madness could be understood well past the point where Jaspers tells us to give up.

Fulford, Thornton, and Graham,[93] however, see Jaspers occupying a crucial and significant place in the evolution of psychiatry as it has veered between physical and psychological explanations of mental disorder. Jaspers was trying to reconcile these two approaches, and he was writing at a time, at the beginning of the twentieth century, when natural scientific approaches to insanity were prominent. Alzheimer and Nissl were describing the brain pathology of Alzheimer's disease; the organism responsible for General Paralysis of the Insane had been discovered; and Kraepelin had outlined his ground-breaking division of the insanities. In response to these developments, Jaspers felt it was important to emphasize the contribution of the human sciences. Laing was working at a time when physical treatments, such as lobotomies, electroconvulsive therapy, and insulin comas, were being employed, but he was also working when new, and, arguably effective, physical treatments, such as anti-psychotic and anti-depressant medication, were being introduced. Rather than trying to reconcile the mental and the somatic, as Jaspers had attempted, Laing was to eventually concentrate exclusively on the psychological.

Later psychiatric theories

Object relations theory

In *The Divided Self*, Laing drew on object relations theory to construct his account of the self. As we have seen, the major exponents of the theory taught and lectured at the Institute of Psychoanalysis when Laing was training there, but it remains unclear as to what extent he had developed his own ideas before he moved to London. Certainly, *The Divided Self* makes extensive reference to the leading practitioners of object relations theory, such as Klein, Fairbairn, Winnicott, and Guntrip. Laing also admitted to the influence of the Berlin analyst, Karen Horney and her notion of the false self,[94] though her work was not mentioned in the book. However, Laing was to claim that he had written *The Divided Self* before he went to the Tavistock and had conceived of his false-self system without being particularly influenced by Winnicott. Rather, he stated that he had been influenced by Heidegger's concept of the authentic and inauthentic.[95]

Object relations theory sought to replace Freud's drive theory with a radically different model which emphasized the primacy of relations with others. In Freudian language, the 'object' is that which is the target of a drive. Object relations theory was concerned with exploring the relationship between real people in the external world and the internal images of them that individuals formed.[96] Thus one might entertain

---

[93] Fulford et al., *Oxford Textbook of Philosophy and Psychiatry*.

[94] Mullan, *Mad to be Normal*, p. 152.

[95] Ibid., p. 152.

[96] Greenberg, J.R. and Mitchell, S.A. (1983). *Object Relations in Psychoanalytic Theory*. Harvard University Press, Massachusetts, Cambridge.

a mental picture of somebody that was at great variance to the way they conducted themselves in real life. Object relations theory sought to examine how these two entities, external and internal 'objects', interacted. Laing was to criticize the use of the term 'objects' in objects relations theory, stating that it was an inappropriate way to describe human beings.[97] Object relations theory has been used and defined in many differing ways, and it is a fruitless enterprise to delineate, or even suggest that there is, one 'true' theory. It has been associated with the work of Melanie Klein, but also with that of W.R.D. Fairbairn, Ian Suttie, Harry Guntrip, and Donald Winnicott.

Melanie Klein

Object relations theory has its origins in the work of Melanie Klein, an Austrian analyst who moved to London in the 1920s. Klein depicted the mental life of the child and adult as being an intricate web of phantasied relations between the self and others, both in the external world and in the internal world of imaginary 'objects'.[98] She maintained that aspects of the internal world, such as feelings or images, could be 'projected' externally, while aspects of the outer world could be 'introjected' into the inner world.[99]

Klein held that the crucial period in life was infancy, when the baby experienced an intolerable conflict between love and hate.[100] The baby tried to resolve this conflict by projecting the aggressive part of him or herself onto the outer world. The infant perceived 'objects' as partial: they were split into the all-good, as represented by the nourishing 'good breast', or the all-bad as represented by the unsatisfying 'bad breast'. The infant projected inner aggression onto the bad breast and lived in the paranoid fear of attack from this imagined monster. As George Makari has observed, Klein's picture of a world of fear and persecution was 'worthy of Hieronymus Bosch'.[101] At a later period, the infant was said to develop a more balanced relation to the mother and to see her as a 'whole' person, made up of good and bad qualities. This attainment of wholeness marked an important stage in the infant's emotional development, but it was also marked by the infant's sudden realization that he or she had entertained violent emotions about their mother. This led to feelings of remorse, guilt, and depression. Klein argued that there was both a 'paranoid position' and a 'depressive position', with the former defending the child against the depressed feelings of the latter. In adult life the individual could swing between these two positions, for example adopting a paranoid view of the world to avoid acknowledging feelings of guilt about their own aggression. Klein saw the process of emotional development in instinctual terms like Freud, but

---

[97] MS Laing A260.

[98] Greenberg and Mitchell, *Object Relations in Psychoanalytic Theory*, p. 130.

[99] Gomez, L. (1997). *An Introduction to Object Relations in Psychoanalytic Theory*. Free Association Press, London, p. 35.

[100] A good short account of the work of Klein, considered in the context of Laing is: Lomas, P., 'Psychoanalysis—Freudian or Existential'. In Rycroft, C. (ed.) *Psychoanalysis Observed*. Constable, London, pp. 119–48.

[101] Makari, G. (2008). *Revolution in the Mind. The Creation of Psychoanalysis*. Duckworth, London, p. 435.

where he had emphasized the sexual drive, she highlighted the aggressive drive. She held that, if this infantile experience was overwhelming, the individual grew up to become schizoid.

As Makari has noted, Klein was not content to just describe the shift from the paranoid to the depressive mode; unfortunately, she claimed to be able to *date* it.[102] The momentous shift occurred, Klein advised, between the fourth and fifth month of life. This claim, which was impossible to prove or disprove, was greeted with incredulity and hostility by many in the psychoanalytic community, and Klein's reputation suffered as a consequence. Some of the earliest criticism of Klein came from Scotland.[103] Ian Suttie, author of *The Origins of Love and Hate*, which Laing had read, objected to the Kleinian picture of the infant as paranoid and aggressive. Instead, Suttie held that the infant had an innately benign and sociable relationship with others, and that negative qualities only emerged if normal development had been impaired by a noxious upbringing. Ian Suttie had been a psychiatrist at Gartnavel in the 1920s.[104] His wife Jane Robertson was also a psychiatrist at Gartnavel and had translated many of the works of Sandor Ferenczi. Suttie quoted with approval Ferenczi's contention that it was the therapist's 'love' that cured the patient. According to Dr Hunter-Brown it was this aspect of Suttie's work that was best known to Glasgow psychiatrists in the 1950s.[105] Fairbairn, too, criticized Klein along similar lines. Further criticism came from Guntrip, who maintained that the Kleinian world was a solipsistic and phantasmagoric one with no essential connection to real people.[106] In opposition to Klein's theory that all the action took place within the child's head, both Fairbairn and Winnicott emphasized the influence of the child's parents as real people rather than objects of fantasy.

Laing found Melanie Klein to be a formidable, dogmatic figure who brooked no dissent from her theories, advising anyone who had the temerity to argue with her to go and see their analyst because they obviously had unresolved problems.[107] Klein, Laing was dismayed to learn, knew nothing about the work of almost any other European thinker apart from Freud.[108] However, he respected her and felt that some of what she was saying resonated with what he had seen clinically, in particular, in his work with psychotic patients. Laing held that in such patients the unconscious became conscious, and he could see evidence of the mental world described by Klein, 'profoundly odd' though it might be, in the 'material' they produced. In *The Divided Self*, Laing did not mention Klein, but he did cite a paper of hers on 'schizoid mechanisms' in the 'References' section.

---

[102] Ibid., p. 436.

[103] Burston, *The Wing of Madness*, p. 49.

[104] Hunter-Brown, *R.D. Laing*, p. 92.

[105] Ibid., p. 92.

[106] Greenberg and Mitchell, *Object Relations in Psychoanalytic Theory*, p.130.

[107] Mullan, *Mad to be Normal*, p. 160.

[108] MS Laing A511/2. R.D. Laing, Review of Charles Rycroft's *Psychoanalysis and Beyond*.

Peter Lomas, a colleague of Laing's at the Tavistock, wrote an essay in which he considered the influence of Melanie Klein on Laing's work.[109] Lomas observed that both Klein and Laing saw 'splitting' as a fundamental psychological mechanism. According to psychoanalytic theory, 'splitting' is a defence mechanism by which a mental structure loses its integrity and becomes replaced by two or more parts.[110] For example, after splitting of the ego, one resulting part-ego is experienced as the 'self'. However, Lomas felt that the similarity between the two theorists ended there, because Laing believed that a person who experienced their ego as split was fighting to maintain his or her identity in the face of an existential threat of destruction. Klein held that such fears arose from fantasy, engendered by the failure to resolve aggressive feelings in infancy. Lomas sided with Laing, contending that Klein paid almost no attention to the actual life circumstances of the person.

Fairbairn

Ronald Fairbairn was educated in Edinburgh where he spent his professional life. He has been seen by Gavin Miller[111] as providing, along with his fellow Scot, Ian Suttie, a particularly Scottish perspective on psychoanalysis, characterized by a philosophy of questioning from first principles the foundations of Freudian theory, and by an emphasis on kinship and community, rather than on the isolated and self-seeking ego of classical psychoanalysis. Miller maintains that this approach was to influence Laing.

Although Fairbairn borrowed some terms from Klein, he changed their meaning, which resulted in his work being quite distinct from hers.[112] Before embarking on his medical career, Fairbairn had studied philosophy and divinity, and this informed his work. He began his psychoanalytic training with a thorough examination of the work of Freud, which he read in the original German. Laing also made efforts to read thinkers in their original language. Fairbairn's objection to Freud's theory was that it was mechanistic, atomistic, and was expressed in a depersonalized language. In a series of papers written in the 1940s, Fairbairn developed his theory which shifted from a Freudian drive model to a relational one.[113] He held that libido was not pleasure-seeking but object-seeking. Pleasure was not the end goal, but a means to its real end: a relation with another person. Where Freud had suggested that the infant was born into

[109] Lomas, P. (1968). 'Psychoanalysis—Freudian or Existential'. In Rycroft, C. (ed.), *Psychoanalysis Observed*. Pelican, London, pp. 116–44. Lomas considered that Laing's concept of 'ontological security' was similar to Klein's terms of 'persecutory anxiety' and 'projective and introjective identification'.

[110] Rycroft, C. (1995). *Critical Dictionary of Psychoanalysis*. Penguin Books, London, pp. 173–4.

[111] Miller, G. (2004). *R.D. Laing*. Edinburgh University Press, Edinburgh; Miller, G. (2008). 'Scottish psychoanalysis. A rational religion'. *Journal of the History of the Behavioural Sciences*, **44**(1), 38–58.

[112] Greenberg and Mitchell, *Object Relations in Psychoanalytic Theory*, p. 152.

[113] Guntrip, H. (1952). 'A study of Fairbairn's theory of schizoid reactions'. *British Journal of Medical Psychology*, **25**, 86–103.

the world unrelated to others and became related only secondarily as they provided him or her with pleasure, Fairbairn held that infants were orientated towards others from the start. Subsequent emotional and mental difficulties were seen, not as deriving from conflicts over pleasure-seeking impulses, but from disturbances in relations with others. A major implication of Fairbairn's work was that all difficulties in living could be traced back to one's parents. If they were not sufficiently emotionally available for the child, then problems ensued in later life. In Fairbairn's scheme no consideration was given to how the particular temperament of the child might have contributed to their emotional problems. He offered an essentially Romantic view of the child, as Laing was to do in his writing.

Fairbairn judged that the most significant relationship in the infant's early life was that with the mother, but relations with others were also crucial. The infant passed from dependence on others to adult mutuality. A disturbance in this process led to a compensatory relation with 'internal objects' and inner fragmentation. As a result, the ego became split, because different parts of the ego related not to others but to 'internal objects'. Energy was drained from the outside world into the inner; a mechanism, which Fairbairn maintained, was fundamental to understanding the schizoid personality. The key elements of the schizoid experience were a sense of emptiness, deadness, and futility. There could also be feelings of being unreal or being cut-off from others. According to Fairbairn, the schizoid person focused on the inner rather than the outer world. They valued the self over others, to whom they showed contempt or indifference. Towards the end of his career Fairbairn became critical of the standard analytic method.[114] He maintained that 'The relationship existing between the patient and analyst is more important than details of technique.'[115]

Laing made extensive notes on Fairbairn's *Psychoanalytic Studies of the Personality*.[116] He was interested in Fairbairn's notion that individuals with schizoid personalities gained the conviction in early life that their mother did not really love and value them as persons in their own right, a notion with which he may have personally identified. It is quite evident from this brief summary of Fairbairn's work that Laing owed a great debt to the Edinburgh analyst's concept of the schizoid personality when he came to formulate his own ideas in *The Divided Self*. Gomez[117] has judged that Fairbairn's work had a far-reaching effect on how psychotherapy was practised. Analysts began to accept that patients needed a genuine relationship with their therapist rather than just merely being given interpretations. Again the influence on Laing's attitude to therapy is clear.

---

[114] Tantam, D. (1996). 'Fairbairn'. In Freeman, H. and Berrios, G.E. (eds) *150 Years of British Psychiatry. Volume II: the Aftermath*. Athlone, London, pp. 549–64.

[115] Fairbairn, W.R.D. (1957). 'Freud: the psychoanalytic method and mental health'. *British Journal of Medical Psychology*, **30**, 53–62.

[116] MS Laing A580 (i).

[117] Gomez, *Object Relations in Psychoanalytic Theory*, p. 79.

D.W. Winnicott

According to Lisa Appignanesi, the work of Donald Woods Winnicott, a paediatrician by training, 'made babies interesting'.[118] Appignanesi sees Winnicott as a Romantic who believed that an infant who enjoyed a relationship with a 'good-enough mother' would develop an authentic and creative self. Winnicott constructed a theory to explain how the self emerged out of its relations with others.[119] He examined the struggle of the self to assert its individuality, whilst at the same time forming relationships with others. Winnicott held that a lack of contact with others or, alternatively, an immersion in the world of others, presented dangers. He observed that classical analytic theory took it for granted that the patient was a 'person': that they had a unified and stable personality which was able to interact with others.[120] This ignored those people who had difficulty being a 'person', because they were psychotic, and those who were unable to interact with others. Winnicott focused on the conditions that enabled the child to see his or herself as separate from others. The mother provided a crucial role in helping the self of the infant to emerge. If maternal provision was inadequate, the infant self might fragment. The infant became overwhelmed by the demands of others and lost touch with his or her own spontaneous needs. This resulted in a split between the 'true self' and the 'false self'. The 'true self' hid away, while the 'false self', which was moulded by maternal expectations, dealt with the outside world. The 'false self' served to protect the integrity of the 'true self'. In adult life, if this strategy failed, the self could fragment into several parts and psychosis developed. The person was unable to maintain a sense of wholeness, coherence, and continuity of the self. Winnicott wrote:

> Psychotic illness is related to environmental failure at an early stage of the emotional development of the individual. The sense of futility and unreality belongs to the development of a false self which develops in protection of the true self.[121]

The true self becomes impoverished from lack of contact with lived experience. Winnicott was proposing an essentialist theory, with the essence being the 'true self'.[122] The true self was the source of what was authentic in a person. Winnicott's ideas would appear to have heavily influenced *The Divided Self*, and initially Laing acknowledged this. In April 1958 he wrote to Winnicott:

> You may or may not remember me. I've written a study (c. 80,000 words) on schizoid and schizophrenic states, in particular trying to describe the transition from a sane to a mad way of being in the world. It draws its inspiration very largely from your writings. May I send it to you?[123]

[118] Appignanesi, L. (2008). *Mad, Bad and Sad. A History of Women and the Mind Doctors from 1800 to the Present*. Virago, London, p. 284.
[119] Winnicott, D.W. (1958). *Collected Papers*. Tavistock, London.
[120] Greenberg and Mitchell, *Object Relations in Psychoanalytic Theory*, p. 191.
[121] Winnicott, *Collected Papers*, p. 286.
[122] Phillips, A. (1988). *Winnicott*. Fontana Press, London.
[123] Rodman, F.R. (2003). *Winnicott. Life and Work*. Perseus Publishing, Cambridge, p. 243.

With some justification, Peter Lomas maintains that Laing's system of the self resembles that of Winnicott.[124] However, Winnicott also contended that there was a pre-split 'real self' to which the individual had to return. Laing had no such concept. In later years, Laing was to deny that he had been particularly influenced by Winnicott. Winnicott, for his part, felt he should have been given more credit for the notion of the false self. Laing argued that many of Winnicott's concepts had long been a part of the Western intellectual tradition.

Other theorists

Originally from a background in the ministry and pastoral counselling, Harry Guntrip became interested in psychoanalysis, but was repelled by Freud's hostility to religion and his mechanistic model of the mind. Guntrip criticized not only Freud, but also the notion that scientific techniques could be applied to humanity. As he wrote:

> Science has to discover whether and how it can deal with the 'person', the 'unique individual', we will dare to say the 'spiritual self' with all the motives, values, hopes, fears and purposes that constitute the real life of man, and make a purely 'organic' approach to man inadequate.[125]

Laing was to express much the same sentiments in his own work. John Bowlby was a major figure in the London psychoanalytic community. His contention that 'maternal deprivation' caused problems for the developing child proved very influential in post-war discussions of parenting. Bowlby drew on ethology and the Darwinian theory of natural selection to present his 'instinct theory'. Fundamental to this was the child's attachment to the mother. Problems arose when the attachment to the mother did not occur or was disturbed. Laing was to claim later that he was not especially interested in ethology, and certainly he makes no mention of Bowlby in his first book, though he did send him a draft manuscript of it. As we have seen from a lecture that Laing gave to divinity students in Dublin, he had reservations about Bowlby's work.[126]

Later psychotherapeutic approaches to schizophrenia

Laing was attracted to the theorists who held that a psychotherapeutic rather than a neurobiological approach was the best way to understand and help patients suffering from schizophrenia. In America, there was an established tradition of treating schizophrenic patients with psychotherapy: it included such writers as Sullivan, Arieti, Federn, Frieda Fromm-Riechmann, Searles, and Rosen. European clinicians from an existential background, such as Binswanger, Minkowski, and Boss also advocated a broadly psychological approach. There were other writers such as Marguerite Sechehave, who, although not formally an existential or psychoanalytical therapist,

---

[124] Lomas, *Psychoanalysis Observed*, p. 126.
[125] Guntrip, H. (1961). *Personality Structure and Human Interaction: the Developing Synthesis of Psychodynamic Theory*. International Universities Press, New York..
[126] MS Laing A154. R.D. Laing: Notes for a lecture at Trinity College, Dublin, 1955.

advocated a type of talking therapy. Laing drew on these traditions and they informed his clinical practice as well as his writing.

Harry Stack Sullivan

Laing had first come across a remark by Harry Stack Sullivan in an article in *Encounter* which he had found intriguing. Addressing a group of young psychiatrists, Sullivan had told them: 'I want you to remember that in our present state of society the patient is right and you are wrong.'[127] On exploring Sullivan's work further, he found that Sullivan had maintained that the close relationship between psychiatry and neurology was a false one, that it was a *misalliance*. The proper subject for psychiatry was disturbances in living, manifest by disturbances in interpersonal relationships, whereas neurology was concerned with pathological lesions of the central nervous system. For Laing, who came across Sullivan's opinion some months after graduating from medical school, this was a revelation.[128] Laing was impressed by Sullivan's emphasis on 'the uniqueness of the individual', not as an object of study. He compared his approach to that of Kierkegaard, Heidegger, and Jaspers.[129] From Sullivan he took the notion that it was only in the context of interpersonal relations that 'personality' existed.[130] Laing was also taken by Sullivan's phrase, 'we are all more simply human than otherwise', and was fond of repeating it. Laing, though, like most people who have tried to read Sullivan's work, found him to have an execrable prose style.

Sullivan was a very influential figure in American psychiatry in the early and mid part of the twentieth century. He ran a unit for male patients with schizophrenia at the Sheppard and Enoch Hospital in Maryland. He was apparently struck by the disparity between *his* patients and those described by his peers who were influenced by the Kraepelinian model of schizophrenia.[131] Sullivan felt that the utterances of his patients were often understandable and that their symptoms could be seen as an adaptation to their circumstances. Laing was later to claim in *The Divided Self* that the patients *he* saw did not resemble those described in contemporary psychiatric textbooks. In this stance he was clearly influenced by Sullivan but it also held polemical value. Laing was implying that he was too sensitive to put patients into Kraepelinian categories: he saw the human being behind the supposedly mad demeanour.

Sullivan argued that when Kraepelin interviewed patients in lecture theatres, he was not, as he contended, demonstrating the symptoms of dementia praecox (or what has since been renamed schizophrenia), but rather showing how institutional life had affected patients' behaviour and communication. The patient's presentation owed more to their adaptation to hospitalization than to underlying illness. Laing was to draw on this Sullivanian concept in *The Divided Self* when he described Kraepelin interviewing a patient in front of a class. For Laing the symptoms were the patient's

---

[127] Mullan, *Mad to be Normal*, pp. 116–7.
[128] Ibid., p. 117.
[129] MS Laing K14.
[130] Ibid.
[131] Greenberg and Mitchell, *Object Relations in Psychoanalytic Theory*, p. 83.

meaningful response to the indignity of being paraded in front of others, or, as Sullivan put it, being made into a 'side-show'.[132]

Sullivan called for a different approach to the subject. The clinician should focus on the person rather than on preconceived formulations and explanations. He felt orthodox methods provided the clinician with an illusory sense of power and knowledge, and duped them into thinking they were being 'objective'. Sullivan held that the clinician needed close personal observation of the patient and that research of real value came from an intimate and detailed study of particular individuals. This was the type of work, of course, to which Laing was to devote his career. Despite his misgivings about Freud, Sullivan was heavily influenced by him, particularly in the early part of his career. Just as Freud had shown that neurotic symptoms were meaningful, Sullivan attempted to demonstrate that psychotic symptoms were comprehensible. Sullivan held that schizophrenia was not the result of some kind of brain malfunction, but was rather a *process* whereby the individual reacted to their social environment, in particular the significant others in their life. Individuals with schizophrenia had a marked disturbance in their ability to relate to other people and this was a result of a whole series of past experiences with others. For Sullivan, patients with schizophrenia could only be understood in the interpersonal context.

Sullivan maintained that the most important therapeutic factor was the relationship between doctor and patient, and this led him to decry those clinicians who adopted a detached and supposedly 'objective' approach to the patient. Sullivan wanted to move away from the approach of his peers who emphasized the importance of diagnostic classification and a neurobiological explanation of patient symptomatology. Sullivan saw psychiatry as the study of interpersonal relations. The personality or the 'self' of the child was formed from the responses of the parents. If the child received critical responses, he or she might block out these unpleasant impressions and, as a consequence, be prone to distorted interpretations of social situations, or what Sullivan called 'parataxic distortions'. If these distortions went uncorrected, the person would increasingly make statements with which others could not agree. The person increasingly lacked what Sullivan calls 'consensual validation'. Sullivan saw the role of the therapist as being to share the patient's frightening world. The therapist was not an *observer* but a *participant*. Once again we see how Sullivan anticipated, if not directly influenced, many of Laing's key ideas.[133]

Other therapists

In *The Divided Self*, Laing referred to the book, *Psychotherapy with Schizophrenics*,[134] which gives a good account of the views of psychoanalytically-minded American psychiatrists in the 1950s on psychological therapy with psychotic patients. The personality of the therapist was held to be of great importance. It was stated that therapy

---

[132] Ibid., p. 83.

[133] A good concise summary of Sullivan's ideas are to be found in Arieti, S. (1955). *Interpretation of Schizophrenia*. Robert Brunner, New York, pp. 33–9.

[134] Brody, E.B. and Redlich, F.C. (1952). *Psychotherapy with Schizophrenics*. International Universities Press, New York.

demanded a rare degree of empathy and sensitivity to communicate with the schizophrenic patient and that it required hundreds of hours of therapeutic work extending over months if not years.[135] As we will see, Laing was to spend many hours with his patients at Gartnavel. Methods of therapy discussed in the book included talking to the patient in a kind of dream language, or using the patient's own language. It was advised that the therapist should let the patient set the pace even though this might mean sitting in silence for hours. Play therapy might be used, on the basis that the schizophrenic patient had regressed to an earlier stage of development and the therapist was actually treating several 'children' of different ages.

Schizophrenic patients were said to possess a heightened sensitivity to non-verbal communication and to be able to pick up on unconscious feelings in the therapist.[136] It was observed that patients with schizophrenia had an uncanny ability to tune into the communications of other schizophrenic patients. Laing was to make a similar point in his portrayal of Miss M., the patient whom he encountered in a refractory ward at Gartnavel and whom he was to describe as his 'mentor' because she decoded the behaviour of other patients.[137]

Frieda Fromm-Reichmann

One contributor to *Psychotherapy with Schizophrenics* was Frieda Fromm-Reichmann. Lauded by some commentators, such as her biographer, Gail Hornstein, as a sensitive and dedicated clinician who talked with her patients rather than inflicting shocks and lobotomies on them, she is damned by the medical historian, Edward Shorter[138] for her use of psychoanalysis to treat psychotic patients and, worse, for creating the concept of 'the schizophrenogenic mother', which led to a generation of women being wrongfully blamed for the mental illness of their offspring. These polarized opinions, of course, mirror the responses to Laing's legacy.

One of the first woman doctors in Germany, Fromm-Reichmann trained in psychoanalysis at the Berlin Institute and saw her work as an intrinsic part of her commitment to Judaism.[139] She was friendly with Martin Buber and tried to base her relationships with patients on his principle of *I and Thou*; that is, treating the patient as a person, rather than an object. She was also influenced by the work of Georg Groddeck, whose concept of 'The It' bore strong similarities to Freud's 'Id'. She was attracted by Groddeck's belief that every patient was potentially salvageable. Fromm-Reichmann was also interested in the writings of Sandor Ferenczi, who, much to the consternation

[135] Redlich, F.C. (1952). 'The concept of schizophrenia and its implications for therapy'. In Brody, E.B. and Redlich, F.C. (eds), *Psychotherapy with Schizophrenics*. International Press, New York, pp. 18–38.

[136] Brody, E.B. (1952). 'The treatment of schizophrenia: a review'. In Brody, E.B. and Redlich, F.C. (eds), *Psychotherapy with Schizophrenics*. International Press, New York, pp. 39–88.

[137] Laing, *Wisdom, Madness and Folly*, p. 122.

[138] Shorter, E. (1997). *A History of Psychiatry. From the Era of the Asylum to the Age of Prozac.* John Wiley and Sons, New York.

[139] Hornstein, G.A. (2005). *To Redeem One Person is to Redeem the World. The Life of Frieda Fromm-Reichmann.* Others Press, New York.

of Freud, had tried to psychoanalyse psychotic patients. In contrast to Freud, who advised that the analyst should be neutral and detached in sessions, Ferenczi maintained that the personality of the therapist was an important factor in therapy. In the 1930s, Fromm-Reichmann fled to America to escape the Nazis. She became a prominent figure in American psychoanalysis and worked with Harry Stack Sullivan, whose interpersonal psychiatry she found attractive. She was to be portrayed in the 1964 novel, *I Never Promised You a Rose Garden* by Joanne Greenberg, who gave a fictional account of her three years in Chestnut Lodge private psychiatric hospital, where she had been admitted with a diagnosis of schizophrenia.[140] Fromm-Reichmann appears as her therapist, 'Dr Fried', a tenacious and imaginative psychiatrist who helps her to recover. The American psychiatrist, Theodore Lidz recalled of Fromm-Reichmann:

> She would, for instance, sit in a patient's urine with him to show there was no difference between them. Or a patient would give his faeces as a gift, and she would take them.[141]

Fromm-Reichmann also had a connection with Gartnavel, in that she provided the foreword to *The Philosophy of Insanity*.[142] This was a reissue of a book by a nineteenth century Gartnavel patient, subsequently identified as James Frame,[143] who described his recovery from insanity and his thoughts on maintaining mental well-being. She had come across the little-known book during her research on patient narratives and was taken with Frame's contention that the difference between the sane and the insane was one of degree not of kind. This fitted with a major tenet of psychoanalysis, and, as we have seen, it was one that Laing echoed in his student essay on 'Health and happiness'. Fromm-Reichmann was also taken with Frame's belief that a bout of insanity did not necessarily leave a person permanently impaired. She was so impressed with the book that she arranged for it to be re-published in order that her students and others could read its optimistic testimony.

Frieda Fromm-Reichmann[144] saw schizophrenia as resulting from early interpersonal trauma. She stated that, if there were problems in forming a therapeutic relationship with a patient with schizophrenia, it was due to the doctor's personality difficulties not to the psychopathology of the patient. This was a statement that Laing was to refer to in *The Divided Self* and one with which he heartily agreed.[145] Fromm-Reichmann took for granted that therapists had abandoned 'the myth' that the utterances of schizophrenic

[140] Appignanesi, *Mad, Bad & Sad*, pp. 315–19.

[141] Lidz, T. (1972). 'Schizophrenia, R.D. Laing and the contemporary treatment of psychosis'. In Boyers, R., Orrill, R. (eds), *Laing and Anti-Psychiatry*. London: Penguin, London, pp. 123–56.

[142] Anon (1947).*The Philosophy of Insanity. By a Late Inmate of the Glasgow Royal Asylum for Lunatics at Gartnavel*. With an introduction by Frieda Fromm-Reichmann M.D. The Fireside Press, London and New York.

[143] Smith, I.D. and Swann, A. (1993). 'In praise of the asylum—the writings of two nineteenth century Glasgow patients'. In De Goie, L. and Vijselaar, J. (eds), *Proceedings of the 1st European Congress on the History of Psychiatry and Mental Health Care*. Erasmus Publishing, Rotterdam, pp. 90–5.

[144] Fromm-Reichmann, F. (1952). 'Some aspects of psychoanalytic psychotherapy with schizophrenics'. In *Psychotherapy with Schizophrenics*, pp. 89–111.

[145] Laing, *The Divided Self*, pp. 35–6.

patients were meaningless. She claimed that psychotic patients sometimes used cryptic and ambiguous types of communication to avoid being misunderstood. Laing also thought that psychotic patients adopted a dissembling style of talking, but he claimed that they did this to avoid being *understood*.

Another book Laing cited in *The Divided Self* was *Progress in Psychotherapy*, which was edited by Frieda Fromm-Reichmann and J.L. Moreno.[146] Fromm-Reichmann wrote that the mental patient should be raised from the ranks of an *object* of therapy to a *partner* of the therapist, and she added that this was one of the central doctrines of existential analytic psychotherapy.[147] She also emphasized the importance of the environment, both in terms of the person's family and the wider culture. Fromm-Reichmann identified what she termed the 'schizophrenogenic mother', whose behaviour was held to alienate her child and induce psychosis. The mother was said to be 'rejecting' and to exhibit 'imperviousness to the feelings of others, rigid moralism concerning sex', and a 'fear of intimacy'. The notion that the mother exercised a toxic effect on her child, which somehow brought about schizophrenia, was a strong one amongst psychotherapists during the mid-twentieth century. It was a notion that Laing was to adopt both in his clinical approach and in his writings, at least in the early part of his career. It will be apparent that there was much in Fromm-Reichmann's approach to therapy that anticipated that of Laing. He was undoubtedly influenced by her, and *The Divided Self* contains no less than eleven references to her work.

Silvano Arieti

In *The Divided Self*, Laing cited *Interpretation of Schizophrenia* by Silvano Arieti, a Professor of Clinical Psychiatry in New York.[148] Arieti concentrated on psychological approaches to schizophrenia, which he felt yielded better results than physical methods. He was critical of Kraepelin, observing that in his writing the patient appeared as a collection of symptoms, not as a person, and that he ignored the social context. Arieti outlined a psychotherapy of schizophrenia which was influenced by Fromm-Reichmann. He advocated listening to the patient for lengthy periods of time, even if the psychiatrist did not understand what was being said. He felt that the clinician's attitude to the patient was even more important than the technique employed. The therapist must have an attitude of positive empathy and their personality was also important. Sometimes the therapist's psychological problems could be used to good effect. Arieti referred to a psychiatrist who felt that 'his childhood fantasy of wanting to rescue people was reactivated when he tried to save schizophrenics from the shock treatment which he considered "a great danger"'.[149] Laing's response to this passage is not recorded, but we know from his autobiography that as an Army psychiatrist he claimed he had taken a patient home with him on leave to help him 'escape'

---

[146] Fromm-Reichmann, F. and Moreno, J.L. (1956). *Progress in Psychotherapy*. Grune & Stratton, New York.

[147] Ibid., pp. 7–8.

[148] Arieti, S. (1955). *Interpretation of Schizophrenia*. Robert Brunner, New York.

[149] Ibid., pp. 451–2.

physical treatment. Arieti's position was typical of how many psychotherapeutically inclined clinicians saw themselves at the time. In the face of colleagues who were prescribing medication and ECT, they felt that they were offering a more humane type of therapy. In addition, it was a widely held belief that, while physical treatments might remove symptoms, psychotherapy dealt with the underlying causes.

John Rosen

Laing was interested in the work of the American analyst John Rosen, who advocated 'Direct Analysis' with schizophrenic patients, and he remembers that it had a remarkable effect on the Department of Psychiatry at Glasgow University.[150] For Laing, Rosen was a therapist who used ordinary language with patients and demonstrated that within the psychoanalytic tradition a method of relating to other people was possible. Others were not so convinced by Rosen's methods. Ivor Batchelor, who became Professor of Psychiatry in Dundee, wrote:

> Rosen's (1953) method of 'direct analysis' of the schizophrenic (a sort of psychiatric all-in wrestling!) is liable to be dangerous in most hands. When it works, its effectiveness is probably due more to the therapist's headlong assault on the patient's social isolation than on his verbal ('oral') interpretations of the patient's symptoms.[151]

Professor Batchelor's comments seem to be borne out when one examines John Rosen's *Direct Analysis*.[152] It is worth looking at it in a little detail, because, as we will see when we come to examine Laing's clinical approach at Gartnavel, he tried to engage directly with his patients' delusions, as Rosen recommended. Rosen re-iterated the orthodox psychoanalytic tenet that the mother was the primary cause of mental illness. He was influenced by Freud's theory that dreams contained a 'manifest content' which protected the dreamer from the 'latent content', the real and perhaps unpalatable message of the dream. Rosen maintained that psychosis was like a dream, or rather a 'nightmare', where the manifest content disguised the latent content. It was the task of the analyst to 'unmask' the 'real content' of the psychosis to the sufferer. Rosen held that the principles of direct analysis were firstly that 'the therapist must be a loving, omnipotent protector and provider', and secondly that 'he must be the idealized mother who now has the responsibility of bringing the patient up all over again' to undo the harm caused by 'unconscious malevolent mothering'.[153] Rosen believed that a 'schizophrenic is always one who is reared by a woman who suffers from a perversion of the maternal instinct'.[154] The therapist made direct interpretations of what was considered the manifest content of the patient's presentation. The therapist might become a figure in the patient's psychosis, but it was important to remember that

---

[150] Mullan, *Mad to Normal*, p. 146.

[151] Batchelor, I. (1958). 'Schizophrenia—a psychotherapeutic approach'. In Ferguson Roger, T., Mowbray, R.M. and Roy, J.R. (eds), *Topics in Psychiatry*. Cassell, London, pp. 57–64.

[152] Rosen, J. (1953). *Direct Analysis. Selected Papers*. Grune Stratton, New York.

[153] Rosen, *Direct Analysis*, pp. 8–9.

[154] Ibid., p. 97.

these figures invariably represented 'the mother'. Rosen gave an example of his intervention with one patient:

> ... after insisting that you are the good omnipotent figure, you force the patient to open his mouth by pressing firmly against his cheeks at the tooth line and when his mouth is forced open, you tell him to drink. '*The milk is warm and good. Not the poison that your mother fed you.*'[155]

Rosen outlined other direct techniques, which included physically restraining the patient, jumping in the air and shouting, imitating the patient's movements, and in the case of a young, long-haired man who thought he was Jesus Christ, manhandling him into a barber's shop and cutting his hair. Rosen described his treatment of a 16-year-old girl called Mary and the case illustrates the psychoanalytic culture of seeing everything in terms of the Oedipus complex as well as the vogue of blaming the mother for the child's mental illness. He writes:

> On November 6, as I continued my pressure towards reality, I called Mary's attention to the fact that in the three weeks that she was in the hospital her mother had not come to see her once. The patient fainted dead away. I should say in all fairness, that the mother had been acting on my orders . . .
>
> M[ary]. My mother didn't come.
> D[octor]. *She will come.*
> M. Why didn't she come during the week?
> D. *That's why you became crazy—on account of your mother.*
> M. I don't know. I'm very stupid.
> D. *No, it's not your fault. It's her fault.*
> M. She was probably very busy out there. We live in Brooklyn.
> D. *I don't like this business of your trying to make believe. During the insanity you went on an imaginary journey.*
> M. I went to hospital.
> D. *I don't mean really. I mean in the imagination. You felt you were all over the world.*
> M. I was an Indian queen.
> D. *If you were the queen, you were married to the king. That way, in your imagination, you could be married to your father. The father is always king.*[156]

There is a grim footnote to Rosen's career, as Masson[157] has reported. He subsequently lost his licence because of his abuse of patients, an aspect of his clinical approach which is clearly apparent in his descriptions of his practice. The term 'direct analysis' had been coined by Paul Federn, whose work *Ego Psychology and the Psychoses*[158] was cited in *The Divided Self* and was admired by Laing's colleague, Thomas Freeman.[159] Federn's explanation of schizophrenia rested on Freud's theory of the ego. Federn felt that there was a weakening in the ego boundary in schizophrenia,

[155] Ibid., p. 21.
[156] Ibid., pp. 134–5.
[157] Masson, J. (1992). *Against Therapy*. Fontana, London.
[158] Ferdern, P. (1953). *Ego Psychology and the Psychoses*. Imago, London.
[159] Freeman, T., Cameron, J.L., and McGhie, A. (1958). *Chronic Schizophrenia*. Tavistock, London.

such that the individual had difficulty in differentiating the self from the outside world. The schizophrenic patient confused external objects with their representations in thought. They also confused thought with action. All this, according to Federn, led to a regression to the ego states of early childhood with an inability to use abstract thought. This led to the emergence of unconscious mental material. Federn held that schizophrenia began, not with the loss of external reality as Freud maintained, but with the creation of a false reality, as a consequence of the breakdown of ego boundaries. The therapeutic task was to demonstrate to the patient that their view of reality was false. This was a task that Rosen seems to have taken on with zealous enthusiasm.

Marguerite Sechehaye

Laing was particularly interested in the work of Marguerite Sechehaye and mentioned three of her books in *The Divided Self*. Madame Sechehaye was not a doctor but a private therapist. She advocated what she called a 'symbolic realization' approach to people suffering from schizophrenia. In two books[160] she described her work with an adolescent girl, apparently suffering from schizophrenia, whom she claimed to have 'cured' by means of her 'symbolic realization' therapy. She gave an overview of her views in her third book, *A New Psychotherapy in Schizophrenia*.[161] The book was based on a series of lectures, which she had been invited by Dr Manfred Bleuler to give to the medical staff of the Burgholzi Psychiatric Clinic in Switzerland.

Sechehaye drew on psychoanalytical and existential theory to fashion her own therapy. She saw the roots of psychosis in infantile emotional trauma. She maintained that this led the victim to constantly renewed efforts to relive the original trauma in order to overcome it. Such people also fled to fantasy, both to try and escape from their pain, but also to make reality subservient to desire. Freudian theory, with its notions of symbolization and displacement, helped decode the patient's communications that emanated from their imaginary world. Unfortunately, Sechehaye conceded, it did not necessarily help to alleviate the suffering of the patient.

Sechehaye advocated that 'the therapist instead of insisting on submission to reality (as he customarily does with the neurotic), will strive to offer him a new reality, such a reality as would have been necessary to avoid the initial, infantile trauma'.[162] The therapist was to adjust reality to meet the needs of the patient. As an example, she described her own treatment of Renee, 'the schizophrenic girl', whom she had seen over a ten-year period. Renee had 'symbolically' used apples to represent breasts. Unlike the patient's real mother who was described as underfeeding her, Sechehaye sought to become the 'good mother' who would adequately nourish the child. Thus reality was to be altered to redress the patient's originally impoverished experience. Sechehaye reported that she said to the patient: 'It's time to drink the good milk from mamma's apples; mamma is going to give it herself to her Little Renee.' The

---

[160] Sechahaye, M.A. (1950). *Autobiography of a Schizophrenic Girl* (trans. Rubin-Rabson). Grune & Stratton, New York; Sechehaye, M.A. (1951). *Symbolic Realization—A New Method of Psychotherapy Applied to a Case of Schizophrenia*. International University Press, New York.

[161] Sechehaye, M.A. (1956). *A New Psychotherapy in Schizophrenia*. Grune & Stratton, New York.

[162] Ibid., p. 7.

therapist was to rely on his or her 'intuition' to determine and decode the symbolic language of the patient. Sechehaye gave a further example of using symbolization in therapy: she produced a baby doll, which she then 'breast-fed' to show the patient that she could have happiness outside her mother's body. She also described adopting a patient's baby language to make contact with them. She cited the example of Eugen Bleuler who created a relationship with a schizophrenic patient by imitating his gestures.[163] As we will see, Laing drew on the work of Sechehaye in his treatment of 'Julie' in *The Divided Self*. In a passage which anticipated Laing's existential perspective, Sechehaye had written:

> Speaking existentially, one might say the schizophrenic had fallen into the world of things, becoming an 'object' for others and for himself. There is still too much tendency to keep him in this mould, classifying him as a schizophrenic and admitting more or less consciously his retreat from the world as a thing to be taken for granted.[164]

It should be clear that Laing was by no means alone in advocating a psychotherapeutic approach to patients with schizophrenia. There was an established tradition in America and Europe, and many of its theoretical assumptions about the nature and treatment of schizophrenia were to be echoed by Laing in his subsequent work. In Glasgow, as we will see, Laing's colleagues applied psychoanalytic thinking to their work with patients suffering from schizophrenia, and in London object relations theory was brought to bear on psychosis. There was also the European existential tradition which we will examine in Chapter 4.

---

[163] Ibid., p. 50.
[164] Ibid., p. 25.

Chapter 4

Laing and existential phenomenology

Introduction

In a famous set-piece in *The Divided Self*, Laing contrasts the standard psychiatric interview technique as exemplified by Emil Kraepelin with what he calls the 'existential-phenomenological construction'.[1] He quotes Kraepelin's account of his interview with a patient before a class of students. Kraepelin begins:

> The patient I will show you today has almost to be carried into the room, as he walks in a straddling fashion on the outside of his feet. On coming in, he throws off his slippers, sings a hymn loudly, and then cries twice (in English), 'My father, my real father!'. . . The patient sits with his eyes shut, and pays no attention to his surroundings. He does not look up even when he is spoken to, but he answers in a low voice, and gradually screaming louder and louder. When asked where he is, he says, 'You want to know that too? I tell you who is being measured and is measured and shall be measured . . .' When asked his name, he screams, 'What is your name?'. . .

Kraepelin considers that the patient is 'inaccessible'. He concludes that the patient had not provided a single piece of useful information and that his talk bears no relation to the context of the interview. Laing objects to this construction of the exchange and maintains that the patient is making a meaningful comment on his situation, albeit in a coded manner. Laing suggests that the patient is actually protesting about being paraded before students and that he is parodying the inquisitorial style of Kraepelin with his need for 'measurement'. Laing contends that the patient's behaviour can be seen in two opposing ways: either as 'signs' of disease, or as 'expressive of his existence'.

If we see the patient's behaviour as signs of disease, then he is the passive victim of a pathological process. However, if we see him from Laing's existential perspective, then he is fully autonomous: he possesses agency for his actions. This is a key concept in Laing's existentialist approach. Individuals are held to be fully responsible for their behaviour and for their mode of being in the world. When this existential principle is applied to mental illness, individuals are considered to make choices as to how they behave and talk. While Laing grants the patient full control over their self, the price is that there can be no mitigating factors, such as biology or heredity, to absolve the patient of responsibility.

---

[1] Laing, R.D. (1960). *The Divided Self*. Tavistock, London, pp. 29–31.

From Laing's point of view, Kraepelin makes no attempt to understand the patient as an individual with his own unique perspective on the situation. Where Kraepelin sees only nonsense in the patient's utterances and behaviour, Laing seeks to find meaning. Again, from an existential perspective, it is held that all the actions of human beings are potentially meaningful. Laing's imaginative 'construction' of what is happening in the interview has a certain plausibility. He has also framed the discussion in dramatic terms so that the two approaches are seen to be in direct conflict. The reader is more likely to identify with Laing's seemingly more humane approach than that of Professor Kraepelin, who, at least in Laing's account, seems deaf to what his patient is trying to communicate. But does Laing's version represent the 'truth' of the matter? Is an approach that tries to *combine* the disease model with the existential one more profitable? Anthony Clare has suggested that Kraepelin was attending to the *form* of the patient's disorder, while Laing was focusing on the *content*.[2] Both aspects are necessary, in Clare's view, to properly understand the patient. Whatever one concludes, Laing has certainly alerted us to the fact that the patient has a point of view and that he cannot be dismissed as *merely* a collection of symptoms and signs. The origins of existential psychiatry grew out of the engagement of a number of European clinicians with the philosophical movements known as existentialism and phenomenology.

Existentialism

Writing in 1958, the American psychotherapist, Rollo May, who was later to befriend Laing, wrote about the definition of existentialism:

> The word is bandied about to mean everything—from the posturing defiant dilettantism of some members of the *avante garde* on the left bank in Paris, to a philosophy of despair advocating suicide, to a system of anti-rationalist German thought written in a language so esoteric as to exasperate any empirically minded reader.[3]

Rollo May was pointing to contemporary perceptions of existentialism, and during this period it enjoyed great cultural prominence. It emerged from the Academy and permeated popular culture. As May indicates, the popular perception of existentialism was shaped by the high profile of French writers such as Sartre, Camus, and de Beauvoir, who, as well as writing philosophical treatises, also wrote novels and plays, which brought existential ideas to a wider audience. May refers to Camus's essay, *The Myth of Sisyphus*, which examined whether suicide was the most appropriate reaction to an absurd world. Finally, he alludes to German philosophy and more specifically to Heidegger, whose writings have certainly 'exasperated' many. This passage illustrates that existentialism was both a popular movement and a serious discipline for professional philosophers. Laing was influenced by the popular and the professional streams of existentialism. As a young man growing up in the mid-twentieth century, he was naturally exposed to the cultural currents of his time, but he also read deeply in

---

[2] Clare, A. (1980). *Psychiatry in Dissent. Controversial Issues in Thought and Practice* (second edition). Tavistock, London.

[3] May, R., Angel, E. and Ellenberger, H.F. (eds) (1958). *Existence. A New Dimension in Psychiatry and Psychology*. Basic Books, New York, pp. 10–11.

Continental philosophy and, as we have seen, he met and conversed with the European émigrés Joe Schorstein and Karl Abenheimer who had personal acquaintance with some of the leading existential thinkers such Heidegger, Jaspers, and Buber. Laing's own book, *The Divided Self*, which dealt with the seemingly narrow subject of phenomenology as applied to mental illness, was to appeal to a wide lay public.

The period from the mid-1940s to the 1960s was the popular heyday of existentialism. Although its philosophical origins were considerably earlier, the popular preoccupation with existentialism grew out of the carnage of the Second World War and the horrors of the Holocaust. There was a questioning of authority and a need to find meaning in an apparently meaningless world. Victor Frankl, a psychiatrist who survived the concentration camps, wrote *Man's Search for Meaning*, in which he put forward his thesis that the most pressing question for human beings was finding a purpose to their life. For many people, existential ideas about the importance of the individual, the absurdity of existence, and the striving for 'authenticity' struck a chord. Many creative writers were judged to offer a broadly existential message—Dostoyevsky, Kafka, and Samuel Beckett—all of whom Laing read and cited in his published work. *Les Tempes Modernes* in France and *Horizon* in Britain provided a platform for existential writers and we know that Laing was familiar with both these publications. The English writer Colin Wilson published *The Outsider* in 1956, which was a popular success. It offered an existential account of the predicament of modern man and took in such writers as Dostoyevsky, Kierkegaard, Nietzsche, Sartre, and Hermann Hesse. It was a book that Laing was apparently very disconcerted to see in print, presumably because it covered the same intellectual terrain he was hoping to occupy.

Overview

Existentialism[4] is a philosophy that takes as its starting point the individual's existence. It begins with the 'individual' rather than the 'universal', and does not aim to arrive at general truths. It holds that self and existence can have no fixed definition: each individual is unique and thus escapes categorization. Kierkegaard introduced the idea of 'authenticity' and contended that there was public pressure to conform to society, which led to 'inauthenticity'. Anxiety in the face of death is considered to reveal the banality and absurdity of life, but it can also reveal that the true nature of our lives is based on the choices we make. Warnock emphasizes that existentialists are primarily interested in human freedom.[5] Man has unique power to choose his course of action. What his freedom of choice amounts to and how it is to be described are central concerns of existentialists. Accepting responsibility for the exercise of freedom is the path to authenticity. Existentialists tend to share an opposition to rationalism and empiricism.[6] Unlike most other philosophies, existential ideas are often expressed through novels and plays, as in the work of Sartre, Camus, and de Beauvoir, while Nietzsche and Kierkegaard had a literary rather than a dry technical style of writing.

[4] Earnshaw, S. (2006). *Existentialism*. Continuum, London; Dreyfus, H.L. and Wrathall, M.A. (eds) (2009). *A Companion to Phenomenology and Existentialism*. Wiley-Blackwell, Oxford.
[5] Warnock, M. (1970). *Existentialism*. Oxford University Press, Oxford.
[6] Dreyfus and Wrathall, *A Companion to Phenomenology and Existentialism*, p. 4.

Writers such as Dostoyevsky, Kafka, and Beckett are considered to be part of the existential tradition.

Origins

Dreyfus has traced the origins of existentialism to the division in Western culture between ancient Greek philosophy and the Judeo-Christian tradition.[7] Greek philosophers held that disinterested theory would reveal objective truth—a set of abstract principles that held for all men, at all places, and at all times. In contrast, the Hebrews held that truth was grasped, not by detached contemplation, but by total commitment to God and that this God was theirs alone, so that the truth was unique to them. Whereas for the Greeks, truth was open to all people because they all had rational souls, for the Hebrews, truth was not universal. Dreyfus maintains that this has produced a 'uniquely conflicted culture' and, to make sense of it, Christian thinkers were 'forced to conceptualize the Hebrew Revelation in Greek philosophical terms'. Saint Augustine and then Saint Thomas Aquinas tried and failed to reconcile this conflict, and by the middle of the seventeenth century, Descartes could 'simply assume that the philosopher's God, who was eternal, infinite, fully intelligible, universal, and good, must be the same as the Judeo-Christian God'.

However, in response to Descartes, there emerged the figure of Blaise Pascal, who has been seen as anticipating existentialism. He rejected Cartesian rationalism, and held that the Judeo-Christian God had nothing in common with that of the philosophers. Further, he maintained that human beings had no essence but rather defined themselves through their cultural practice. Whereas Greek philosophy spoke of human beings achieving harmony between the body and soul, Pascal held that these two aspects were incompatible. He regarded human beings as consisting of an essential paradox, a contradiction between mind and body. Dreyfus sees Kierkegaard as the heir of Pascal's thought.

Carroll[8] has also traced the origins of existentialism and offers a slightly different path to that sketched by Dreyfus, but which, nevertheless, can be seen as complementary. Carroll sees existentialism as having its roots in Renaissance humanism, which introduced the idea that man occupied a central place in the universe. It was the individual man, not some divine hierarchy or even a socially constructed hierarchy, that was of primary importance. He traces this tradition of 'individualism' through to the seventeenth century and Calvinism, which held that a man's soul and the quality of it was to be decided, not by his fellow citizens, but by himself, 'the lonely individual in relation to his God'. This led to introspection and an emphasis on the inner man. Carroll sees the tradition continuing through the nineteenth century with the Romantic movement, which saw the individual as being in conflict with a society intent on the repression of the spirit of its citizens. A high value was placed on the individual's own feelings and inner sensations. Carroll places existentialism, with its notion of the

[7] Dreyfus, H.L. (2009). 'The roots of existentialism'. In Dreyfus, H.L. and Wrathall, M.A. (eds), *A Companion to Phenomenology and Existentialism*. Wiley-Blackwell, Oxford, pp. 137–61.

[8] Charlesworth, M. (1976). *The Existentialists and Jean Paul-Sartre*. George Prior, London. From an interview with John Carroll, pp. 10–11.

primacy of the self and of the individual as the centre of human value, firmly in the Romantic tradition. Carroll emphasizes that existentialism has roots in Calvinism and Romanticism, and both these traditions had a marked effect on Laing.

John Macquarrie's existentialism

John Macquarrie, the Scottish religious philosopher who was part of the discussion group that Laing attended in Glasgow in the 1950s, wrote an excellent guide to existentialism.[9] In his book, *Existentialism*, he mentions Laing as someone who brought an existential approach to psychiatry. It is worth considering Macquarrie's book in some detail, as the ideas expressed in it are likely to be similar to those that Laing was exposed to during his time in Glasgow. Macquarrie begins his work by admitting that existentialism is difficult to define and this, he holds, is partly because a certain elusiveness is built into existentialism itself. It is a philosophy that denies that reality can be neatly packaged into concepts or systems, and, for example, Kierkegaard protested against the all-inclusive system of Hegelian philosophy. Our experience and our knowledge are always fragmentary. Existentialism focuses on the notion of particularity: it rejects any notion of universal principles. Decisions are individual and particular, not based on universal laws. There is no core doctrine to which existentialist philosophers subscribe, and Macquarrie prefers to describe existentialism as a 'style of philosophy'. The term 'style' is pertinent, because it has been argued that Laing brought a particular *style* to his interactions with patients.[10] Rather than rigidly following textbook guidelines on psychotherapy, he brought his personal way of being in the world to the clinical encounter.

Macquarrie writes that the basic characteristic of existentialism is that it begins from man rather than nature. It is concerned with man in the whole range of his existing: thinking, feeling, and acting. It denies that there is a 'nature' or 'essence' of man. As Sartre had famously contended, man's existence precedes his essence. Sartre continued:

> We mean that man first of all exists, encounters himself, surges up in the world—and defines himself afterwards. If man, as the existentialist sees him, is not definable, it is to begin with he is nothing. He will not be anything until later, and then he will be what he makes of himself.[11]

Macquarrie identifies several recurring themes in existentialist philosophy. These are freedom, decision, and responsibility. By taking free and responsible decisions 'man becomes authentically himself'.[12] But this freedom of choice generates a deep sense of dread in the face of a universe completely lacking in order and direction.

---

[9] Macquarrie, J. (1973). *Existentialism*. Pelican Books, London.

[10] Heaton, J. (2000). 'On R.D. Laing: style, sorcery, alienation'. *The Psychoanalytic Review*, **87**, 511–26.

[11] Sartre, J.P. (1958). 'Existentialism is a humanism'. In Kaufmann, W. (ed.) (1958), *Existentialism from Dostoyevsky to Sartre*. Meridian Books, Cleveland and New York, p. 290.

[12] Macquarrie, *Existentialism*, p. 4.

In this context Macquarrie refers to the Scottish 'personalist' philosopher John Macmurray and his notion of the 'self as agent', which he states is a central theme in existentialism, in contrast to traditional Western philosophy, which at least since the time of Descartes has concentrated on the 'self as subject'. Macquarrie feels that one limitation of existentialism is that it tends to focus on the individual and ignore the fact that the individual is part of a community. There are exceptions, and he cites Martin Buber, whose work greatly influenced Laing.

Macquarrie also identifies the themes of guilt, alienation, despair, and death in the philosophy of existentialism, themes which are not often treated in traditional philosophy. He claims that the greatest contribution of existentialist philosophy is its focus on the emotional life of human beings. He writes:

> Where philosophy has been dominated by the narrower kinds of rationalism, the changing feelings, moods, or affects that appear in the human mind have been considered irrelevant to philosophy's tasks, or even a hindrance in the way of the ideal of objective knowledge. But the existentialists claim that it is precisely through these that we are involved in our world and can learn some things about it that are inaccessible to a merely objective beholding. From Kierkegaard to Heidegger and Sartre, the existentialists have provided brilliant analyses of such feeling states as anxiety, boredom, nausea, and have sought to show that these are not without their significance for philosophy.[13]

Where existentialists agree

Despite their many differences, all existential thinkers share a common approach: it is the individual human being who is of central importance and it is the 'lived experience' of the individual that is the foundation of all knowledge.[14] This entails the rejection of all abstract, systematic thought in favour of the singular and particular experience of the individual. Lived experience is held to be the only valid criterion of truth. Karl Jaspers maintained: 'I cannot verify anything save through my personal being, and I have no other rule than this personal being itself.'[15] As Earnshaw has observed, existentialist thought in the twentieth century reflected many of the themes of the period: the notion of indeterminism of science; the renunciation of metaphysical system-building; and ideas of subjectivity and freedom. Although it has often been considered to be an atheistic doctrine, existentialism has attracted many religious thinkers, such as Nikolai Berdyaev, Paul Tillich, Rudolf Bultmann, Karl Barth, and Martin Buber, all of whom Laing had read. In contrast, Sartre put the case for unbelief. As he wrote in *Existentialism and Humanism*:

> The existentialist . . . finds it extremely embarrassing that God does not exist, for there disappears with Him all possibility of finding values in an intelligible heaven. There can no longer be any good a priori, since there is no infinite and perfect consciousness to think it. It is nowhere written that 'the good' exists, that one must be honest or must not lie, since we are now upon the plane where there are only men. Dostoyevsky once wrote 'If God did

[13] Ibid., p. 5.

[14] Charlesworth, *The Existentialists and Jean Paul Sartre*, p. 9.

[15] Quoted in Charlesworth, *The Existentialists and Jean Paul Sartre*, p. 9.

not exist, everything would be permitted'; and that for existentialism, is the starting point.[16]

Laing and individual existential thinkers

All existential philosophy is an attempt to say: 'What way can a man live—in his most essential aspects'.[17]

When we approach Laing's understanding of existentialism, we have to remember that he was reading the great exponents through the cultural lens of the mid-twentieth century, and the reputation of and response to some of these thinkers has changed since then. For example, the standard guide to Kierkegaard during this period was Walter Lowrie, who was responsible for the first English translations of the Danish philosopher, and he also wrote a biography that Laing read. Lowrie is considered by later scholars to have missed the ironic aspects of Kierkegaard's work, and, in particular, his use of pseudonyms to provide what he called 'indirect communication'.[18] Whereas in the 1950s Kierkegaard was seen as the archetypal existentialist, later decades have seen him as a post-modernist and as a critical social theorist.[19] The main authority on Nietzsche in the English-speaking world during this period was Walter Kaufmann, who wrote *Nietzsche: Philosopher, Psychologist, Antichrist*, which appeared in 1950.[20] Kaufmann saw 'the will to power' as the core of Nietzsche's thought, but also contended that it was inseparable from his idea of 'sublimation'. Kaufmann portrayed the will to power as an apolitical, existential principle in which the individual sought to overcome the self and achieve self-transcendence. Kaufmann's views were very influential in the English-speaking world in the 1950s, but recent scholarship has challenged his emphasis on the centrality of the will to power in Nietzsche's philosophy.[21] This is not to say that later scholars necessarily provide a superior reading of philosophical texts than their predecessors, but only to stress that each era sees historical figures in the light of their own preoccupations. In the case of Heidegger, the extent of his Nazi sympathies was not so well documented when Laing was writing *The Divided Self* and only really began to be uncovered from the 1960s onwards.[22]

We also have to remember that Laing did not view these philosophers in a dispassionate light. Nor did he approach their work in a dry, scholastic manner. Rather, they

[16] Sartre, *Existentialism and Humanism*, p. 33.

[17] MS Laing K14. R.D. Laing: Notebook and partial diary covering Laing's stay at the military hospitals at Netley and Catterick, January 1952 to June 1953.

[18] Poole, R. (1998). 'The unknown Kierkegaard: twentieth century receptions'. In Hannay, A. and Munro, G. (eds), *The Cambridge Companion to Kierkegaard*. Cambridge University Press, Cambridge, pp. 48–75.

[19] Westphal, M. (1999). 'Kierkegaard'. In Critchley, S. and Schroeder, W.R. (eds), *A Companion to Continental Philosophy*. Blackwell, Oxford, pp. 128–38.

[20] Kaufmann, W. (1974) *Nietzsche. Philosopher, Psychologist, Antichrist* (fourth edition). Princeton University Press, Princeton.

[21] Behler, E. (1996). 'Nietzsche in the twentieth century'. In Magnus, B. and Higgins, K.M. (eds), *The Cambridge Companion to Nietzsche*. Cambridge University Press, Cambridge, pp. 281–322.

[22] Steiner, G. (1992). *Heidegger* (2nd edn.). Fontana Press, London.

were his intellectual heroes, particularly Kierkegaard and Nietzsche, whom he dubbed respectively 'the knight of faith' and 'the Anti-Christ'. These two thinkers represented to Laing the opposing sides of the argument he was having with himself about belief and unbelief. He took a great interest in their life stories, and felt personally affronted if they were attacked by others. For example, he became disenchanted with Jaspers and Jung when he read their criticisms of Nietzsche. He was annoyed with Jock Sutherland, the Tavistock psychoanalyst, when he dismissed the writings of Kierkegaard as showing signs of 'psychopathology'.

When Laing came to write *The Divided Self*, he was not aiming to produce a text-book of philosophy; rather he was trying to understand extreme mental conditions and develop an effective therapy. He used everything he had gleaned from his voracious reading and this included not only existential philosophy, but also psychoanalysis, sociology, and literature. If we look at the number of specific references to individual philosophers in *The Divided Self*, we find that Sartre receives the most attention, but there are also considerations of Kierkegaard, Heidegger, and Buber. Nietzsche, for all the interest Laing maintained in him throughout his life, receives only one mention.

At the beginning of *The Divided Self*, Laing writes:

> . . . this study is not a direct application of any established existential philosophy. There are important points of divergence from the work of Kierkegaard, Jaspers, Heidegger, Sartre, Binswanger, and Tillich, for instance.[23]

He continues:

> To discuss points of convergence and divergence in any detail would have taken me away from the immediate task. Such a discussion belongs to another place. It is to the existential tradition, however, that I acknowledge my intellectual indebtedness.[24]

Laing of course has a point here. He was trying to describe clinical conditions, not explicate the theoretical aspects of existential philosophy. However, some may view his stance as a convenient way to avoid difficult questions, and philosophers, such as Eric Matthews, whose critique will be considered later in the chapter, have found weaknesses in Laing's philosophical approach. This does raise the fundamental question as to what extent philosophical ideas can be applied to clinical practice. This dilemma was not unique to Laing, and, for example, Jaspers faced similar difficulties and attracted criticism concerning his understanding of phenomenology. As Fulford and colleagues have suggested, the problem lies less with individual philosopher–psychiatrists than with the nature of mental illness itself.[25]

Soren Kierkegaard

Of all the existential thinkers, Soren Kierkegaard seems to have been the most important to Laing and the one that he referred to most often in his diaries, interviews, and books.

---

[23] Laing, *The Divided Self*, p. 9.

[24] Ibid., p. 9.

[25] Fulford, K.W.M., Thornton, T. and Graham, G. (2006). *Oxford Textbook of Philosophy and Psychiatry*. Oxford University Press, Oxford.

In *Wisdom, Madness and Folly*, Laing describes, in dramatic, Damascene terms, his life-changing encounter with the work of the Danish philosopher. Laing had discovered the work of Kierkegaard in the Govan Hill Public Library when he was still an adolescent. The first major work he read was *Concluding Unscientific Postscript*, which he described as 'one of the peak experiences of my life'.[26] Laing claimed that he read it through, without sleeping, over a period of 34 hours. We can see why Kierkegaard exercised such a fascination over Laing.

Kierkegaard, like Laing, was an elitist who saw himself as an 'exceptional' individual, above and apart from the dim, conformist masses.[27] He lambasted the establishment, whether it was the Church, university professors, or the local press. He felt the natural sciences were entirely inappropriate to the understanding of human beings and that they had nothing to say about the spiritual dimension of life. From a Protestant background, Kierkegaard was intensely concerned with the concept of sin, as was Laing. Kierkegaard has been described as 'a kind of poet' and he certainly brought a literary sensibility to the practice of philosophy.[28] His use of multiple pseudonyms can be seen, in Laingian terms, as a series of 'false' selves created as a means of hiding the 'true' self. Kierkegaard cut a singular figure in the streets of Copenhagen, where, with stooped back and ill-fitting clothes, he could be seen, in the words of the Scottish poet, Iain Crichton Smith, 'daily taking his cramped stroll'. He was misunderstood and later ridiculed by his peers. Kierkegaard lived in the shadows of madness, melancholia afflicting both himself and his father. Indeed he had written that he wanted to enter a madhouse 'to see if the profundity of madness' would not 'disclose the solution to life's riddle'.[29]

Kierkegaard's writings, then, anticipated many of Laing's preoccupations: the creative individual in conflict with society; the notion of multiple selves; the absolute primacy of the spiritual over the material; and the rejection of 'scientific' explanations of man. Kierkegaard's background had some similarities to that of Laing: both were brought up in the Protestant faith, both suffered from low spirits, and both had melancholy fathers. Kierkegaard's persona was also attractive to Laing, in that he was an outsider, mentally and spiritually troubled, and was unappreciated by the dullards and dimwits of his day. Kierkegaard thus easily attained membership of Laing's 'awkward squad', his select group of creative misfits, who teetered on the edge of madness and who challenged the complacency of the *bourgeoise*.

In his notebooks, Laing considered Kierkegaard's personality. He felt that he was 'a queer fish' and definitely 'schizoid'.[30] He mused on Kierkegaard abandoning his fiancée, Regine, whom Laing, in psychoanalytic terms, equated both with the world

---

[26] Mullan, B. (1995). *Mad to be Normal. Conversations with R.D. Laing*. Free Association Books, London, p. 94.

[27] Garff, J. (2005). *Soren Kierkegaard. A Biography* (trans. Kirmmse, B.H.). Princeton University Press, Princeton.

[28] Mackey, L. (1971). *Kierkegaard. A Kind of Poet*. University of Pennsylvania Press, Philadelphia.

[29] Quoted in Thompson, J. (1974). *Kierkegaard*. Gollancz, London, p. 59.

[30] MS Laing K14.

and with the mother figure.[31] He was intrigued by Kierkegaard's inability to sustain a relationship with a woman, a feature of his personality, Laing noted, that he shared with Nietzsche, who also remained single all his life.[32]

Kierkegaard's work

Existentialism has traditionally been seen as originating in the nineteenth century with Kierkegaard.[33] Much of Kierkegaard's writing was taken up with the analysis of emotional and mental states: 'fear and trembling', 'sickness unto death', 'anxiety', 'despair', and 'melancholy'. Kierkegaard explored themes which subsequently became central to existential thought: freedom, authenticity, angst, alienation, the individual as 'becoming' rather than 'being', the self as 'exception', responsibility for one's self, one's existence, and the necessity to 'choose' one's life.[34]

Kierkegaard kept extensive journals, which Laing read and which seemed to have influenced him when he came to write his *own* personal diaries. In a revealing entry, written when he was 23 years old, Kierkegaard expressed his existential credo:

> What I really lack is to be clear in my mind *what I am to do*, not what I am to know, except in so far as a certain understanding must precede every action. The thing is to understand myself, to see what God really wishes *me* to do: the thing is to find a truth which is true *for me*, to find *the idea for which I can live and die*. What would be the use of discovering so-called objective truth, of working through all the systems of philosophy and of being able, if required, to review them all and show up the inconsistencies within each system;— what good would it do me to be able to develop a theory of the state and combine all the details into a single whole, and so construct a world in which I did not live, but only held up to the view of others;—what good would it do me to be able to explain the meaning of Christianity if it had *no* deeper significance *for me and for my life* . . .[35]

As we have seen, Laing expressed very much the same sentiments in his diaries, and emphasized the individual basis of adopting or choosing a philosophical perspective on life.

Kierkegaard was in conflict with his society, which he saw as adopting a superficial, unengaged Christianity. Instead he wished to emphasize what being an authentic Christian involved. He wrote: 'One does not prepare oneself to become attentive to Christianity by reading books or by world-historical surveys, but by immersing one-self deeper in existence.'[36] Kierkegaard was critical of 'the public' or 'the crowd', because its members had allowed others to decide how they should live.

Kierkegaard envisaged three ways of life. The 'aesthetic' way of life involves following one's inclinations and interests. In the 'ethical' way of life, the individual concentrates on helping others. The 'religious' way of life transcends both the 'aesthetic' and the

---

[31] MS Laing K12. R.D. Laing: Notebook 1951–1952, p. 95.

[32] Mullan, *Mad to be Normal*, p. 253.

[33] Honderich, T. (1995). *The Oxford Companion to Philosophy*. Oxford University Press, Oxford, pp. 257–61 and 442–5; Gardiner, P. (1988). *Kierkegaard*. Oxford University Press, Oxford.

[34] Robinson, D. and Zarate, O. (2003). *Introducing Kierkegaard*. Icon Books, Cambridge.

[35] Dru, A. (ed.) (1938). *The Journals of Soren Kierkegaard*. Oxford University Press, London, p. 15.

[36] Quoted in Charlesworth, *The Existentialists and Jean Paul Sartre*, p. 11.

'ethical' and seeks to go beyond what obligation demands. Later existentialists, such as Camus or Sartre, did not share Kierkegaard's religious outlook, but they were influenced by his emphasis on the individual and lived experience. They also sided with him in his criticism of abstract, speculative thought, which Kierkegaard held served to objectify people and to classify and generalize what was unique and particular. Kierkegaard proclaimed that Hegel's identification of abstract truth with reality was an illusion. 'Truth exists', he wrote, 'only as the individual himself produces it in action'.[37]

In 1843 Kierkegaard published *Either/Or* which portrayed two views of life: the aesthetic or hedonistic, and the ethical. The decision as to which to choose is seen as a personal one and not the result of philosophical deliberation. The following year he published *The Concept of Dread*. In 1846 he published the book that had so impressed Laing, *Concluding Unscientific Postscript to Philosophical Fragments*. The main target was Hegel, whose work was seen as taking the lived experience and subsuming it into a grand 'System'. A scientific approach to matters of personal development was inappropriate. It abstracted a person from their own existence. Kierkegaard remarked: 'One thing always escaped Hegel: what it was to live.'[38]

Against Hegel's concept of 'absolute consciousness', in which all conflicts are reconciled, Kierkegaard insisted on the irreducibility of the individual, of their subjective and personal world. He objected to what he saw as Hegel's theory that in the future the concerns and crises of humanity will be resolved in an all-encompassing objective understanding of the universe. Individuals have to decide ethical questions for themselves: questions which arise out of the unique circumstances of their lived situation. Appeals to an impersonal, objective system are misguided. In opposition to Hegel's 'system' built on rationality, Kierkegaard argued for the essential absurdity of the human condition.

Kierkegaard held that there was a dynamic relation between ethics and subjectivity. A person was 'the ethically existing subject' but this was an aspect of our existence that needed to be developed if we were to realize our full potential as individuals. Life inevitably throws up ethical questions, but we may lack a sufficiently developed sense of ourselves to answer them. How do we attain this? How do we become an individual? Kierkegaard answered that we do this by engaging with life and making choices. This forges our personal identity, enabling us to become an 'existing individual'. However Kierkegaard added a religious dimension to this. An individual also had to make 'a leap of faith' to believe in Christ and lead a committed spiritual life. Without this we experience *angst* or dread and anxiety when we realize that life based on fortune or human love is unsatisfactory. We need to commit ourselves to an 'ethico-religious' life, which involves a relation with God.

In 1849 he published *The Sickness unto Death* which saw despair as a problem with the self or spirit.[39] Kierkegaard begins the book:

> *Despair is a sickness of the spirit, of the self, and so can have three forms: being unconscious in despair of having a self (inauthentic despair), not wanting in despair to be oneself, and wanting in despair to be oneself.*

---

[37] Quoted in May et al., *Existence*, p. 12.

[38] Dru, *The Journals of Soren Kierkegaard*, p. 175.

[39] Kierkegaard, S. (2004). *The Sickness unto Death*. Penguin Books, London.

> The human being is spirit. But what is spirit? Spirit is the self. But what is the self? The self is a relation which relates to itself . . . A human being is a synthesis of the infinite and the finite, of the temporal and the eternal, of freedom and necessity. In short a synthesis.[40]

The commonest form of despair is one in which people fail to recognize the condition in themselves or mistake it for the opposite. In a spiritless society that has taken over the role of the spirit, individuals are unable to attain true selfhood or a genuinely spiritual life. Instead they chase distractions, or they may fall into madness or lead a life of hedonism. The solution to despair is faith: becoming a self as defined by a transcendent power. Laing was to cite *The Sickness unto Death* in *The Divided Self* and to claim that one could not understand schizophrenia without understanding despair.[41]

The Kierkegaardian scholar, Roger Poole thought *The Divided Self* owed much to the Danish philosopher.[42] He maintained that *Concluding Unscientific Postscript*, with its emphasis on taking the concepts of the person, the individual, and subjectivity with absolute seriousness, was a founding text for Laing's first book. *The Concept of Dread*, with its analysis of the various types of despair, was also important, particularly Kierkegaard's concept of 'shut-up-ness', whereby an individual takes refuge in silence to avoid communicating with anyone in the outside world. Laing drew on *The Sickness unto Death*, with its description of the multiplicity of selves, to develop his concept of the 'false-self system' in *The Divided Self*. He commented: 'The false self is one way of not being oneself.'[43]

Poole writes:

> By suggesting that there is a division between an implied 'true self' (an intelligible self, which is threatened by implosion of other identities and is therefore struggling for survival) and a series of 'false selves', which threaten the true self; and by proposing on top of this that there might be division between the embodied and the unembodied self, Laing has absorbed the Kierkegaardian insights while moving out beyond them to apply them in modern psychiatric practice.[44]

In contrast, John Heaton, has been somewhat critical of his former colleague's understanding and use of Kierkegaard's concept of despair. Heaton examined Kierkegaard's seemingly obscure statement 'The self is a relation which relates to itself.' It was a statement Laing puzzled about in his notebooks, exclaiming: 'If only I knew what K. meant by "a relationship which relates itself to itself"'.[45] Laing felt that Kierkegaard's definition neglected the self's relation with other people, a dimension which Heidegger, Sartre, and Buber had all emphasized. Laing pondered the relationship between self

---

[40] Ibid., p. 43.
[41] Laing, *The Divided Self*, p. 39, n. 1.
[42] Poole, R. (2005). 'R.D. Laing's reading of Kierkegaard'. In Raschid, S. (ed.), *R.D. Laing. Contemporary Perspectives*. Free Association Book, London, pp. 99–112.
[43] Laing, *The Divided Self*, p. 100, n. 1.
[44] Poole, *Laing's Reading of Kierkegaard*, p. 105.
[45] MS Laing K12, p. 100.

and others, and tried to reconcile the views of Kierkegaard with other existential thinkers:

> Knowledge of other people, and of oneself, cannot be teased apart. From the beginning your life, everything we do, is in relationship to other people. Withdrawal from other people can only be understood in terms of that fact, that it is a withdrawal from other people. Other people are everywhere: it is impossible to posit oneself to oneself, unless in some relationship with others. Thus the self's relationship to itself must be understood in terms of the person's relationship with other people, and the person's relationship with others cannot fully be comprehended without understanding how the self stands with itself.[46]

However, Heaton links Kierkegaard's statement about the self to the philosophical notion of spirit. He writes:

> Kierkegaard . . . goes on to point out that a relation which relates to itself must either have established itself or been established by something else . . . there are two forms of authentic despair. If the human self were self-established there would be only one form, not wanting to be oneself, wanting to be rid of oneself. But in humans there is the despair of wanting to be oneself.[47]

Heaton maintains that Kierkegaard's notion of the self is different from that of Laing, whom he feels has reified the self. For Kierkegaard, the self is a *relation,* and not an entity which can be anchored in the body. Heaton feels that Laing was attempting the impossible task of reconciling philosophical concepts of the self, as exemplified by Kierkegaard's existential approach, with psychological concepts of the self, as exemplified by Winnicott's object relations theory.

Friedrich Nietzsche

Nietzsche appealed to Laing for many of the same reasons that Kierkegaard was an inspiration to him. Nietzsche was the lone outsider, who rejected academia and religious authority. He was an elitist who looked down on the masses whom he called 'the herd'. But there were other reasons why he appealed to Laing. Nietzsche outlined a psychology, that emphasized man's endless capacity to deceive himself and others, a topic that fascinated Laing. Nietzsche's account of human psychology anticipated and influenced psychodynamic theory. Nietzsche contrasted the deities, Apollo and Dionysus, whom he maintained represented, respectively, the forces of order and excess. In Laingian terms, these two forces could be seen as representing the conflict between psychiatric reason and the exuberance of madness. They also spoke to Laing of the division in his own mind between sober industry and unrestrained creativity. Laing had ambitions to write a book on Nietzsche, which he never realized, but he did go on to adopt the aphoristic style of the German thinker in his later work, such as *Sonnets.* In fact Laing, who always attended to the quality of his own writing,

---

[46] MS Laing K15. Notebook, begun 12 March 1953.
[47] Heaton, J. (1991). 'The divided self: Kierkegaard or Winnicott?' *Journal of the Society for Existential Analysis,* **2**, 30–7.

was attracted to Nietzsche's dazzling literary style.[48] He was later to state that Nietzsche had influenced the writing of *The Divided Self* and also *The Politics of Experience*.[49]

In an interesting essay entitled, 'The hero as outsider', Hollingdale considers the legend of Nietzsche. He was the 'proud and lonely truth-finder', whose mental breakdown was idealized as an 'ascent' to a realm above and beyond the concerns of the mundane world. Hollingdale writes:

> The Nietzsche legend is the modern legend of the isolate and embattled individual: the hero as outsider. He thinks more, knows more, and suffers more than other men do, and is as a consequence elevated above them. Whatever he has of value he has created out of himself, for apart from himself there is only 'the compact majority', which is always wrong. When he speaks he is usually misunderstood, but he can in any case be understood only by isolated and embattled individuals such as himself.[50]

Laing seems to have been very swayed by the 'legend' of Nietzsche, which incorporated many of the elements he prized. The legend also influenced how Laing conducted himself and how he saw himself, and, indeed, how his admirers came to see him: the psychiatrist who looked into the depths of the soul and *felt* too much and *saw* too much.

In his book, *The Discovery of the Unconscious*, Henri Ellenberger allocates Nietzsche a significant role in the birth of dynamic psychiatry and portrays him as a master-psychologist, who anticipated many of the ideas of Freud. Nietzsche was the great advocate of the 'unmasking' psychology. He wished to show that man was a self-deceiving being, who also deceived his fellow-men. Man's actions and utterances were shaped by unconscious lies. For Nietzsche, the unconscious was an arena of confused thoughts, emotions, and instincts, but it was also an arena for the re-enactment of past stages of the individual and of the species. Modern civilization demanded that man renounce the gratification of his instincts, thus making him ill. Civilization induced individuals to turn against themselves. An important part of Nietzsche's conception of psychology was his emphasis, not only on the aggressive, but also the self-destructive instincts. For Nietzsche, sublimation was an important mechanism, whereby evil actions became good ones. Nietzsche also described the mechanism of repression. Ellenberger considers that Nietzsche was the common source of Freud, Adler, and Jung.

Nietzsche's work

Nietzsche believed that the conceptual framework of Western civilization, based on the tenets of Christianity, was fundamentally flawed and was careering towards a profound crisis. This involved what he called 'the death of God', or rather the gradual loss of belief which had begun to pervade Western culture. Nietzsche prophesied that this development would usher in a new era of nihilism, by which he meant that, at the

---

[48] For an account of the literary character of Nietzsche's philosophy, see Nehamas, A. (1985). *Nietzsche. Life as Literature.* Harvard University Press, Cambridge, Massachusetts.

[49] Mullan, *Mad to be Normal*, p. 97.

[50] Hollingdale, R.J. (1996). 'The hero as outsider'. In Magnus, B. and Higgins, K.M. (eds), *The Cambridge Companion to Nietzsche*. Cambridge University Press, Cambridge, pp. 71–89.

same time as individuals were beginning to recognize their freedom, there was a simultaneous breakdown in the order of meaning, brought about by the collapse of belief in a transcendental power that gave life its purpose.[51] Nietzsche sought to understand and to remedy the impending crisis. He was hostile to most traditional explanations of morality, which he held fostered weakness and robbed life of its vitality. Instead, Nietzsche advocated what he called a 'transvaluation of all values', that would lead to the overthrow of the old order of Christian submissiveness and joylessness.

In his first book, *The Birth of Tragedy*, published in 1872, Nietzsche theorized that Greek tragedy was based on the relationship of two principles, represented by Apollo and Dionysus.[52] Apollo was associated with order and beauty, while Dionysus was associated with frenzy and excess. Nietzsche saw these two principles as analogous to dreams and drunkenness. Whereas he associated Apollo with 'measured restraint', 'freedom from wilder emotions', and 'philosophical calm', he saw Dionysus in these terms:

> . . . we shall gain an insight into the nature of the *Dionysian*, which is brought home to us most intimately perhaps by the analogy of *drunkenness*. It is either under the influence of the narcotic draught, which we hear of in the songs of all primitive men and peoples, or with the potent coming of spring penetrating all nature with joy, that these Dionysian emotions awake, which as they intensify, cause the subjective to vanish into complete self-forgetfulness . . . Under the charm of the Dionysian not only is the union between man and man reaffirmed, but Nature which has become estranged, hostile, or subjugated, celebrates once more her reconciliation with her prodigal son, man . . . Now, with the gospel of universal harmony, each one feels himself not only united, reconciled, blended with his neighbour, but as one with him; he feels as if the veil of Maya had been torn aside and were now merely fluttering in tatters before the mysterious Primordial Unity.[53]

Such passages were to exercise a powerful influence on Laing, especially when he came to write *The Politics of Experience and the Bird of Paradise*. Nietzsche maintained that Socrates had led Western culture to favour the Apollonian over the Dionysian perspective on life. Nietzsche criticized contemporary culture's reliance on reason and its optimistic belief in the power of science. This had produced individuals who were blind to the Dionysian aspect of reality, to the overwhelming and dynamic character of life. Laing recalled:

> The distinction which I first came across, between *Dionysian* and *Apollonian*, was a major distinction, in my mind, that separated two types of mind, and two types of my own mind.[54]

In *Human, All Too Human, a Book for Free Spirits*, published in 1878, Nietzsche contended that 'free spirits' were those individuals who had freed themselves from cultural conditioning. The book introduced his aphoristic style for the first time. In *Daybreak: Thoughts on Moral Prejudice*, published in 1881, Nietzsche expanded on his

[51] Critchley, S. and Schroeder, W.R. (eds) (1999). *A Companion to Continental Philosophy*. Blackwell Publishing, Oxford.

[52] Nietzsche, F. (1995). *The Birth of Tragedy* (trans. Clifton Fadiman, P.). Dover Publications, New York.

[53] Ibid., pp. 3–4.

[54] Mullan, *Mad to be Normal*, p. 98.

critique of Christian morality which he had begun in the previous book. He outlined a psychological account of the motivations and consequences of adopting a Christian world view. Nietzsche held that the Christian concepts of sin and the afterlife were psychologically harmful. Such concepts devalued life in favour of another realm, which Nietzsche maintained did not exist. By dwelling on their own sinfulness and by allowing themselves to be tormented by the prospect of eternal damnation, Christians incurred heavy emotional and psychological damage. They were taught to be ashamed of their 'sinful' bodies. Their consciousness of their own guilt led them to try and find others who were more sinful than they were, and, as a consequence, Christians were excessively judgemental of others. Nietzsche held that Christian morality insisted on absolute conformity and that this punished the individual, especially those of a superior cast of mind.

It was in his next book, *The Gay Science* of 1882 that Nietzsche made his famous statement: 'God is dead'. Significantly, it is a madman who announces the death of God. Nietzsche has a madman tell a group of scientific atheists at a marketplace, '*We have killed him*—you and I! We are all his murderers.'[55] In *Thus Spake Zarathustra* (1883–5), Nietzsche described the emergence of exceptional individuals whose independence of thought and creativity raised them above the common run of humanity. These were the 'higher types' who stood out from 'the herd'. Nietzsche distinguished between what he called 'master' and 'slave' moralities, and maintained that the latter had come to dominate the former. This suited 'the herd' but was oppressive to the exceptional or 'higher types'. Charlesworth[56] considers that Nietzsche's philosophy is elitist, in that it is only a select few who are capable of bearing the burden of the death of God and making their own values. The vast majority of people, the 'herd', are incapable of this. Laing, of course, would not have had a problem with Nietzsche's distinction between the gifted few and the uninspired many. More sympathetically, Magnus and Higgins maintain that *Zarathustra* can be read as the chronicle of a character's development towards spiritual maturity.[57] As such, it represents a modern tale of a spiritually sensitive individual, grappling with nihilism and the crisis in values brought about by the collapse of Christianity.

In his 1887 book, *Toward the Genealogy of Morals: A Polemic*, Nietzsche reiterated his critique of Christianity as a 'slave' morality, but he also criticized the modern scientific world view, which he held was also based on faith, in this case, faith in 'truth'. It encouraged individuals to curtail their desires in pursuit of 'truth'. Warnock remarks:[58]

> . . . Nietzsche regarded 'objectivity' as the main enemy of understanding. For him objectivity meant the myth that there are hard, identifiable facts in the world, about which hard definite statements can be made . . . Against this view he argued that all concepts which we employ in describing the world and predicting its behaviour are imposed upon it by ourselves. We have a choice about what view of the world to adopt . . . 'Our very sense perceptions', he says, 'are altogether permeated with valuations . . .'

---

[55] Nietzsche, F. (2006). *The Gay Science*. Dover Publications, New York, p. 90.

[56] Charlesworth, *The Existentialists and Jean Paul Sartre*, p. 20.

[57] Magnus, B. and Higgins, K.M. (eds) (1996). *The Cambridge Companion to Nietzsche*. Cambridge University Press, Cambridge.

[58] Warnock, M. (1970). *Existentialism*. Oxford University Press, Oxford, pp. 13–14.

Laing was to be critical of the so-called 'objective' gaze of clinical psychiatry and its reliance of 'facts' to support its judgements about patients. He maintained that how we approached the clinical encounter and how we behaved during it shaped what we saw. In one of Nietzsche's last books, *The Antichrist* published in 1895, he mounted his most savage attack on religion. While he admired Jesus Christ, he vehemently rejected Christianity. He wrote:

> ... philosophy is ruined by the blood of theologians. The Protestant minister is the grand-father of German philosophy, Protestantism itself is the latter's *peccatum originale*. Definition of Protestantism: the partial paralysis of Christianity—and of reason.[59]

In the book, Nietzsche called for 'the transvaluation of all values', by which he meant values derived from Christianity. He regarded them as life-denying and ener-vating, and called for their overthrow. Laing recalled his exposure to this idea, though he wrongly attributed it to *Thus Spake Zarathustra*:

> ... *the transvaluation of all values*. For someone like me who had this great propensity to be devout, if I could be, just be given the chance to justify, the nerve with which he rejected that, and my horrified terror at what the destiny of thinking in this way might turn out to be if one thought these things as far as he did.[60]

In a notebook written in the 1950s, Laing commented: 'After Nietzsche, after that fine spirit, how could I shelter for comfort from anything in anything?'[61] Laing was interested in the fact that Nietzsche eventually went mad. As a young man, Laing had read *The Madness of Nietzsche* by E.F. Podach.[62] Podach wanted to rescue Nietzsche from somatically-minded psychiatrists who maintained that the philosopher's mental breakdown could be seen as an example of a typical medical 'case' and could be explained purely in terms of brain disease. Instead, Podach contended that Nietzsche should be seen as an individual and that his mental disintegration should be seen in the context of his personal and philosophical struggles. Podach aimed to 'apprehend the meaning and the significance' of Nietzsche's life 'as a whole', and he referred to the Swiss existential psychiatrist, Ludwig Binswanger, who stated that a man's creative work was a part of his 'inner life story'. Podach held that 'certain basic forces' of Nietzsche's 'true self were released by morbid factors', which although of causal sig-nificance could not explain these basic forces.[63] Podach's views, of course, would have struck a chord with Laing, who disliked what William James had called 'medical mate-rialism', the tendency to reduce creativity and spirituality to manifestations of brain dysfunction.

Laing claimed to have examined Nietzsche's asylum case notes and concluded that the philosopher did *not* suffer from general paralysis of the insane, as many had affirmed. Whether he was referring to the actual case notes or to the extensive excerpts

---

[59] Nietzsche, F. (2000). *The Antichrist* (trans. Lodovici, A.M.). Prometheus Books, New York, p. 11.

[60] Mullan, *Mad to be Normal*, p. 98.

[61] MS Laing A622.

[62] Podach, E.F. (1974). *The Madness of Nietzsche* (trans. Voight, F.A.). Gordon Press, New York.

[63] Ibid., pp. 14–15.

of them in the book by Podach is not clear. These excerpts certainly provide the strong suggestion that Nietzsche had *some* form of brain disease as evidenced by the descriptions of his increasingly poor memory, disorientation, and outbursts of unprovoked aggression. More recent commentators have agreed with Laing that Nietzsche did not suffer from general paralysis of the insane, and, instead, have suggested manic-depressive illness with later vascular dementia, or fronto-temporal dementia.[64]

In his notebooks Laing observed:

> Nietzsche's tragedy—He lived out existential 'truth' which he recognised as destructive. He yet said that 'truth' is merely the lie that enables a particular species to survive. But he did/could not believe the 'lie' himself. But to reject the 'lie' is that not to be already—mad?[65]

In this we see Laing exploring the association between sanity and conforming to the mores of society. Does conforming equate with sanity? Do those who rebel possess a more profound insight into the nature of reality, or are they courting madness? Laing later remarked:

> Nietzsche had absolute contempt for '*The Lie*', as he called it. The last words that he wrote . . . were 'I deny the Lie'. Then after that it's silence. 'I deny the Lie'. That sense of demystification, right into our physiological system, our flesh and blood and the way that our body operates, embedded in this mass of confusion that is put over as the truth.[66]

Here Laing was referring to Nietzsche's pronouncements throughout his last book, *Ecce Homo*, in which he inveighed against the 'lie'. Nietzsche maintained that Western civilization was built on a lie, and declared:

> The *lie* of the ideal has hitherto been the curse on reality, through it mankind itself has become mendacious and false down to its deepest instincts—to the point of worshipping the *inverse* values to those which alone could guarantee it prosperity, future, the exalted *right* to a future.[67]

As we have seen, Laing was extremely disconcerted as a child to learn that Santa Claus did not exist, and thereafter appears to have been pre-occupied with the subject of lies and subterfuge for the rest of his life.

Martin Heidegger

For Laing, Martin Heidegger does not seem to have occupied the same role of philosopher-hero as did Kierkegaard and Nietzsche. Heidegger's life did not lend itself to legend, at least what was known about it when Laing was reading his work in the 1950s. Heidegger seemed to have spent most of his career living and lecturing in Freiburg, in Germany,

---

[64] Cybulska, E.M. (2000). 'The madness of Nietzsche: a misdiagnosis of the millennium?' *Hospital Medicine*, **61**, 571–5; Orth, M. and Trimble, M.R. (2006). 'Friedrich Nietzsche's mental illness—general paralysis of the insane vs. frontotemporal dementia'. *Acta Psychiatrica Scandanavica*, **114**, 439–45.

[65] MS Laing K14.

[66] Mullan, *Mad to be Normal*, p. 97.

[67] Nietzsche, F. (1979). *Ecce Homo* (trans. Hollingdale, R.J.). Penguin Books, London, p. 34.

and the only external event of note in his life was his notorious involvement with the Nazis, which was not the behaviour expected of Romantic heroes. However, recent biographies have painted a more complicated picture.[68] From lowly rural origins, Heidegger was repelled by his exposure as a student to city living, which he perceived as superficial and frivolous. Brought up in the Catholic Church, he was critical of modernist culture which he perceived as Godless. As a young academic, Heidegger made a rather gauche impression in the middle-class environment of the university, and, even in the 1920s when he had become successful and was regarded by his peers as the 'secret king of philosophy', he could be mistaken for the janitor by staff who did not know him personally. After he married, Heidegger had a clandestine affair with his student Hannah Arendt, a brilliant Jewish woman who was later to become a major political theorist and cultural commentator, publishing *On the Origins of Totalitarianism* in 1951 and *The Human Condition* in 1958. Later in his career when he was barred from university teaching as a result of his involvement with the Nazis, Heidegger suffered a mental breakdown and spent time in the Haus Baden sanatorium under Dr Victor Gebsattel, a follower of Ludwig Binswanger, whose existential analysis had been inspired by Heidegger's early work. It is possible that Laing knew some of the details of Heidegger's life story from his mentor Joe Schorstein, who had been personally acquainted with the German philosopher.

Born in Messkirch, Germany in 1889, Martin Heidegger originally studied theology at Frieburg, before changing his course to study philosophy, natural sciences, and the humanities. His Habilitation dissertation was on the medieval Scottish theologian Dun Scotus, a figure who greatly influenced one of Laing's favourite poets, Gerard Manley Hopkins, and whom we will consider in more detail in Chapter 6. In his biography of Heidegger, Rudiger Safranski vividly depicts the intellectual culture of early twentieth century Germany. Many of the figures with whom Heidegger was acquainted produced work that was to greatly influence Laing. For example, in 1918 Heidegger became an assistant to the founder of modern phenomenology, Edmund Husserl, and ten years later succeeded him to the chair of philosophy in Frieburg. In 1920 Heidegger began his friendship with Karl Jaspers, and the two men devised plans to found a new journal which would challenge the academic philosophical establishment. In 1923 Heidegger met Rudolf Bultmann and subsequently lectured on his work concerning hermeneutic readings of the New Testament. Laing was to refer to Bultmann in *The Divided Self*.

Heidegger's major work was *Being and Time*, which was published in 1927.[69] The central task of the book was to discover the meaning of being.[70] Laing had written: 'In this work, Heidegger undertook a phenomenological analysis of what he called

[68] Safranski, R. (1999). *Martin Heidegger. Between Good and Evil* (trans. Osers, E.). Harvard University Press, Harvard (originally published in German in 1994); Ott, H. (1994). *Martin Heidegger. A Political Life* (trans. Blunden, A.). Fontana Press, London (originally published in Germany in 1988).

[69] Heidegger, M. (1962). *Being and Time* (trans. Macquarrie, J, and Robinson, E.). Blackwell, Oxford.

[70] Dreyfus, H.L. and Wrathall, M.A. (eds) (2007). *A Companion to Heidegger*. Blackwell Publishing, London.

"Dasein," as a first step towards being able to ask the fundamental ontological question—the question of being, which in his view had been unasked, and had become almost unaskable, since pre-Socratic times.'[71] Heidegger maintained that the core of the human mode of existence was to be found in our always already existing in the world. Heidegger used the term *Dasein* or 'being-there' to describe the mode of being that is distinctive of human life. The fundamental mode of 'being-in-the world' is action. Social relations play an important role in constituting who we are. We understand ourselves and the world through others who also exist in the world: we inhabit a shared world. *Dasein* is not a subject that is isolated in its own sphere; it is in-the-world and inevitably bound up with others.[72] Human existence is essentially being-in-the-world, but it is also being-*with*. For each of us, our own being is an issue, and the way we deal with this issue determines the nature of our existence. Heidegger denied that there was a fixed human essence. Heidegger's philosophy differed from both naturalism, which held that consciousness originated from the world, and idealism which held that the world was constructed from consciousness.[73] Instead he offered a third way: one must begin with our being-in-the-world, because we do not perceive ourselves, and *then* the world, or the other way around: we do not perceive the world *then* ourselves. We experience the two simultaneously. When psychiatrists came to draw on Heidegger's philosophy, it was his concept of being-in-the-world that they found most useful in their work.[74] In *The Divided Self* and *The Self and Others*, Laing utilizes this concept to describe the experiences of people suffering from schizophrenia and schizoid conditions.

Heidegger emphasized the distinction between 'authenticity' and 'inauthenticity', a concept he borrowed from Kierkegaard. In fact Heidegger borrowed heavily from Kierkegaard, though he barely acknowledged this in his published work. Those who did not have a true understanding of the nature of their existence, Heidegger deemed to lead inauthentic lives. They could achieve an authentic existence by experiencing *angst*, which Heidegger defined as an awareness of the precariousness of a life whose goals and values do not arise out of one's own existence. *Angst* enables us to see the existential structure of our life and we then achieve an authentic recognition of our freedom. Heidegger also maintained that if one adopted the opinions and behaviours of everyone else, instead of taking an independent stance, one was guilty of inauthenticity. Heidegger designated other people as the 'they'. The individual had to guard against being submerged by the 'they' who represented averageness and were wary of the exceptional. Being submerged by the 'they' was alluring because one did not have to take responsibility for one's self. One had to avoid this temptation if one wanted to retain authenticity. However, Carman has argued that such an account of Heidegger's

[71] MS Laing A116-7. Laing, R.D. (1960). 'The development of existential analysis'. A paper submitted to RMPA, December 1960, p. 15.

[72] Schatzi, T.R. (2007). 'Early Heidegger on sociality'. In Dreyfus, H.L. and Wrathall, M.A. (eds), *A Companion to Heidegger*. Blackwell Publishing, London, pp. 233–47.

[73] Safranski, *Martin Heidegger*, p. 154.

[74] Burston, D. and Frie, R. (2006). *Psychotherapy as a Human Science*. Duquesne University Press, Pittsburg.

concept of authenticity introduces an evaluative element which judges being inauthentic and conformist as somehow bad, in comparison to the supposedly superior qualities of being authentic and not following the crowd.[75] Heidegger, he maintains, did not mean to use the terms in this way, but he concedes that the inconsistent definitions of them in *Being and Time*, lends some support to depicting authenticity and inauthenticity in such an evaluative way.

Heidegger's work offered a critique of objectivization. Human life cannot be captured by a theoretical, objectivizing approach. Human life must be allowed to *reveal* itself. Lafont has argued that *Being and Time* sought to bring about a paradigm shift that would demonstrate that philosophy was hermeneutics. She writes:

> . . . Heidegger generalizes hermeneutics from a traditional method of interpreting authoritative texts . . . to a way of understanding human beings themselves . . . to be human is not primarily to be a rational animal, but first and foremost to be a self-interpreting animal.[76]

Safranksi's biography of Heidegger is very valuable in placing Heidegger in his cultural and historical setting.[77] He observes that Heidegger's philosophy of angst or anxiety as expressed in *Being and Time* should be seen in the context of the general mood of crisis in the 1920s. For example, Freud's pessimistic account of the evolution of human society, *Civilisation and its Discontents,* appeared in 1929. Safranski maintains that cultural commentators of the time expressed unease and a sense that they were living in a deteriorating and alienated world. *Being and Time* fitted into this general mood of crisis, but it differed from the majority of publications by not offering a solution or therapy. In this Heidegger resembled Freud who also refused to offer 'consolation' to humankind.

However, in later years, Heidegger engaged in discussions with psychiatrists about philosophy and therapy.[78] He had been approached by the Swiss psychiatrist Medard Boss who wanted help in understanding Heidegger's thinking. Heidegger, for his part, was keen for his philosophical ideas to reach beyond the academic community and in particular to people in need of help. Out of this grew the Zollikon Seminars.

Heidegger met with Boss and about fifty to seventy psychiatrists in the latter's home in Zollikon, Switzerland for a series of seminars which took place regularly between 1959 and 1969. One of Heidegger's explicit goals in the seminars was to break the hold of 'the dictatorship of scientific thinking'; he felt that psychoanalysis and scientism were becoming the dominating theoretical influences in Europe.[79] He wanted to

[75] Carman, T. (2007). 'Authenticity'. In Dreyfus, H.L. and Wrathall, M.A. (eds), *A Companion to Heidegger*. Blackwell Publishing, London, pp. 285–96.

[76] Lafont, C. (2007). 'Hermeneutics'. In Dreyfus, H.L. and Wrathall, M.A. (eds), *A Companion to Heidegger*. Blackwell Publishing, London, pp. 265–84.

[77] Safranski, *Martin Heidegger*, pp. 152–3.

[78] Heidegger, M. (2001). *Zollikon Seminars. Protocols, Conversations, Letters* (Boss, M., ed.; trans. Mayr, F. and Askay, R.). Northwestern University Press, Evanston, Illinois.

[79] Askay, R. (2001). 'Heidegger's philosophy and its implications for psychology, Freud, and existential psychoanalysis'. In Heidegger, M. (2001). *Zollikon Seminars. Protocols, Conversations, Letters* (Boss, M. ed.); (trans. Mayr, F. and Askay, R.). Northwestern University Press, Evanston, Illinois, pp. 301–16.

encourage psychiatrists to develop 'meditative thinking' in their approach to medical science, their practice, and themselves.

Laing recalled that he encountered Heidegger through his reading of Sartre's *Being and Nothingness*.[80] The first work that he read by Heidegger was *Being and Time*, which he was to discuss in *The Self and Others*. Laing remembered: 'This made me very thoughtful indeed. There hadn't been a text that I read that seemed to be so contemporarily to the point to me than *Being and Time*.'[81] Laing began reading Heidegger when he was working at the neurosurgical unit at Killearn. At the same time he met Joe Schorstein, who was heavily imbued with the work of Heidegger. The philosophy of Heidegger was also debated in the Schortsein/Abenhiemer discussion group. Laing recalled there were arguments over the correct understanding of Heidegger's *mit sein* in *Sein und Zeit*, and that he had argued over this with John Macquarrie, who was working on the translation at the time.

Jean-Paul Sartre

Of all the major existential thinkers that he studied, Jean-Paul Sartre was the only one that Laing actually met, although he did see both Martin Buber and Paul Tillich when they lectured in Glasgow. Some commentators, such as Douglas Kirsner, have maintained that he was a seminal influence on Laing,[82] and Sartre's work is certainly referred to repeatedly in *The Divided Self* and *The Self and Others*. Laing was later to recall that Sartre's early work was a 'gate-opener' to phenomenological philosophy, and in particular to the writings of Hegel, Husserl, and Heidegger.[83] For Laing, with his ambitions to be a European thinker, Sartre would have been an immensely attractive figure: he was a public and *engagé* intellectual, the co-editor of *Les Temps Modernes*, a philosopher, novelist, and playwright, and he was also a *bon viveur* who held forth to admiring audiences in the cafes and bars of Paris's Left Bank.

Laing had been influenced by one of Sartre's early works, *The Psychology of the Imagination*, in which the French philosopher argued that the defining feature of the imagination lay in the ability of the human mind to imagine *what is not* the case.[84] Sartre went on to contrast the 'imaginary self' with the 'real self'. In *The Divided Self*, Laing drew on this distinction to describe how individuals with schizoid personalities are split between an inner, imaginary world in which they are omnipotent and free, and the outside world where they are subject to a plethora of constraints and influences.[85]

In 1943 Sartre published his most important philosophical work, *Being and Nothingness*, a book which Laing read in the original French when he was in the Army. Laing stated that it was through reading Sartre's *Being and Nothingness* that he was introduced to the philosophy of Hegel and Husserl. *Being and Nothingness* has come

---

[80] Mullan, *Mad to be Normal*, p. 97.

[81] Ibid., p. 110.

[82] Kirsner, D. (1976). *The Schizoid World of Jean-Paul Sartre and R.D. Laing*. University of Queensland Press, Queensland.

[83] Charlesworth, *The Existentialists and Jean Paul Sartre*.

[84] Sartre, J.P. (1972). *The Psychology of the Imagination*. Methuen, London.

[85] Laing, *The Divided Self*, pp. 88–90.

to be regarded as the 'textbook of existentialism'.[86] Sartre argued that men were free to choose how they lived their life; how they responded to moral questions; and how they related to others. A key consideration in the book was the nature of consciousness. Sartre argued that human consciousness belonged to a different ontological category than that of the physical world. He held that conscious beings have 'being-*for*-themselves', whereas the objects of our consciousness have 'being-*in*-themselves'.

Sartre sought to explain the relation between these two entities, indeed, to explain and describe '*being* in the world'. Sartre started from the standpoint, which he had taken from Heidegger, that an individual's consciousness was already engaged with the external world and was modified in countless ways by this engagement. Thus an impersonal or 'scientific' approach to human consciousness was misguided from the start. However, Matthews has detected a contradiction at the core of Sartre's concept of being:

> Sartre thus first (correctly) recognises that an existential, or a concrete, view of our place in the world requires that we see our own being, not as that of a 'for-itself' or consciousness which is distinct in nature from the 'in-itself' of objects, but as the 'union of man with the world' which Heidegger had called 'being-in-the-world'. But then he almost immediately reintroduces the separation of the 'for-itself' from the 'in-itself'. The result is that he sees the self as entirely empty, as something to be invented by our absolutely free choices of action, not only undetermined but even unaffected by what we have been in the past, or by our present physical or other situation . . . This is not a genuinely 'existentialist' view of human beings, but a reversion . . . to a Cartesian view of the essential human being as disembodied and so outside the material world, timeless and placeless and unaffected by the chances of time and place.[87]

For Sartre the most important characteristic of consciousness was that it was separated from the world of things by a gap, or what he called 'Nothingness'. We were first made aware of this gap when we realized that we were able to lie or make false claims about the world of things. If it were not possible to make untruthful assertions about the world, then 'bad faith' would not be possible. Bad faith was a key concept in Sartre's work and was defined as a lie to oneself, by which a person sought to escape the responsible freedom of being-for-itself.[88] Sartre's concept of bad faith grew out of his belief that there was a tension between our freedom and the elements of the situation we find ourselves in that we cannot change. The human response to this tension was often one of bad faith. As Matthews explains it: 'Bad faith refers to the cultivated illusion by which we seek to conceal from ourselves the uncomfortable ambiguity of our position—that we must and can choose, and yet the only real choices we can make are those presented to us by the situation in which we happen to find ourselves.'[89]

[86] Warnock, M. (1969). 'Introduction' to *Being and Nothingness* by Jean-Paul Sartre (trans. Barnes, H.E.). Metheun, London, p. viii.

[87] Matthews, E. (2006). *Merleau-Ponty*. Continuum, London, p. 87.

[88] Sartre, *Being and Nothingness*, p. 629.

[89] Matthews, E. (1996). *Twentieth Century French Philosophy*. Oxford University Press, Oxford, p. 68.

Laing made use of the concept of bad faith in *The Divided Self*, where he defined it as the 'ways of pretending to oneself that one is not "in" what one is doing'.[90]

Matthews has highlighted the problem of what he calls the 'complete individualism' of Sartre's existential philosophy, which has difficulty in explaining the being of other people. Other people have an ambivalent status, in that we do not have access to their consciousness, but they clearly have a 'being-in the-world' which is distinct from inanimate objects. We attribute self-consciousness to them. In this context, Sartre gives the example of the Look, and describes the situation of someone eavesdropping by putting his ear to the keyhole. Initially he is only conscious of himself, but when he hears footsteps he is suddenly aware of himself as seen by another: as an eavesdropper. He becomes a 'being-for-others'. As Sartre observed: 'By the mere appearance of the Other, I am put in the position of passing judgment on myself as on an object, for it is as an object that I appear to the Other.'[91] For Sartre, the relationship between human beings is necessarily one of conflict. Each individual resists being turned into an 'object' by the other, and this is achieved by denying that the other has consciousness and turning *them* into an object. Thus the stage is set for a battle that no one can win. As Matthews observes, Sartre's picture of relations between human beings is 'incredibly bleak', and leaves no room for community.

Laing was interested in Sartre's discussion of 'being-for-others' and it informed his description of schizoid and schizophrenic experience in *The Divided Self*. He wrote:

> . . . if one experiences the other as a free agent, one is open to the possibility of experiencing oneself as an *object* of his experience and thereby of feeling one's own subjectivity drained away. One is threatened with the possibility of becoming no more than a thing in the world of the other, without any life for oneself, without any being for oneself.[92]

In a notebook, Laing commented:

> Sartre's destruction of solipsism is I think absolute: it has general validity. The original, immediate experience of being an "object", which is to know that one is being looked at by another subject—to be turned to stone—Solipsism is absolutely destroyed.[93]

In *The Self and Others*, Laing discussed Sartre's play *Huis Clos* (In Camera) in which three characters find themselves trapped with each other for eternity in Hell, represented by a room with no windows or doors. They are condemned to exist only as the objects in the mind of others: each character is a 'being-for-others', rather than a 'being-for-themselves'. They have lost the freedom to determine their existence, and they find, in the famous words of the play: 'L'enfer, c'est les autres' (Hell is other people). For Laing the play was about 'the agony of the failure to sustain one's identity when the project of one's life is such that it has to be an identity based on collusion'.[94]

In *Being and Nothingness*, Sartre criticized Freud's theory of the unconscious and went on to describe what he called 'existential psychoanalysis'. He felt that Freudian

---

[90] Laing, *The Divided Self*, p. 102.

[91] Sartre, *Being and Nothingness*, p. 222.

[92] Laing, *The Divided Self*, p. 49.

[93] MS Laing K14.

[94] Laing, R.D. (1961). *The Self and Others*. Tavistock, London, p. 102.

theory reduced man to a 'bundle of drives'.[95] He objected to the notion that individual human beings could be understood by 'abstract, universal laws'.[96] Sartre outlined the tenets of existential psychoanalysis:

> The *principle* of this psychoanalysis is that man is a totality and not a collection. Consequently he expresses himself as a whole in even his most insignificant and his most superficial behaviour. In other words there is not a taste, a mannerism, or a human act which is not *revealing*.
>
> The *goal* of psychoanalysis is to *decipher* the empirical behaviour patterns of man . . . Its *point of departure* is *experience*.[97]

Existential psychoanalysis held that there were no 'givens', such as hereditary dispositions or fixed character. Sartre held that *existence* preceded *essence*. Human beings existed before they became strong, weak, charming, or repellent. Man was free to choose his path. He was a dynamic and perpetually searching being. Existential psychoanalysis sought to determine 'the *original* choice'—the original choice a person made in the face of the world about his position in the world. Further, individuals could change their choices—they could adopt a different attitude to an unalterable past. Sartre held that existential psychoanalysis was 'a method destined to bring to light, in a strictly objective form, the subjective choice by which each living person makes himself a person; that is, makes known to himself what he is'.[98]

Existential analysis differed from psychoanalysis in that it rejected the concept of the unconscious. Man was not the passive plaything of unconscious forces. Further, Sartre maintained that, contrary to psychoanalytic teaching, there was not a uniform way of interpreting psychic events which could be applied to all individuals at all times: for example, faeces did not always symbolize gold, nor pincushions, breasts. Existential psychoanalysis was a new development and it had 'not yet found its Freud'.[99]

Laing felt that *Being and Nothingness* was an attempt to cover the same ground as Freud, but that it emphasized the importance of the relationship between subject and object.[100] Douglas Kirsner has described *The Divided Self* as composed of Sartre's existentialism blended with object relations theory, minus the concept of the unconscious.[101] Kirsner maintained that object relations theory was incompatible with Sartre's philosophy, which held that there is no human nature and no essential self, but he allowed that Laing's false-self systems could be understood as examples of Sartrean self-deception.

Sartre's existential perspective differed from that of Albert Camus. Laing was interested in the dispute between Sartre and Camus. The two had famously fallen out when Camus's book *The Rebel* received a hostile review in Sartre's journal *Les Temps Modernes*.

---

[95] Sartre, *Being and Nothingness*, p. 557.

[96] Ibid., p. 559.

[97] Ibid., p. 568.

[98] Ibid., p. 574.

[99] Ibid., p. 575.

[100] Laing, *Mad to be Normal*, p. 366.

[101] Kirsner, D. (2005). 'Laing and philosophy'. In Raschid, S. (ed.) *R.D. Laing. Contemporary Perspectives*. Free Association Books, London, pp. 154–74.

Laing took the side of Sartre because he felt that Camus's book explicitly came out against the very basis of existentialism.[102] It maintained that there was an 'essence' common to all human beings and that this formed the basis for a genuine community. Sartre maintained that there was no essence and that the essential relationship between human beings was one of conflict.

Laing was actually to meet Jean-Paul Sartre in Paris in November 1963.[103] He had sent Sartre his English translation summaries of the latter's *The Critique of Dialectical Reason* but initially received no reply. However, when his partner, Simone de Beauvoir, read and recommended *The Divided Self*, Sartre decided it was worth his while to respond. Laing and his colleague David Cooper went on to provide an English language précis of some of Sartre's writings in their *Reason and Violence. A Decade of Sartre's Philosophy 1950–1960*, which appeared in 1964.[104] In order to seek approval for the book, Laing had gone to meet Sartre in Paris and had taken his ex-girlfriend Marcelle Vincent along with him. Laing describes their meeting at the Palais Royal Hotel:

> We talked solidly, he talked mainly, for about six hours solid. He set the pace. Every 20 minutes or so he would order whatever he was drinking, double dry martinis. I was drinking whisky. The energy he had was quite amazing as was the sustained *engagement* that he had which was quite remarkable . . . I never met anyone comparable to him in that quality of brilliance and absolute concentration.[105]

Laing recalled that Marcelle 'said the thing that most impressed her was that he [Sartre] treated me as a complete equal, and he did'.[106] Characteristically, Laing added: 'In a way I took it for granted that he would'. At the meeting Sartre agreed to write a foreword to *Reason and Violence*.[107] In it, Sartre thanked the authors for their faithful translation of his work and went on to praise their existential approach to psychiatric illness, which mirrored that of his own. The foreword is worth quoting as it gives a clear account of the existential perspective on mental disturbance:

> Like you, I believe that one cannot understand psychological disturbances *from the outside*, on the basis of a positivistic determinism, or reconstruct them with a combination of concepts that remain outside the illness as lived and experienced. I also believe that one cannot study, let alone cure, a neurosis without a fundamental respect for the person of the patient, without a constant effort to grasp the basic situation and relive it, without an attempt to rediscover the response of the person to that situation, and—like you,

---

[102] Laing discusses the dispute in an undated letter to Marcelle Vincent, written during his time at Catterick and quoted in Mullan, *Creative Destroyer*, pp. 86–8.

[103] Clay, *R.D. Laing*, p.107.

[104] Laing, R.D. and Cooper, D. (1964). *Reason and Violence. A Decade of Sartre's Philosophy 1950–1960*. Tavistock, London.

[105] Mullan, *Mad to be Normal*, p. 364.

[106] Ibid., p. 355.

[107] Cohen-Solal, A. (2005). *Jean-Paul Sartre. A Life*. The New Press, New York.

I think—I regard mental illness as the 'way out' that the free organism, in its total unity, invents in order to be able to live through an intolerable situation.[108]

In this passage we see the dismissal of 'positivistic determinist' approaches to psychiatric conditions, the emphasis on seeing the patient as a person, the attempt to see the situation from the sufferer's point of view, and the contention that a person in some way 'chooses' or 'invents' their mental illness in response to untenable life circumstances. This was, of course, how Laing approached psychiatric disorder.

Although he was very influenced by Sartre, Laing was later to deny that his work was a direct descendant from that of the French philosopher. He commented:

. . . Sartre was writing out of the same tradition that I'd been immersed in and swimming in for some while, and I felt that rather than being a lineal descendant, Sartre was a big vessel afloat in the same ocean that I was trying to keep afloat in myself.[109]

Other philosophers

Laing was also interested in other writers loosely associated with existentialism, such as the French religious philosopher, Simone Weil, the French phenomenologist, Maurice Merleau-Ponty, the German theologian, Paul Tillich, the Scottish personalist thinker, John Macmurray, and the Russian religious philosopher, Nikolai Berdyaev. He also read Max Scheler's *On the Phenomenology and the Theory of Sympathy*. Called 'the Catholic Nietzsche', Scheler was a German philosopher who attempted to apply Husserl's phenomenology to ethics, culture, and religion.[110] Laing was very taken by the work of Martin Buber and recorded his responses to it in his notebooks. He also referred to Buber in *The Divided Self* and *The Self and Others*.[111] Buber was an Austrian religious philosopher who played a prominent role in the early Zionist movement. In his classic book, *I and Thou*, Buber maintained that the word 'I' had two very different meanings, depending on its relation to a 'thou' or a 'him/her'.[112] In the sphere of the 'I–Thou', 'I' is expressed with one's whole being and expects reciprocity. In the sphere of 'I–Him/Her', 'I' is expressed with a part of one's being: it is the sphere of utilitarian relationships. As Burston and Frie have commented, whereas Kierkegaard, Nietzsche, and early Heidegger were 'radical individualists' who saw the community and the individual as *necessarily* in conflict, Buber disagreed.[113] He emphasized that human existence was intrinsically relational in character.

---

[108] Sartre, J.P. (1974). 'Foreword' (trans. Sheridan Smith, A.M.) to Laing, R.D., Cooper, D.G. *Reason and Violence. A Decade of Sartre's Philosophy 1950–1960*. Pantheon Books, New York.

[109] Laing in interview with Charlesworth, in Charlesworth, *The Existentialists and Jean Paul Sartre*, p. 49.

[110] Honderich, T. (ed.) (1995). 'Scheler, Max'. In *The Oxford Companion to Philosophy*. Oxford University Press, Oxford, p. 800.

[111] Laing, *The Divided Self*, p. 208; and *The Self and Others*, p 88 and p. 99.

[112] According to Burston and Frie, *Psychotherapy as a Human Science*, p. 163, 'thou' is a mistranslation: it should be simply 'you'.

[113] Ibid., pp. 167–8.

Phenomenology

> Scientific psychology, at its very inception, is an inescapable dilemma. In order to study its subject, man, it has to turn man into a thing, an object. It has to objectify man. Henceforth, all its data are referrable to *man as object* . . . As Science studies 'objects', as if it believed that the only knowledge, in the proper sense, is a knowledge of objects, then the trick is to turn everything into an object and then to study it. The world does contain 'things' and objects. Consciousness consists of its objects. But these are a whole class of bastard pseudo-objects—objects only as concepts, corresponding to no real objects, only imaginary objects, shadows, taken to be substantial—thus Freud's ghostly mental hydraulics of ego, superego, id . . . it is not possible to start off from a neutral position, and thereby imagine that we describe only things as they are.[114]

In *The Divided Self*, Laing described his approach as 'existential-phenomenological'.[115] In the middle decades of the twentieth century, there was debate as to whether existentialist philosophy and phenomenology belonged together or were even compatible with each other.[116] In 1973 Macquarrie[117] had observed that most existentialists were phenomenologists, though there were many phenomenologists who were not existentialists. Phenomenology seemed to offer existentialists the most appropriate methodology to investigate human existence. Dreyfus and Wrathall contend that nowadays the two disciplines have largely merged into a common canon of works and a way of doing philosophy.[118] They are both concerned with providing a description of human existence that is not distorted by scientific pre-suppositions. Such scientific concepts and categories may fail to capture the world as it presents itself to us in experience. Both disciplines hold that what it is to be human cannot be reduced to a set of facts, because human beings transcend such an approach.

The term phenomenology was used by Kant to describe the study of phenomena or appearances, as opposed to the 'things in themselves', which he held lay behind the appearances. Hegel had used the term in 1807 in his *Phenomenology of Mind*, a book which Laing had read and to which he referred in *The Divided Self*. Hegel used the term to describe the many manifestations of mind or spirit as it unfolded itself. More pertinently, 'phenomenology' refers to a method of enquiry elaborated by the German philosopher Edmund Husserl as a development of his teacher Franz Brentano's conception of 'descriptive', as opposed to 'genetic', psychology. Also of influence was Wilhelm Dilthey, who contended that the techniques of the natural sciences were inappropriate in the study of man and that a more descriptive approach should be adopted.[119] Phenomenology begins from an exact, attentive inspection of one's mental processes,

---

[114] MS Laing A233, Love and nihilism, p. 1–4.

[115] One of Laing's guides was Ferm, V. (ed.) (1958). *A History of Philosophical Systems*. Rider, New York.

[116] Dreyfus, H.L. and Wrathall, M.A. (eds) (2009). *A Companion to Phenomenology and Existentialism*. Wiley-Blackwell, Oxford, p. 1.

[117] Macquarrie, *Existentialism*, p. 8.

[118] Dreyfus and Wrathall, *A Companion to Heidegger*, p. 5.

[119] Ibid., p. 2.

in which all assumptions about causes or their wider significance are eliminated. For Husserl, phenomenology was the study of the structures of consciousness. Objects outside consciousness were to be 'bracketed off' in order to allow one to systematically describe the contents of consciousness in terms of their essential structures.[120] Husserl believed that philosophy could be established as a rigorous science that would discover the structures common to all acts.

When Laing first discovered the work of Husserl, he was both encouraged that he recognized his own ideas, but also disconcerted that Husserl had worked out these ideas in such a profound and sophisticated manner. He concluded that he would have to master the phenomenological method for himself if he wished to do serious work.[121] Laing was interested in Husserl's concept of 'bracketing off' one's pre-conceived ideas in order to provide a pure description of the contents of the mind. Laing felt that this served to undermine psychiatrists who contended that they were merely providing 'descriptions of diseases', because what they were claiming were simple 'descriptions' actually contained the assumption that what was being described was a 'disease', i.e. they were value-laden.[122]

Dreyfus and Wrathall have given a lucid account of how Heidegger's work differed from that of Husserl.[123] Heidegger rejected Husserl's focus on consciousness and held that the purpose of phenomenology was not to discover the structures of consciousness, but to make manifest the structure of our everyday being-in-the-world. He was interested in worldly relations rather than mental contents. Sartre, too focused on existential, worldly relationships, but sought to account for these relationships by focusing on consciousness in a manner similar to Husserl. Merleau-Ponty extended Heidegger's work to study our bodily experience of the world in perception.

Karl Jaspers felt that phenomenology had a distinctive role as a methodology in psychopathology.[124] Edmund Husserl's work promised to be a new 'rigorous' science of psychological experience. There has been recent debate[125] as to whether Jasper's phenomenology corresponds with that of Husserl. There were certainly important differences between the two. Jaspers' phenomenology was partly empirical while Husserl's was entirely a priori. Both Husserl and Jaspers agreed, however, that phenomenology was descriptive not explanatory. Like Husserl, who had talked of 'bracketing' off one's own pre-conceptions, Jaspers emphasized the need to avoid pre-supposing any particular theory when describing conscious life. Phenomenology, as Jaspers used the term, was limited to the description and understanding of mental states, as opposed to explanations of the kind provided, for example, by neurophysiology. Bracken and Thomas maintain that Jaspers' phenomenology focused on the description of the subjective world of the patient, rather than attending to the meaning

---

[120] Ibid., p. 2.
[121] MS Laing K14.
[122] Mullan, *Mad to be Normal*, p.112–13.
[123] Dreyfus and Wrathall, *A Companion to Heidegger*, p. 3.
[124] Fulford, *Textbook of Psychiatry*.
[125] Bracken, P. and Thomas, P. (2005). *Postpsychiatry*. Oxford University Press, Oxford.

of their experiences.[126] They suggest that the appeal of Husserl's work to Jaspers was that it seemed to offer a clear and accurate account of human subjectivity: it seemed to pave the way for a scientific underpinning of psychology and psychopathology.[127] Further, they maintain that Jaspers and Husserl, at least in his early years, adopted an essentially Cartesian approach, which saw the mind as separate from the body and the meaningful world around it. As Matthews has shown, Husserl was to adopt a more critical attitude towards Descartes in his later work.[128] In *The Crisis of European Sciences and Transcendental Phenomenology*, Husserl developed the notion of the 'life-world' or *Lebenswelt*, which was the 'pre-given', everyday world that is the basis for all our theoretical constructions in science and philosophy. Husserl contended that Descartes' position was untenable because, in the words of Matthews: 'it is not possible to conceive of oneself as a disembodied soul while adopting the stance of the life-world, since our ordinary experience of ourselves is of a mind–body-unity actively engaged with the world around us'.[129] The Cartesian view of the 'soul' was based on an unquestioned scientific construction of the world. A more radical perspective would lead to an awareness that our ordinary, lived experience takes precedence over the theoretical constructions of science.

During the 1950s and 1960s, when Laing was wrestling with existential ideas, English academic departments were dominated by analytic and linguistic philosophy, and many of their practitioners viewed existentialism with distaste. The lack of sympathy between Continental and English philosophy was described well by Charlesworth:

> Both sides view each other with mutual incomprehension. For English philosophers Existentialism is bad poetry, completely un-rigorous and wilfully obscure. For the Continental philosophers on the other hand English philosophy is philistine, logic-chopping, word-mongering, trivial, with no reference to life as it is really lived.[130]

As recent scholars have observed, the divide between Continental and Analytic philosophy has been exaggerated.[131] Matthews has emphasized that both traditions, each in their own way, attempt to get back from the abstractions of traditional metaphysics to what Husserl called the 'things themselves', i.e. the concrete realities we actually experience.[132] Analytic philosophers examine how we actually use words, while phenomenologists study the immediate experience on which our concepts are based. Laing was very interested in language and was alive to how words could be used in the clinical encounter to avoid seeing the patient as a person.

---

[126] Ibid., p. 121.

[127] Ibid., p. 120.

[128] Matthews, E. (2002). *The Philosophy of Merleau-Ponty*. Acumen, Chesam.

[129] Ibid., p. 29.

[130] Charlesworth, *The Existentialists and Jean Paul Sartre*, p. 28.

[131] Critchley, S. and Schroeder, W.R. (ed.) (1999). *A Companion to Continental Philosophy*. Blackwell Publishing, Oxford.

[132] Matthews, E. (2009) *Broken Brains and Broken Minds*. Talk to Scottish Psychiatry and Philosophy Group, 30th September 2009.

Existential-phenomenological psychiatry

When Laing set out to learn about existential-phenomenological psychiatry,[133] he turned to the European pioneers in the field, such as Minkowski, Binswanger, and Boss, little of whose work was available in English. Undeterred, and, in characteristic fashion, he read their work in the original French and German.

Eugene Minkowski

Laing was particularly interested in the Russian psychiatrist, Eugene Minkowski. He made notes on his writings[134] and referred to him several times in his first book. He even used a quotation from Minkowski at the beginning of *The Divided Self*.[135] The quotation expressed what Laing was trying to do in his own writing: 'I give you a subjective work, however a work which aspires with all its might to objectivity.'[136] Laing considered that Minkowski made 'the first serious attempt in psychiatry to reconstruct the other person's lived experience' and that his 'carefully documented phenomenological investigations' were 'an important contribution to psychiatry'.[137] Born of Jewish parents in 1885 in St Petersburg, and completing his medical studies in Warsaw and Munich, Minkowski went on to work with Eugen Bleuler in Zurich, where he developed an interest in schizophrenia.[138] Migrating to France in 1915, he became one of the founders of the journal *L'Evolution Psychiatrique*, which attempted to combine psychoanalysis with the philosophy of Henri Bergson and the phenomenology of Edmund Husserl. His 1927 book *La Schizophrenie* ushered in a new approach to schizophrenia.[139] Minkowski maintained that schizophrenia represented 'a loss of a vital contact with reality', a concept to which Laing referred in *The Divided Self*.[140]

Laing was also impressed by Minkowski's contention that the psychiatrist drew on their personal response to the patient when deciding on the diagnosis. Laing held that 'Minkowski became one of the first to make explicit the use of inter-personal disjunction

---

[133] See Weigert, E. (1949). 'Existentialism and its relation to psychotherapy'. *Psychiatry*, 21, 399–412; Spiegelberg, H. (1972). *Phenomenology in Psychology and Psychiatry*. Northwestern University Press, Evanston; Halling, S. and Dearborn Nill, J. (1995). 'A brief history of existential-phenomenological psychiatry and psychotherapy'. *Journal of Phenomenological Psychology*, 26(1), 1–45. Van Deurzen, E. and Arnold-Baker, C. (2005). *Existential Perspectives on Human Issues. A Handbook for Therapeutic Practice*. Palgrave Macmillan, London.

[134] MS Laing A258. E Minowski. Le Temps Vecu.

[135] Laing, *The Divided Self*, pp. 90, 150 and 158.

[136] Ibid., p. 12.

[137] Laing, R.D. (1963). Minkowski and Schizophrenia. *Review of Existential Psychology and Psychiatry*, 3, 195–207. Henri Ellenberger credits Minkowski with producing 'the first paper on clinical phenomenology'. Ellenberger, F.H. (1970). *The Discovery of the Unconscious. The History and Evolution of Dynamic Psychiatry*. Basic Books, New York, p. 843.

[138] Shorter, E. (2005). *A Historical Dictionary of Psychiatry*. Oxford University Press, Oxford, pp. 179–80.

[139] Ellenberger, *The Discovery of the Unconscious*, p. 850.

[140] Laing, *The Divided Self*, p. 150.

or conjunction as a diagnostic instrument.'[141] In *The Divided Self*, Laing was to emphasize this point: 'I suggest, therefore, that *sanity or psychosis is tested by the degree of conjunction or disjunction between two persons where the one is sane by common consent* [italics in original].'[142] Whilst he lauded Minkowski as a psychiatric pioneer, Laing felt that were limitations to his work:[143] First, his attempts at a phenomenological technique were compromised by his tendency to bring in his own judgments and attributions. As we will see in the final chapter when we consider *The Divided Self*, Laing was also vulnerable to this charge. Secondly, Laing felt that Minkowski was unable to see that the schizophrenic patient existed within a social system; a point that Laing was to make repeatedly in his own work.

Ludwig Binswanger

Ludwig Binswanger is considered as one of the foremost existential therapists of his era.[144] Laing was to cite eight of his works in *The Divided Self*, but made only brief mention of him in the actual text. Binswanger trained as a psychiatrist under Bleuler and Jung at the Burgholzli Hospital in Zurich, before becoming the director of the Bellevue Sanatorium in Kreuzlingen. In contrast to the situation in Germany and Switzerland where there is continued interest in Binswanger, his work is now little known in American and British psychiatric circles and only a fraction of it has been translated into English.[145] Laing, unlike most of his contemporaries, was prepared to read Binswanger's original German texts. Binswanger was one of the first Swiss followers of Freud, but developed reservations about certain aspects of his work. He argued that Freud's application of a natural sciences model to the study of man was misguided; however he felt that it did serve to expose the crisis in psychiatry that resulted from using such a model. He considered that Freud's work reinforced the Cartesian divide between the 'inner' and 'outer' world. Binswanger turned to the work of Heidegger who opposed such a division and instead put forward the concept of unity: that we are 'beings-in-the-world'. Binswanger developed what he termed *Daseinanalyse* or Existential Analysis.[146] It was a synthesis of psychoanalysis, phenomenology, and existential concepts, especially as outlined by Heidegger, though the latter was to claim that Binswanger had misunderstood his philosophy.[147] Laing had read Binswanger's key 1942 work, *Basic Forms of Knowledge of Human Existence*, in which he examined the different ways that human beings could live their lives with others.[148] This could involve solitude, using others for one's own ends, or genuine love and friendship of another. In his discussion, Binswanger also brought in Buber's concept

[141] Laing, *Minkowski and Schizophrenia*, p. 196.

[142] Laing, *The Divided Self*, p. 37.

[143] Laing, *Minkowski and Schizophrenia*, p. 207.

[144] One of the best English-language accounts of Binswanger is contained in Burston and Frie, *Psychotherapy*, pp. 174–85.

[145] Ibid., p. 175.

[146] May et al., *Existence*, pp. 120–1.

[147] Askay, *Heidegger's Philosophy*.

[148] Laing, *Existential Analysis*, pp. 27–8.

of the I–Thou relation. Binswanger examined what he called the 'world designs' of his patients, or the particular way they construed their existence. His approach to therapy involved a move from the Freudian focus on the intrapsychic to examining the interpersonal dimension. Phenomena that were considered to be manifestations of inner mental processes by classical psychoanalysis were now interpreted as having been formed in the interpersonal field. As Burston and Frie observe, Binswanger's emphasis on the importance of relatedness led to the conclusion that the *loss* of relatedness to others was the core problem in severe mental disorders, a view that Laing fully endorsed.[149]

Laing was particularly interested in Binswanger's most famous case description, that of 'Ellen West'. Laing made extensive notes on the case and drew on them when he came to write about Ellen West in *The Voice of Experience*.[150] Ellen West was the pseudonym of a patient who was admitted in the early part of the twentieth century to Kreuzlingen Sanatorium. Binswanger and Eugen Bleuler made a diagnosis of schizophrenia and considered that she was a hopeless case. Three days after her discharge home, she committed suicide. She was just 33 years old. In his notes of commentary on the case, Laing adopted a critical stance towards Binswanger's clinical skills.[151] Although Binswanger's report initially appeared to be a detailed account of a patient, Laing commented contemptuously that it was not up to the standard of a first year psychiatrist. He felt that Binswanger had no grasp of interpersonal interaction, and that he gave no details as to how Ellen interacted with her family. As Laing eloquently observed: it was like watching a film of a football match in which all but one player had been erased. He complained that Binswanger had buried the young woman under a 'mountain of verbal rubble'.[152] One of the factors that distinguished Laing from existential therapists like Binswanger was that he was able to write about his patients in accessible and engaging prose. When he came to write about Binswanger's famous case in *The Voice of Experience*,[153] Laing stated that it demonstrated psychiatric diagnostics taken to the point of absurdity. Binswanger exhibited all the qualities, such as being distant and objectifying the patient, that he was supposedly trying to avoid.

Medard Boss

Laing was also influenced by the Swiss psychiatrist, Medard Boss,[154] whose work was cited in *The Divided Self*. Boss trained in Zurich and worked with Eugen Bleuler and Carl Jung at the Burgholzli. He met Freud and in 1925 was analysed by him over the course of thirty sessions.[155] However, he became disenchanted with psychoanalysis

[149] Burston and Frie, *Psychotherapy as a Human Science*, p. 182.

[150] Laing, R.D. (1982). *The Voice of Experience*. Allen Lane, London, pp. 53–62.

[151] MS Laing A713. R.D. Laing. A Critique of Binswanger's Ellen West. MS Laing, R.D. Laing. A229/A. The Case of Ellen West.

[152] Ibid., p. 21.

[153] Laing, *The Voice of Experience*, pp. 54–62.

[154] Condrau, G. (1991). 'Obituary of Medard Boss'. *Journal of the Society for Existential Analysis*, **2**, 60–1.

[155] Askay, *Heidegger's Philosophy*. Also Burston and Frie, *Psychotherapy as a Human Science*, p. 185.

and found himself in sympathy with Binswanger's critique of Freud's work.[156] As we have seen, Boss turned to Heidegger to help clarify his thinking about existential analysis. The first book by Boss to reflect his interest in Heidegger was *Meaning and Content in Sexual Perversion*, which was published in 1947. It presented a phenomenological study of sexual deviancy and drew on six case studies. Both this work and Boss's next two books *Analysis of Dreams* and *Psychoanalyse und Daseinanlytik* were cited by Laing in *The Divided Self*. Boss was critical of Freud, and maintained that his theory did not fit with the empirical data he presented. Boss suggested that when Freud was not theorizing, his clinical approach was unwittingly existentialist. Boss's main book, written in close cooperation with Heidegger, was entitled *Existential Foundations of Medicine and Psychology* and was a Heideggerian examination of the use of the natural scientific method in medicine and psychiatry.[157] Boss aimed to humanize medicine by giving it a new existential foundation. Like Heidegger, Boss opposed Descartes' division of human beings into mind and matter. This Cartesian divide had justified the introduction of a natural science methodology to the study of human beings. While this paradigm had brought about great advances in medicine, it had its limitations; in particular it neglected the existential aspects of what it was to be human. Following Heidegger, Boss stated that humans and the world required each other for their very being: human beings existed only insofar as they related to self, others, and the world. In neurotic and psychotic patients, these relations were disturbed and constricted. By means of existential analysis, Boss sought to uncover how modifications in a person's being-in-the-world led to pathological experiences.

Existence

In one of his 1950s notebooks, Laing complained that existential analysis was ignored by British psychiatry.[158] He cited several reasons for this: the key works were in foreign languages, translations were variable, and the terms were unfamiliar to English speakers. However, in 1958 there appeared a book entitled *Existence. A New Dimension in Psychiatry and Psychology* by Rollo May, Ernest Angel, and Henri Ellenberger.[159] This made several key European works, such as Binswanger's case history of Ellen West, available in English for the first time; it was a book that Laing read and cited in *The Divided Self*. In a stirring introductory chapter to *Existence*, Rollo May declared:

> Existentialism, in short, is the endeavour to understand man by cutting below the cleavage between subject and object which has bedevilled Western thought and science since shortly after the Renaissance.[160]

---

[156] Stern, P.J. (1979). 'Introduction to the English Translation'. In Boss, M., *Existential Foundations of Medicine and Psychology* (trans. Conway, S. and Cleaves, A.). Jason Aronson, Northvale, pp. ix–xxii.

[157] Boss, M. (1979). *Existential Foundations of Medicine and Psychology* (trans. Conway, S. and Cleaves, A.). Jason Aronson, Northvale.

[158] MS Laing A258. R.D. Laing: Notes and drafts on Eugene Minkowski, c. 1960. p. 19.

[159] May et al., *Existence*.

[160] Ibid., p. 11.

May identified Kierkegaard and Nietzsche as the pre-eminent thinkers of the nineteenth century and averred that their startling psychological insights had been translated by Freud into the language of the natural sciences. He felt that, despite its undoubted value, psychoanalysis placed too much emphasis on what he called 'technical reason'. It was a matter of 'crucial significance' that existential psychotherapy had been created to counter this tendency. May asserted that existential psychotherapy stood for 'defining neurosis in terms of what destroys man's capacity to fulfil his own being'.[161] Further, it was based on the assumption that it was possible to have a science of man which did not 'fragmentize man and destroy his humanity at the same moment it studies him'.[162] The book stated that there was no standard system or method of existential psychotherapy. Henri Ellenberger wrote about the concept of 'existential neurosis', which he defined as an individual's inability to see meaning in life. Such people were deemed to lead an 'inauthentic' existence.[163] Ellenberger ended with an extract from the writing of Professor Manfred Bleuler, the son of Eugen Bleuler. Manfred Bleuler's observations about therapy with people suffering from schizophrenia contain many of the principles that Laing would later articulate in his work:

> Existential analysis treats the patient's utterances quite seriously and with no more prejudice or bias than in ordinary conversation with normal people . . . Existential analysis refuses absolutely to examine pathological expressions with a view to see whether they are bizarre, absurd, illogical or otherwise defective; rather it attempts to understand the particular world of experience to which these experiences point and how this world is formed and how it falls apart.[164]

In addition to the *Existence* volume, Laing read other English language accounts of existential psychiatry. For example, he was familiar with the work of Gregory Zilboorg, who, as well as writing *A History of Medical Psychology*, was also a practising psychiatrist and drew on existential theory in his clinical work. Laing noted that Zilboorg used existential analysis with psychotic patients and saw therapy as an attempt to recapture a sense of unity with life. Zillboorg had argued against large statistical studies of clinical populations in favour of in-depth longitudinal studies of individual patients, which was, of course, the approach that Laing adopted in *The Divided Self*.[165]

Laing on existential analysis

> The patient before me is another human being: another mortal man. He is terrified of the dark: or, he feels unreal: or, he is impotent: or he has ulcerative colitis. Very well: the question is: to what extent, or in what way is this 'symptom' an outcome of his *existence*: that is, of the basic way he has chosen to live with others and with himself in the face of his own death.[166]

---

[161] Ibid., p. 35

[162] Ibid., p. 36.

[163] Ibid., p. 119.

[164] Quoted in ibid., p. 124.

[165] MS Laing A694. Laing made notes on Zilboorg, 'Affective reintegration in the schizophrenias'. *Archives of Neurology and Psychiatry* (1930).

[166] Laing, *Existential Analysis*, p. 23.

This extract is taken from a paper Laing delivered to the Royal Medical Psychological Association in December 1960, and in it he gives his clearest and most comprehensive account of what he means by existential analysis.[167] The paper reflects Laing's views on the leading practitioners of existential therapy and is worth considering in some detail. He begins by stating that, in the nineteenth century, there were two major trends of philosophical thought: the speculative; and that based on the natural sciences. The existential thinker emerged as a reaction to these two philosophies. To the speculative philosopher he says, and here Laing quotes Feuerbach: 'Do not wish to be a philosopher in contrast to being a man ... do not think as a thinker ... think as a living, real being ...'[168] To the natural scientist, he says, 'Do not wish to be a scientist in contrast to being a man.'

Laing maintains that the existential thinker has a passion for wisdom, rather than for a particular subject, and wisdom is discovered through decision and action. The existential thinker is not irrational, his intention is to articulate the 'existence' that each person 'is'. This is done in opposition to the impersonal abstractions of certain types of philosophy and to technology that turns a man into a thing.

Laing concedes that the language of existential thought can be difficult to understand. He tells his London audience:

> It requires an extra effort of goodwill, on the part of older educated Englishman, because many of the propositions of existential thought are not verifiable by the criteria that some influential English philosophers have recently taught.[169]

Here Laing is alluding to Analytic philosophers and their critique of Continental philosophy. Laing goes on to consider what it is to be a human being:

> It involves taking responsibility for whatever one chooses to do in whatever situation one is in. One is in the world, but one knows that one was not always in the world and that one will not always be in the world. As a result of these considerations a person has to decide how to live one's life.

As Laing states:

> Shall I eat, drink and be merry, shall I glorify God, shall I stick it out as best I can, fortifying myself as best I can against the encroachments of disease and decay, of doubts about the point of it all, shall I seek solace or satisfaction: shall I turn to the scent of roses, or to prayer, or to other people? And so on.[170]

Laing next draws on Heidegger and Sartre: '*My existence* is my way of being-in-the-world.' If another person relates to my existence rather than regarding me as an object, then this is, according to Laing, an *existential* relation. Existential psychiatry aims to relate to the patient's way of being-in-the-world.

Laing outlines what he called the basic phenomenological step:

> Existential psychiatry should not be regarded as an *application* of preconceived philosophical speculations to empirical data. Its use of philosophy is to discard preconceptions,

---

[167] Ibid.

[168] Ibid., p. 3. Laing does not give a reference for this quotation from Feuerbach.

[169] Ibid., p. 4.

[170] Ibid., p. 5.

or at any rate to make one aware of what they are. One of its basic intentions is to discard any preoccupations which prevent one seeing the individual patient in the light of his own existence. That is, it attempts to understand the patient's complaints in his terms, as well as in our terms.[171]

Laing states that in medicine, one's own experience is the crucible of all clinical judgement. In existential psychiatry, the clinician goes one step beyond this, so that he takes into account not only his experience of the patient but the patient's experience of him. Laing claims that existential analysis is more than just our everyday 'common sense' understanding of others. It involves an attempt to understand the patient's being-in-the-world systematically and not simply by flashes of intuition. Furthermore, it is an attempt to do so in a critical way which tests the validity of its propositions. It is a 'scientific discipline'—it is existential science, not natural science.

However, the process is hazardous as Laing explains:

> Obviously, the psychiatrist may not step into the patient's experience, he may simply step through the looking-glass into his own projected fantasy, and if he does, there are few signposts to bring him to his senses. It is hazardous also because he lacks at present the security and assurance of well worked out criteria of variability comparable to those that natural science has been able to develop in its relatively long history.[172]

The core difficulty, then, for the existential analyst is that there is no accepted technique for trying to understand another person's being-in-his-world. It is no use looking to the natural sciences for the answer because they are not directly concerned with human experience and do not possess the appropriate techniques.

Laing goes on to consider the leading theorists in the field. Jaspers, he states, was the first to introduce phenomenology in his book, *General Psychopathology* in 1913. The work of Eugene Minkowski represented a half-way stage between the phenomenology of Jaspers and existential analysis. Minkowski regarded Jaspers' work as mere cataloguing of types of mental phenomena. He wanted to go further and discover whether there was a basic structural alteration in the whole fabric of a patient's experience. Laing points out that, whereas clinical description categorizes *our* experience of the patient, phenomenology of the Jaspers or Minkowski type tries to enter *the patient's* experience of himself and his world. Psychiatric research that ignores these phenomenological considerations, Laing judges, may be fatally flawed.

Laing continues:

> The initial and basic phenomenological step—from cataloguing the patient's behaviour (verbal or otherwise) as observable by the psychiatrist to the construction of the basic structures of the patient's being-in-his-world—has itself important consequences. To single out one: if the basic disturbance is on this experiential level, it means that 'signs' and 'symptoms' in the usual sense may not correlate very closely with the phenomenological level. For instance, 'thinking' which appears to us as pathological may be undisturbed per se.

---

[171] Ibid., p. 6.
[172] Ibid., p. 7.

> If language is a mirror of the world, language may be a distorted mirror, but alternatively, it may be an adequate mirror reflecting the image of a distorted world . . .[173]

Laing notes that the term, 'phenomenology' is used differently by different authors, such as Husserl, Jaspers, Minkowski, Heidegger, Binswanger, Boss, and Sartre. He observes that existential analysis began with Martin Heidegger's *Being and Time* which was published in 1927. Laing claims that existential analysis does not investigate states of consciousness or inner worlds; rather it is concerned with 'the entire structure of a person's being-in-the world'. Laing emphasizes that existential analysis does not represent a particular 'school' within psychiatry, but is, instead:

> . . . the synthetic unity of what were previously the antithetical approaches of the psycho-logical and the physical. This antithesis is now abolished. A human *being* is intrinsically somatic . . . One can see the person as a body, but also, one must see the body as a person. Physical person and personal body are two ways of seeing the same being.[174]

And here Laing makes reference to *Structure of Behaviour* by the French existential phenomenologist, Maurice Merleau-Ponty, who had likewise argued against mind–body dualism. Laing's statement is interesting because, in his writings, he tended to neglect the somatic aspects of human beings. Eric Matthews has argued that this neglect undermined Laing's account of psychosis in *The Divided Self* and that a con-sideration of the work of Merleau-Ponty made good this 'philosophical deficit'.[175] Matthews argues that, whereas Merleau-Ponty emphasized the unity of mind and body, Laing presented 'the neuro-physiological and the human-meaning account of behaviour as mutually exclusive'. By doing so, he ruled out the possibility that brain disturbance could have any relevance to the understanding of psychosis. In contrast, Merleau-Ponty stressed that we should see all human behaviour as part of human 'embodied' subjectivity, and thus he left open the possibility that neurobiological factors might well play a role in mental illness, at least in certain individuals. In *The Divided Self*, Laing was to use Merleau-Ponty's observation that what we see on someone's face is a *smile*, something with human meaning, not the 'contraction of the circumoral muscles'.[176] As Matthews points out, in the spirit of Merleau-Ponty, a smile is not only something with human meaning, but also a set of contractions of facial muscles. If our muscles were not functioning, we could not smile.

Laing ends his paper by stating that existential psychiatry can claim to be 'the present heir to the central tradition in psychiatry'. He contends that it has influenced many therapists who would not designate themselves as primarily existentialists. He cites: Silvano Arieti, Henry Ey, Marguerite Sechehaye, Eugene Minkowski, Frieda Fromm-Reichmann, Gregory Zilboorg, Karen Horney, Edith Weigert, Henricus Rumke, and Manfred Bleuler. The work of majority of these therapists is discussed in *The Divided Self*.

---

[173] Ibid., p. 14.

[174] Ibid., p. 33.

[175] Matthews, E. (2005). 'Laing and Merleau-Ponty'. In Raschid, S. (ed.) *R.D. Laing. Contemporary Perspectives*. Free Association Books, London, pp. 79–98.

[176] Laing, *The Divided Self*, p. 32.

The Divided Self

We will conclude this chapter by examining Laing's account of existential-phenomeno-logical psychiatry in *The Divided Self*, but because it was originally intended as a companion volume to *The Self and Others*, it is important to consider the latter book as well. In a manuscript entitled 'Reflections upon an Ontology of Human Relations' and written in 1954, Laing wrote:

> In the absence of an adequate ontology of human relatedness and thus of man as a whole, the empirical science of the interpersonal process is chaotic. Brilliant observations and insights there are but the whole framework in which they are incorporated requires to be restructured and brought into line with an adequate idea of man ... such an ontology does not seem to me to exist ... [177]

It was Laing's ambition to provide just such an ontology; *The Divided Self* and *The Self and Others* represented his attempts to do so. The first two chapters of *The Divided Self* are entitled respectively 'The existential-phenomenological foundations for a science of persons' and 'The existential-phenomenological foundations for the understanding of psychosis'. In them Laing outlines his approach:

> Existential phenomenology attempts to characterize the nature of a person's experience of the world and himself. It is not so much an attempt to describe particular objects of his experience as to set all particular experiences within the context of his whole being-in-the world. [178]

Laing felt that the very language that psychiatrists used to talk about their patients immediately put them at a remove from them. The technical language of psychiatry or psychoanalysis split human beings up verbally. Such language placed man in isolation from his being-in-the world and from his relation to others. It also broke him up into bits, such as 'ego', 'superego', and 'id'. The enterprise to elicit 'psychopathology' was flawed from the outset, because it made certain assumptions which served to objectify the person. As a result, Laing argued, it was unable to understand that a person's disorganization represented a failure to achieve a 'specifically personal form of unity'. Psychopathological terms were abstract and ignored the interpersonal. Here Laing brought in Buber's concept of *I* and *Thou*, and stressed that it was crucial to recognize that each individual was at the same time separate from others, but also related to them. For Laing this was 'an essential aspect of our *being*'. He insisted that the proper focus of study was man's *existence*, his *being-in-the world*. Laing writes:

> Unless we begin with the concept of man in relation to other men and from the beginning 'in' a world, and unless we realize that man does not exist without 'his' world nor can his world exist without him, we are condemned to start our study of schizoid and schizophrenic people with a verbal and conceptual splitting that matches the split up of the totality of the schizoid being-in-the- world. [179]

---

[177] MS Laing A113. R.D. Laing, Reflections upon the ontology of human relations, p. 10.
[178] Laing, *The Divided Self*, p. 15.
[179] Ibid., p. 18.

Laing contended that 'man's being' could be seen from different points of view, for example, as a person or as an organism. How one saw man determined how one related to him and how one conceived of him. Laing maintained it was a common illusion that we somehow increased our understanding of a person if we could translate a personal understanding of him into the impersonal terminology used to describe organisms, and here he referred to John Macmurray's concept of the 'biological analogy'. In a celebrated passage Laing writes:

> ... people who experience themselves as automata, as robots, as bits of machinery, or even as animals ... are rightly regarded as crazy. Yet why do we not regard a theory that seeks to transmute persons into automata or animals as equally crazy?[180]

For Laing, existential phenomenology attempted to reconstruct the patient's way of being himself in his world, and this might be done by focusing on the patient's way of being with the therapist. When the patient came to see the psychiatrist, he brought to the meeting 'his existence, his whole being-in-his-world'. One had to grasp how the patient experienced *his* world. The therapist must try to transpose himself into another strange and alien world. Only by doing so could he hope to understand the patient's 'existential position'. In subsequent chapters, Laing attempted to describe the existential positions of the patients he had encountered in his clinical work.

The Self and Others

In this book, Laing devoted two chapters to existential theory: 'Existential position as a function of the action of the self' and 'Existential position as a function of the action of others'. Laing examined the concept of alienation and how individuals could find themselves in 'false' positions, either because they had put themselves there or because they had been put there by others. He contrasted being in a false existential position with 'authenticity', which he defined as being 'true to oneself, to be what one is, to be "genuine"'.[181] He added: 'The intensification of the being of the agent through self-disclosure, through making patent the latent self, is the meaning of Nietzsche's "will to power"'.[182] For Laing, an action was genuine if one was oneself in it.

Laing drew on Heidegger's essay 'On the essence of truth'[183] to discuss how we judged if a person was behaving in an authentic manner, or whether they were lying, pretending, or equivocating. Heidegger had contrasted the natural scientific concept of truth with that of pre-Socratic thinking. Whereas the former held that truth was a correspondence between what goes on in the mind and what goes on in the world, the latter maintained that truth was 'literally that which is without secrecy, what discloses itself without being veiled'.[184] Laing maintained that this latter notion of truth helped us to read another's 'existential position': whether they were being true to themselves

---

[180] Laing, *The Divided Self*, p. 22.
[181] Laing, *The Self and Others*, p. 118.
[182] Ibid., p. 118.
[183] Heidegger, M. (1949). 'On the essence of truth'. In Heidegger, M., *Existence and Being* (Introduction, Brock, W.). Gateway, South Bend, Indiana, pp. 292–324.
[184] Laing, *The Self and Others*, p. 120.

or whether they were concealing something. Laing borrowed Heidegger's analogy about the difference between a genuine and counterfeit coin. Heidegger had maintained that both coins were 'real', but we were able to tell them apart. Laing argued 'when a man's words, gestures, acts, disclose his real intentions, one can say that they are genuine and not counterfeit'.

In the same passage, Laing continued his discussion of authenticity. He maintained that problems began if a person was unable to 'reveal' his 'true' self, or when others were unable to see it when he did. Such a person might turn in 'partial despair' to 'false-modes of self-disclosure'. By doing so, they would be in 'bad-faith'. Perhaps the person did not realize that they were in this false position. If this was the case, Laing judged that they would be in 'that supreme despair which is, as Kierkegaard says, not to know he is in despair'.[185] They would have lost the starting point to launch themselves into life. Here Laing is giving a fairly straightforward existential account of inauthenticity, which brings in not only Heidegger but also Sartre's concept of bad faith and Kierkegaard's concept of despair. Guy Thompson has maintained that the question of the relationship between truth and authenticity was central to Laing's existential approach.[186] Thompson expressed surprise that both Binswanger and Boss ignored this crucial existential concept, which he held was of the utmost relevance to clinical practice. He credited Laing with being the only existential analyst who recognized its importance.

We have seen that Laing was widely read in the literature of existentialism, phenomenology, and existential psychiatry. From this he attempted to construct his own version of existential psychiatry. Such an endeavour was a bold and difficult undertaking. At times, Laing succeeded brilliantly in providing a clear and accessible account of existential philosophy and demonstrating its application to the clinical situation. However, as we will see when we come to consider the individual patients who appeared in Laing's published work, his employment of existential theory did not always unlock the mystery of madness and, at times, it obscured it.

---

[185] Laing, *The Self and Others*, p. 122.
[186] Thompson Guy, M. (1998). 'Existential psychoanalysis: a Laingian perspective'. In Marcus, P. and Rosenberg, A. (eds), *Psychoanalytic Versions of the Human Condition*. New York University Press, New York, pp. 332–61.

Chapter 5

Laing and religion

A burning concern of Laing throughout his life was religion. It informed his approach to medicine, to psychiatry, and to his very existence. But the subject was also agonizing, and fraught with uncertainty. Did God exist? Or was the concept a relic from an earlier, more credulous age? Should he side with Kierkegaard, 'the knight of faith', or with Nietzsche, 'the Anti-Christ'? If there was a God, how should one conduct oneself? Should we strive to love our neighbour, or was this an impossible demand? Were we born in sin and in need of salvation from a higher authority? Was God, not man, the ultimate judge of our actions? How could human suffering be reconciled with a benevolent deity? Was the world everything that was the case, or was there another dimension, a transcendental realm? Laing was tormented by these questions, and read countless books, not only by Christians, but also by Jewish, Buddhist, and Hindu authors. He was fascinated by mysticism and studied the work of Dionysius the Aeropagite, Meister Eckhart, and Jacob Boehme.

Peter Sedgwick[1] has portrayed the later Laing as merely dabbling in Eastern religion and mysticism. In Sedgwick's version, Laing is seen as a dilettante, who was so swayed by the West's voguish and superficial flirtation with the East that he deserted radical politics and retreated to Ceylon in order to meditate and disengage from the problems of society. In fact, Laing was fully immersed in matters of faith from an early age, and he was also very knowledgeable about world religions. Politics was always of secondary interest to him, and in a choice—to use 1960s parlance—between seeking change from within or from without, Laing always chose the former. Laing was of course living through a period when there were many secular currents, in science, philosophy, and psychoanalysis, that sought to undermine if not refute the claims of religion. Laing was well aware of the arguments against a spiritual conception of the world, and, in his notebooks and debates with others he tried to resolve the conflict. As a psychiatrist, the most pressing question for Laing was the nature of madness: was it the result of impaired bodily mechanism, or was it a sign of a troubled soul? As he was fond of pointing out, the definition of the word 'psychiatry' was 'healing of the soul'. Time and again, in his accounts of his patients, Laing sought a spiritual interpretation of their plight.

There were several facets in Laing's response to religion. First, he considered the place of faith in the evolution of human history: were spiritual factors still valid, or were they irrelevant in the modern world? Second, was religion a force for repression in society? In Laing's eyes, this was the version of Christianity held by those in authority, the parents, the teachers, and the Sunday school preachers, who sought to crush

---

[1] Sedgwick, P. (1982). *Psychopolitics*. Pluto Press, London.

the human spirit. Laing's hero, William Blake, had portrayed this type of Christianity as a Chapel with '"Thou shalt not writ" over the door'. Laing also had strong ideas as to what constituted the religious life, and, like Kierkegaard, he was critical of those who did not live it: those who went to Church on Sunday but failed to follow the Christian code for the rest of the week. For Laing, to be religious was to believe in a higher reality and to seriously engage with it. In later years, Laing was to claim that modern man had lost touch with the divine, and he was to contend that some forms of madness could be seen as an attempt to re-connect with the holy. Rather than being evidence of pathology, the experience of psychosis might be a spiritual journey, which offered the traveller a glimpse of the transcendental. Another aspect of Laing's response to religion was his interest in biblical exegesis: he grappled with religious texts in an attempt to decode their meaning and to reconcile their apparent contradictions. Laing was brought up in the Presbyterian tradition, which placed great importance upon education and life-long learning. Continuous study of the scriptures and the understanding and interpretation of church doctrine were embodied in several statements of faith and catechisms. The discipline of hermeneutics, of course, grew out of the interpretation of religious texts, and Laing was to use the skills he developed in studying the Bible and other Christian texts to examine the 'sacred' texts of psychiatry, by Kraepelin, Bleuler, Jaspers, and Binswanger.

Religious upbringing

Laing provided many descriptions of his religious upbringing in his notebooks, essays, and books. In a revealing article, entitled 'Religious sensibility', he wrote:

> I grew up, theologically speaking, in the 19th century: lower middle class Lowland Presbyterian, corroded by 19th-century materialism, scientific rationalism and humanism. The books were Darwin's *Origins of Species*; Haeckel's *Riddle of the Universe*. The figures were Voltaire, John Stuart Mill, Thomas Huxley. I listened to and later partook in long arguments on the existence or non-existence of God, the veracity of the Old and New Testament narratives.[2]

It is worth pausing to consider the intellectual figures Laing mentions in this passage in a little detail. The *Origins of the Species*, which appeared in 1859, outlined Darwin's theory that evolution developed randomly by the process of natural selection. Darwin's theory seemed to imply that God was not necessary for the emergence of life, that there was no Grand Designer in the background with a master plan. The nineteenth century witnessed fierce arguments as to whether religion or science offered the more accurate explanation of the world. Ernst Haeckel was a German biologist and philosopher who promoted and popularized the work of Darwin. In *The Riddle of the Universe at the Close of the Nineteenth Century*, which was published in English in 1901, Haeckel used the *Origin* as ammunition to attack entrenched religious dogma.[3] He claimed that the immense progress of science, particularly evolutionary theory, in the preceding hundred years had widened the conflict between science and revelation. He complained

---

[2] Laing, R.D. (1970). 'Religious sensibility'. *The Listener*, 23 April, p. 536.
[3] Haeckel, E. (1992). *The Riddle of the Universe* (trans. McCabe, J.). Prometheus Books, New York.

that 'metaphysical' philosophy had not taken account of the great advances in science which had been made during the nineteenth century. Voltaire, one of the leading French Enlightenment thinkers, attacked organized religion and promoted Deism, a philosophy which held that God was revealed by reason and by observation of the natural world, rather than by miracles, consulting sacred texts, or by a 'leap of faith'. John Stuart Mill, the English utilitarian philosopher, wrote *Three Essays on Religion*, in which he argued that it was impossible that the universe was governed by an omnipotent and loving God, but he conceded that it was likely that a less powerful benign force was at work in the world.[4] The biologist, Thomas Huxley was known as 'Darwin's bulldog' because of his combative advocacy of the theory of evolution; he played a significant role in the debates about science and religion that took place in late Victorian England. As Laing observes, his early attitudes to religion were heavily influenced by nineteenth century thought. When he came to study medicine and psychiatry, the great arguments between science and religion informed his response to human suffering. Was biology or faith the answer?

Laing's parents were nominally Church of Scotland. Presbyterian theology typically emphasized the sovereignty of God, maintained a high regard for the authority of the Bible, and stressed the necessity of grace through faith in Christ. Laing started reading the Bible at home when he was 10 or 11 years old and he remembered being rather self-conscious because an excessive interest in religious matters was frowned upon. He recalled arguing with his father each evening about the existence of God. Laing's father claimed he was not an atheist and his favourite saying was 'God is man's idealised expression of his own image'. In retrospect, Laing felt this was 'pure atheism'.[5] A Christian ethos prevailed at the various educational institutions Laing attended, and, in addition, he also went to a Presbyterian Sunday School.[6] As a pupil he struggled with Christian teaching. In a series of unpublished sketches,[7] Laing described his adolescent concerns about religion. He felt that initially he was imbued with an orthodox Christian faith but that doubts set in when he was 14. At this time he was exposed to a teacher at Hutchesons' Grammar School who was a 'free thinker' and who questioned the existence of God. Laing recalled: 'this was the first time I ever heard such sacrilegious and blasphemous views expressed'.[8] He went home and told his parents about these provocative opinions, but found that his mother would not commit herself on the matter and that his father had a 'disturbing' attitude to religion.

Rebellion against religious authority

As Laing observed of the change in his beliefs during his adolescence: 'The rot had set in.' His naive childhood faith was eroded and he became tormented by doubts. He still believed in his heart, but not with his mind. Laing re-read the Bible, but also Voltaire.

---

[4] Mautner, T. (2005). *A Dictionary of Philosophy*. Penguin, London.

[5] MS Laing K1, Elements for an Autobiography by R.D. Laing, p. 53.

[6] MS Laing A343. R.D. Laing: Diary, p. A.

[7] MS Laing A522. Autobiographical Sketches, November 1977.

[8] Ibid.

He looked at one of the few books his father had read, *Religion without Revelation* by Julian Huxley,[9] the biologist and grandson of Thomas Huxley. Julian Huxley held that there was no separate supernatural realm: all phenomena were part of one natural process of evolution. A change of emphasis from a God-centred to an evolutionary-centred religion was required. Huxley believed that man had to discard the notion of a personal, 'imaginary God' and accept full responsibility for himself. Man was the 'highest entity' and the Kingdom of Heaven lay within each individual.

The adolescent Laing expressed his concerns to the head of the Scripture Union, a Christian organization which ran summer camps for school children:

> I was riddled with doubts after a year. At the next camp when I was a 'trust leader' and ostensibly 'saved', I confided some of my doubts to 'The Boss'. Who moved the stone? . . . In Luke there are two men, In Matthew there are two angels. And what about Voltaire? And what about the suffering of children, and the war and the Jews, and is all this the Infinite Mercy of God? I was a fool, said 'The Boss'. But these are natural questions. Where are they answered?[10]

Here we see Laing analysing the different books in the Bible and being troubled by their apparent contradictions. He had read a book entitled, *Who Moved the Stone?*, which highlighted biblical inconsistencies.[11] We also see Laing trying to equate Christian teaching with contemporary events. Laing was a school boy during the Second World War, and, like a great many, he tried to make sense of the carnage and the concentration camps. He tried to understand how such terrible things were possible in a world presided over by a supposedly compassionate God. He found his superior to be of no help. When Laing recounted this episode in *Wisdom, Madness and Folly*, he made himself sound more sophisticated. He claimed that he told 'The Boss': 'The trouble with Jesus . . . was they got Him too young. He didn't have time to mature like the Buddha'.[12]

Laing continued to seek out people to discuss religion. When he was 18 he had debates with an ex-Jesuit novitiate about Saint Thomas' *Summa Theoligica*. But they did not get very far because, as Laing admits:

> I kept casting up contemporary French 'existentialism' which I was now imbued with (1945–6). Neither of us could find the connection between Aquinas's version of the ontological proof and 'The Plague'.[13]

In Camus's novel *The Plague*, the priest Father Paneloux gives a sermon in which he tries to justify the ways of God in the face of the plague, which is decimating the population of the town.[14] Paneloux argues that the townspeople deserve the plague because of their sinful and ungodly ways. God has not willed the plague; he has withdrawn his

[9] Huxley, J. (1940). *Religion without Revelation*. Watts & Co., London.

[10] MS Laing K1, p. 47.

[11] Mullan, *Mad to be Normal*, p. 230.

[12] Laing, *Wisdom, Madness and Folly*, p. 68.

[13] MS Laing K1, p. 54.

[14] Camus, A. (1960). *The Plague* (trans. Gilbert, S.). Penguin Books, London (originally published in French, 1947). pp. 81–3.

compassionate protection. The priest proclaims: 'No earthly power, nay, not even . . . the vaunted might of human science can avail you to avert that hand once it is stretched towards you'. Here Paneloux is asserting that medicine is powerless, and the novel dramatizes the conflict between scientific and religious approaches to human afflic-tion. It was a conflict that tormented the young Laing. Paneloux concludes his sermon by saying that people should still rejoice because God is leading them onto a righteous path: 'this same pestilence which is slaying you works for your good and points your path'. The will of God was 'unfailingly transforming evil into good'. Laing had a great deal of difficulty in accepting Paneloux's argument, which attempted to justify the existence of God in the face of the terrible suffering of humanity. Laing mentions Saint Thomas of Aquinas, the great mediaeval Catholic theologian, who sought in his *Summa Theologica* to provide proofs of the existence of God. Aquinas held that God's existence could be demonstrated by reason on the basis of logical argument. Laing pondered whether this was a better response to the question of the existence of God, than that of Panleoux. Was an argument based on logic, rather than the declaration that God was essentially good, more compelling? Again, Laing was not so sure. As he observed, the arguments of Paneloux and Aquinas were not compatible, which made Laing even more confused.

During this period Laing read extensively, and adopted various positions along the spectrum from belief to unbelief. It is probably impossible as well as unnecessary to construct an exact chronology of the various positions Laing held as he battled with these questions. Suffice it to say that he examined a great many viewpoints and experi-mented with numerous ideas. At one stage, he argued himself out of Christianity and concluded that he was an atheist. He commented:

> For years thereafter, whatever I might have been, I could no longer call myself a Christian, I became a dialectical historical materialist. Along with Nietzsche, George Bernard Shaw, HG Wells, I did not believe in God. The Christian story was a MYTH. It was no more true than other myths.[15]

Nietzsche, or the 'Anti-Christ' as he styled him, was an important figure to Laing, as we have seen. Nietzsche had written:

> In Christianity, neither morality nor religion comes in touch at all with reality. Nothing but imaginary *causes* (God, the soul, the ego, spirit, free will—or even non free-will); noth-ing but imaginary *effects* (sin, salvation, grace, punishment, forgiveness of sins). Imaginary beings are supposed to have intercourse (God, spirits, souls) . . . an imaginary *psychology* (nothing but misunderstandings of self, interpretations of pleasant or unpleasant general feelings . . .[16]

George Bernard Shaw was a socialist, as was H.G. Wells, and both believed that society could be improved by the application of human reason. Wells had studied biology under Thomas Huxley in London and evolutionary theory informed his work. He portrayed man as a biological entity with a precarious hold on his environment.

---

[15] MS Laing A522.

[16] Nietzsche, *The Antichrist*, pp. 17–18.

In the light of his reading of atheistic texts, Laing's outlook changed. He swore. He took a less inhibited attitude towards sex. He records:

> I did not feel guilty or ashamed even of smoking or of consuming alcohol. I sang bawdy songs. I went to pubs. I got drunk. I sang hymn tunes to blasphemous words. I was defiant. I regretted having wasted so much of my time for so many years on superstition. I looked forward to the adventure of free thought. I felt I had a lot of ground to catch up on.[17]

Laing went through a period of resenting his Christian upbringing, of being exposed to what seemed a fairy tale. He resented, too, that it had impinged so heavily on his consciousness. He wrote: 'I wanted to exorcise myself of all that. So I took to psychoanalysis (for this, and other reasons)'.[18] And yet the revolt against God was not straightforward. Laing continued to be beset by doubts. He asked of religion:

> Is it all mumbo-jumbo? Is it destroyed by a psychoanalytic interpretation? Is it all totally economically culturally anthropologically conditioned? Is it a way of speaking about the profoundest Truth?[19]

Despite his atheistic leanings during this period, Laing was still drawn to religious thinkers, such as Pascal and Kierkegaard. He read Paul Tillich and decided he was a Christian atheist. Laing also went through a stage of what, in retrospect, he called, 'Neoplatonic Christianity',[20] a creed which held that there must be a higher form of reality than what we perceive with our senses. Laing was attracted by the idea that the love of knowledge could be a way of liberating the soul. The notion of a secret doctrine revealed only to initiates would also have appealed to Laing's elitist tendencies. In the final sketch of his account of his adolescent protest against God, Laing commented wryly on himself as a religious rebel:

> It was not lost on my pals and me, that we were a comic lot, and a bore often to ourselves as well as to others, that we should be unable to get out of our systems conflicts we regarded as invalid.
>
> We no longer seemed to believe in God, but we still reacted against him.
>
> Here we were, standing God knows where, on planet earth, hurling drunken howls of protest, abuse and defiance at absolutely infinitely nothing. We must be really daft.[21]

Enlightenment secularism and Marcelle Vincent

In another memoir, Laing contrasted his religious outlook with that of some of his atheistic contemporaries:

> I remember vividly how startled I was to meet for the first time, when I was 18, people of my age who had never ever opened a Bible. The stories of Jacob, Joseph, Samuel and all the others were further from them than I am now from the mythological systems of the pre-Aztec inhabitants of Mexico.

---

[17] MS Laing A 522.

[18] Ibid.

[19] Ibid.

[20] Mezan, P. (1972). After Freud and Jung, Now Comes R.D. Laing. *Esquire,* **77,** 92–7; 160–78.

[21] MS Laing A 522.

> For the first time in my life, I could see myself being looked at rather as I imagine a native may see himself looked at by an attentive, respectful anthropologist. I could see myself regarded with incredulity by an 18 year-old French girl, a student from the Sorbonne, as some idealistic barbarian still occupied by issues of religious belief, disbelief or doubt, still living before the Enlightenment, exhibiting in frayed but still recognisable form the primitive thought forms of the savage mind.[22]

The 18-year-old French girl was his then-girlfriend, Marcelle Vincent and, in another account of her, Laing wrote:

> She was the first entirely secular person I had ever met . . . Marcelle had never even read the Bible. She had only the foggiest ideas of Abraham, Isaac, Joseph and the rest. She regarded the Bible as simply Judaic mythology of which she had never made a special study. She was amazed that I had ever seriously believed any of it . . . She could not understand how I seemed in odd moments still to take some of that sort of thing, in some sense seriously.[23]

These two extracts demonstrate that Laing was well aware of how religion was viewed by non-believers. He eloquently described how those who saw themselves as heirs to the Enlightenment perceived those who still believed in God. Laing found himself pulled by both camps: the European intellectual tradition he so admired and to which he craved to belong; and the older, supposedly 'primitive' world of the Bible, which had peopled his youthful imagination.

Christian social activism and George MacLeod

As a young man, Laing was interested in the Iona Community and came to know its leader, the charismatic Reverend George MacLeod, as well as his lieutenant, Penrys Jones.[24] In his book, *We Shall Rebuild*, MacLeod outlined the credo of the Iona Community.[25] He pointed to the failure of the Church to adapt to the modern world, and declared that there was a need to find forms of faith and life which held together the individual and the community. Social problems were to be tackled by the active involvement of concerned Christians. MacLeod's organization held meetings in Community House in Clyde Street in the centre of Glasgow, and they attracted large crowds, eager to hear politicians, intellectuals, and religious leaders clash over their prescriptions for alleviating the ills of society. In fact the 1950s were to represent the last era when the Church of Scotland engaged in a prominent manner in political and cultural debate in Scotland.[26] Laing attended these meetings, where Communists did theoretical battle with Christians.[27] MacLeod, preacher, visionary, and social crusader, influenced Laing, and gave him advice, for example, as to whether serving in the British Army was compatible with Christianity (it was).[28] MacLeod is described by his

---

[22] Laing, 'Religious Sensibility'. *The Listener*, 23 April, p. 536.

[23] MS Laing A522.

[24] Mullan, *Mad to be Normal*, p. 88.

[25] MacLeod, G. (1944). *We Shall Rebuild*. Iona Community, Glasgow.

[26] Ferguson, R. (1990). *George MacLeod. Founder of the Iona Community*. Collins, London, p. 239.

[27] Mullan, *Mad to be Normal*, p. 88.

[28] Mullan, *Mad to be Normal*, p. 126.

biographer as a 'cosmic mystic' and an 'evangelical', who believed in his heart that he had been set free by Jesus Christ.[29] Further:

> He believed in conversion, in the direct intervention of God, and in miracles. He also believed in a cosmic God who was in and through all things, yet had revealed his nature as being that of suffering Love for individual persons.[30]

MacLeod tried to bring together the theological, the philosophical, and the practical. This endeavour was very much in keeping, not only with what is claimed to be characteristic of the Scottish temperament, but also with Laing's own outlook.

Doubts as an adult

Laing's diaries as a young man reveal that he continued to be tormented by issues of belief and unbelief:

> No matter what you do you cannot escape: you may forget, or seek to forget, for a minute, or an hour, a day or a week but the outcome is the same. This wretched unblessed misery will continue until you acknowledge this 'thing' or person which is called 'God'.[31]

His later notebooks are full of references to God. He asked himself:

> Was the fact that he believed in God, evidence of His existence? The great assumption/ necessity that what one believes (in) must exist! I believe in God. Therefore God must exist . . . God must exist—our being demands it. But why should our demands be met?[32]

Laing was deeply troubled by the thought that his belief in God might be entirely misguided, built upon a lie, an illusion, or a fantasy. But, then, how would he know? Laing returned, as he often did, to his experience of finding out as a child that Santa Claus did not exist:

> The fear of being deceived, by others, by myself, by God, this dread of getting it all wrong, of discovering later that I had been up a gum tree, had squandered my life in trivial illusions, I had been so cowardly or so stupid to take to be true has never left me. It remains one of my major attachments. After my shame at my own gullibility and naivety over Santa Claus at the age of five (I can remember remembering that incident all through my childhood and later, and that sense of fear & shame), and my torture over whether I believed in God: whether I did, whether I should, whether I should and didn't. I tried hard to become an atheist because I thought I should not believe in Him if he was the delusion, the 'paradigm' delusion of the human race & I proved to be graced with belief.
> O Lord if thou exist, if it be Thy Will please let me know you do . . .[33]

Laing continued to be unsettled by the problem of reconciling the existence of God with the miseries of the world. As a doctor, how could he account for the suffering he

---

[29] Ferguson, *George MacLeod*, p. 193.

[30] Ibid., p. 206.

[31] MS Laing K14. R.D. Laing: Notebook and partial diary covering Laing's stay at the military hospitals at Netley and Catterick, January 1952 to June 1953.

[32] Ibid.

[33] MS Laing A535. On the *Lancet* paper, 'Patient and Nurse', Laing has written these comments, possibly when drunk.

saw, alongside his belief in a beneficent God? How could he reconcile the apparently arbitrary nature of death and destruction with idea of a just God? He wrote:

> I used to condemn God—on the grounds of his injustice. Or rather, I felt that the unhelped, and apparently unblamed suffering & wretchedness of the world reduced to an absurdity any idea or conviction that this was the creation of a just God. Despite all the sophistry about the origin of evil, there seemed no help for the conclusion that ultimately God was responsible for all this: and a just God could not be responsible for such injustice; and God, if he exists must be just—ergo, God could not exist.[34]

Laing went through intense periods of doubt and uncertainty as he struggled with these questions, but he could find no easy answer. In one notebook entry he described his spiritual journey:

> I used to have a simple faith. Then I had a simple un-faith. Now I can hardly distinguish between hope and despair. Now one has to resort to tortuous expressions, ambiguous phrases, paradoxes of dialectic, which, to an outsider, must appear mere verbal gymnastics . . . We are born into a world in which the battle has been lost. We are exiles from Paradise.[35]

Laing's ex-lover Marcelle Vincent observed that he would often consider how little he attended to the voice of God and how little trust he had in Him.[36] Laing remembers George MacLeod having contempt for those who thought that all that was involved in being a Christian was going to Church on a Sunday. Rather, he maintained, one had to fully live the life of a Christian.[37] Laing felt this way too. His great hero Kierkegaard also inveighed against the hypocrisies of Christendom. However there were problems in unreservedly following the precepts of Christianity. As we have seen in Chapter 2 when we considered his paper on Paul Tillich, Laing was perplexed by the Christian command, 'Thou shalt love thy neighbour as thyself .' In a notebook he wrote:

> How can I love my neighbour as myself. I don't love myself though God I'm conceited enough—and who is my neighbour. Is he the North K[orean]. on whom I, yes I—and you—are dropping Napalm bombs. I certainly don't hate the N. Korean—I suppose I don't really recognise his existence—but if I did would I love him?[38]

He wondered about the nature of this love. Was it a feeling, an instinct, or a drive? He did not *feel* any love for his neighbour; he did not *act* as though he felt any love. Surely society could not function if everyone followed this precept? Perhaps such an experience existed on a transcendental plane, but what was that?[39] In *The Divided Self*, Laing again referred to the concept of loving one's neighbours, but at this point he concluded that one could not love them, if one did not first know and understand them.[40]

---

[34] MS Laing K16. R.D. Laing: Notebook, July 1953 to August 1962.

[35] MS Laing K15. Notebook, begun 12 March 1953.

[36] Mullan, B. (1997). *R.D. Laing. Creative Destroyer*. Cassell, London, pp. 65–88.

[37] Mullan, *Mad to be Normal*, p. 211.

[38] MS Laing K14.

[39] Ibid.

[40] Laing, *The Divided Self*, p. 35.

Calvinism and the question of sin

Laing set out his own spiritual outlook in a passage that demonstrated how seriously he took religion:

> Spiritual life for me begins with the conviction of sin. I am not justified. And I cannot myself make myself just. As an organism and as a social being, the only absolute I face is my own death. But I do not experience my biological death, but nevertheless I am convicted absolutely of my sin and this is phenomenologically not just another relative term—another condition of my finitude—a product of environment, of brain rhythms—of a malignant growth of my superego.[41]

The notion of sin preoccupied Laing. He defined it as follows: 'Sin is the unasked, uninvolved experience of the wrath of God of absolute condemnation.'[42] The concept of sin was an important aspect of Presbyterianism, as was the notion of being 'justified'. Those who were of the 'Elect' had been chosen by God and their salvation was guaranteed: they were 'justified'. The centuries' old doctrine of Calvinism emphasized the notion of predestination, which stated that an individual could not know or influence their salvation.[43] Significantly, James Hogg's satirical critique of Calvinism was called, *The Private Memoirs and Confessions of a Justified Sinner*. George MacLeod believed that gospel truth was obscured by rigid theological systems like Calvinism. He observed: '. . . Calvinism was probably a justified protest against the raging romantic subjectivism of the Celtic character . . . Calvinism is now a concept of mind, but its virus still lurks in the marrow of our psyche'.[44]

MacLeod saw Calvinism as a necessary reaction against the 'raging, romantic' Celt, and Laing could be said to embody these two cultural stereotypes: within him battled the ghosts of John Knox and Ossian. However, the social historian Calum Brown cautions against stereotyping the Scots and points out that Calvinism has been used to explain features as diverse as 'their glumness, their aggression to succeed in worldly affairs, and their Rabelaisian qualities'.[45] Despite Brown's understandable caution, in the case of Laing, it could be argued that he embodied all these diverse features: he was melancholic, highly ambitious, and prone to excess.

In this context it is useful to look at a book that Laing knew well and from which he took the term 'the divided self'.[46] This is *The Varieties of Religious Experience* by the American psychologist, William James, who greatly influenced Laing. In the chapter entitled 'The Divided Self', James wrote about the struggle to unify the self amidst a sea of conflicting impulses, temptations, and feelings. In a passage which could be describing Laing, he writes:

> Unhappiness is apt to characterise the period of order-making and struggle. If the individual be of tender conscience and religiously quickened, the unhappiness will take the

---

[41] MS Laing K16.

[42] Ibid.

[43] The poet Alasdair MacLean has remarked that the dour Scots aimed to 'eliminate Purgatory by getting it over while we're still alive'. Quoted in Brown, C. (1987). *The Social History of Religion in Scotland Since 1730*. Methuen, London, p. 8.

[44] Ferguson, *George MacLeod*, p. 193.

[45] Brown, *The Social History of Religion*, p. 9.

[46] Mezan, *After Freud*, p. 171.

form of moral remorse and compunction, of feeling inwardly vile and wrong, and of standing in false relations to the author of one's being and appointer of one's spiritual fate. This is the religious melancholy and 'conviction of sin' that have played so large a part in the history of Protestant Christianity. The man's interior is a battle-ground for what he feels to be two deadly hostile selves, the one actual, the other ideal.[47]

Sutcliffe has attempted to understand Laing's religious and personal difficulties in the context of the breakdown of traditional Presbyterianism in mid-twentieth century Scotland.[48] This breakdown, he contends, produced disquiet and anguish amongst many individuals as the seemingly fixed identity of the Scottish Presbyterian self began to crumble in the face of the revolt against parental authority and the increasing secularization and pluralization of Scottish society. Sutcliffe sees Laing's emotional turbulence and his lack of ease in his chosen profession of psychiatry as a consequence of the conflict he experienced between the values instilled by his traditional upbringing or 'the religion of my fathers', and the wider cultural changes to which he was exposed as a young man.

Religion and science, psychoanalysis, psychology, philosophy, and psychiatry

'You are an artist, Ronnie: and also a scientist. You're done for, unless you become a [Christ]Xian'.

'You'll never be a good psychiatrist unless you're a Xian, and if you are a good psychiatrist— it doesn't matter anyway'.

'You'll never be a Xian, Ronnie, until you are physically sick'.

I wish I could remember all the wise, silly, brilliant—but always arresting—remarks that George MacLeod made to me about myself . . .[49]

In his notebooks Laing mused over these remarks. MacLeod highlighted the contradictions Laing was struggling to reconcile between his spiritual beliefs and his scientific aspirations. For Laing, religion and natural science seemed to offer opposing perspectives on the world:

'All corruption will come from the nat[ural]. sciences'. Perhaps if I don't take the easy way out, I may help to resolve the new consciousness of the dualism between nat[ural]. Sc[ience] & "_____ this that I don't know what to call. God?[50]

Here we see Laing grappling with the conflict between science and religion, but he is unsure and uncertain about the spiritual aspect. The quotation is by Kierkegaard and is taken from his journals.[51] Kierkegaard felt that the natural sciences were used

---

[47] James, W. (1902). *The Varieties of Religious Experience*. Longmans, Green, and Co., London, pp. 170–1.

[48] Sutcliffe, S. (2010). 'After "The Religion of My Fathers": The quest for composure in the "Post-Presbyterian" self'. In Abrams, L. and Brown, C.G. (eds), *A History of Everyday Life in Twentieth-Century Scotland*. Edinburgh University Press, Edinburgh, pp. 181–205.

[49] MS Laing K14.

[50] Ibid.

[51] Kierkegaard, S. (1938). *The Journals of Soren Kierkegaard* (ed. and trans. Dru, A.). Oxford University Press, London, p. 181.

inappropriately to 'explain' God, and, in the same journal entry, he mocked the notion of staring down a microscope to discover the origin of consciousness. Kierkegaard's example of the microscope appealed to Laing, capturing as it did the misapplication of scientific technique to the mysteries of humanity. Laing commented on science and religion: 'Scientific knowledge, alone is not illusionary and thus can say nothing about the object of belief. The belief can be "explained" without recourse to the necessity of postulating the reality of the object believed.'[52] In another notebook entry, Laing identifies two conflicting attitudes to spiritual experience. The first is the scientific one as represented by psychoanalysis, and the other is the religious one, to which Laing gives a decidedly Kierkegaardian colouring with his reference to 'despair':

> There are only two choices. Either deny the validity of the experience i.e. it is not really what it is (seems to be)—once one introduces 'seems' it is invalidated: one explains: one cures oneself—or goes to an analyst by whose 'love' one is cured—or one accepts it for what it is; and seeks an adequate 'cure' which is in despair and hope to pray for forgiveness and redemption: or rather for the strength to accept forgiveness.[53]

The entry reflects Laing's sceptical attitude to psychoanalysis, at least in its treatment of spiritual matters, and it is clear he favoured the religious approach. In another notebook entry, he expressed what he saw as the essential difference between religion and psychoanalysis: 'It is true that a sense of the presence of God will not save one from neurosis or insanity, but sanity and the possibility of mature genital relationship will not save anyone from estrangement from God and damnation.'[54] Gavin Miller has argued that Scottish psychoanalysts, such as Fairbairn and Suttie, distinguished themselves from Freud by incorporating Christianity into analytic thinking in order to create what Miller calls a 'rational religion'.[55] They saw the human personality as being forged by communion with others: communion was seen as the essence of Christianity. Miller sees Laing as being part of this tradition. For example, the preparation and sharing of food is considered to be an integral part of communion, and the 'Rumpus Room' experiment, conducted by Laing and his colleagues at Gartnavel Hospital, specifically tried to encourage deeper personal relations amongst patients and staff by involving them in making tea and cakes for each other. In a passage from *Wisdom, Madness and Folly*, in which he recalls the Glasgow hospital, Laing emphasizes the benefits of human communion:

> In Gartnavel, in the so-called 'back wards', I have seen catatonic patients who hardly make a move, or utter a word, or seem to notice or care about anyone or anything around them year in and year out, smile, laugh, shake hands, wish someone 'A Guid New Year' and even dance . . . The intoxicant here is not a drug, not even alcoholic spirits, but the celebration of a spirit of fellowship.[56]

---

52 MS Laing K14.
53 MS Laing K16.
54 MS Laing A223. R.D. Laing: Love and Nihilism, p. 5.
55 Miller, G. (2008). 'Scottish psychoanalysis. A rational religion'. *Journal of the History of the Behavioural Sciences*, **44**(1), 38–58.
56 Laing, *Wisdom, Madness and Folly*, pp. 31–2.

As well as criticizing Freudian psychoanalysis, Laing also attacked behavioural psychology's perspectives on religion: 'The spiritual is not another variable, or aspect, to be taken into consideration, to be added on to psychology, it is not another type of stimuli matched to a particular receptor organ. It is not another level to be integrated with a psychological substratum.'[57] Laing also condemned linguistic philosophers who had attempted to dissolve metaphysical questions by contending that they were merely problems of language. As he wrote in a spirit of defiant exasperation:

> Is this experience [of sin] valid or invalid? Who can answer for me? . . . It forces me to use words such as 'existence' and ontology—it forces me to say that in me there is a co-incidence—meeting between what is uniquely me, and being other than I. Wittgenstein can go to hell. I am going to keep my disease.[58]

Laing also drew on existential philosophy to support a religious outlook:

> Religion is said to take for truth what one desires to be true. And so it is called an illusion. God is the most absolute and fundamental desire that a man can have when he is living in all authenticity. In such a case a man can say truly, 'God is the name of my desire' . . . One cannot betray God without betraying oneself.[59]

In *The Self and Others* Laing again drew on existentialism, this time to explain the attractions of religion. Commenting that it seemed to be a universal human desire to want to occupy a place in the world of at least one other person, he wrote: 'Perhaps the greatest solace in religion is the sense that one lives in the Presence of an Other.'[60]

Albert Schweitzer

Laing questioned the underlying assumptions of psychiatry and its attitude towards the sacred. In his notebook, he made the following amused observation:

> Schweitzer wrote his thesis to show that Christ in terms of modern psychiatry was not insane. What I hope to do is to prove that in terms of modern psychiatry he was insane![61]

Albert Schweitzer, whom Laing's father had actually met, was a German theologian and physician, who had written a book, entitled *The Psychiatric Study of Jesus*, in which he attempted to refute those who had claimed the Jesus was mad.[62] In an earlier book, *The Quest for the Historical Jesus*, which appeared in 1906, Schweitzer had undermined the view of a Jesus who spoke of a Kingdom of Heaven that was to be achieved gradually on earth. Schweitzer held that this was a modern construction of liberal Protestantism. Instead, he claimed that a historical examination of the evidence revealed a Jesus who expected the imminent end of the world and who believed himself to be appointed by God as the ruler of a supernatural Kingdom which was about

---

[57] MS Laing A223, p. 2.
[58] MS Laing K16.
[59] MS Laing K14.
[60] Laing, *The Self and Others*, p. 128.
[61] MS Laing K14.
[62] Schweitzer, A. (1975). *The Psychiatric Study of Jesus. Exposition and Criticism* (trans. Joy, C.R.). Peter Smith, Gloucester, Mass (originally published in German in 1913).

to appear.[63] An unexpected consequence of Schweitzer's book was that it led some to conclude, that if Jesus really did believe such things, then this was evidence of deranged thinking.

In the wake of *The Quest for the Historical Jesus*, four books appeared which concluded that the Man from Nazareth was insane. All agreed that Jesus suffered from 'paranoia'. They also claimed that he suffered from hallucinations, ideas of reference, and delusions of grandeur. Schweitzer was appalled at this development and set out to refute such suggestions. In defending Jesus, Schweitzer placed him in the context of his time and pointed out that his beliefs were typical of his era. The control of the world by evil spirits, the coming of the Messiah and his Kingdom, the resurrection, and the transfiguration of nature were all part of late Jewish Messianic dogma. Schweitzer drew on the psychiatric authorities of *his* time to argue that the picture Jesus presented did not meet the criteria for a diagnosis of insanity. In particular, he cited the work of Kraepelin on the paranoiac form of dementia praecox to demonstrate that Jesus did not suffer from this condition. Schweitzer observed that hallucinations were also found in people who were not mentally ill.

The point that Laing was making in his notebook entry about Jesus was that modern psychiatry, as exemplified by Kraepelin, had no understanding of spiritual experience and dismissed it as evidence of mental pathology. In another observation in the same notebook, Laing wrote:

> The great realities of Faust no longer exist—there is no God, no Devil, no Damnation, no Salvation. A man who experiences these 'realities' is ipso facto mad. Madness is the nearest modern category to damnation.[64]

In *The Divided Self*, Laing was to write:

> The schizophrenic is desperate, is simply without hope. I have never known a schizophrenic who could say he was loved, as a man, by God the Father or by the Mother of God or by another man. He either *is* God, or the Devil, or in hell, estranged from God.[65]

Laing felt that spiritual experience was not taken seriously in his time. Laing pondered whether there was a spiritual realm and observed: 'There is nothing of God in the dull, prosaic normality of the objective world order.'[66] He felt most people were oblivious to the spiritual and wrote: 'There must be very few people in the country, phil[osophers] included who have any feeling for the meaning of "transcendental"'.[67] People who admitted to spiritual experiences would be dismissed as madmen. Laing contended that psychiatry could be used to invalidate religious experience. If the experience of the divine could be taken as evidence of insanity, was the reverse true? Was madness a sign of communion with God? In *The Divided Self*, Laing wrote:

> . . . the cracked mind of the schizophrenic may *let in* light which does not enter the intact minds of many sane people whose minds are closed. Ezekiel, in Jaspers' opinion, was schizophrenic.[68]

---

[63] Ibid., Joy, C.R., Introduction, pp. 17–26.
[64] MS Laing K14.
[65] Laing, *The Divided Self*, p. 39.
[66] MS Laing K14.
[67] Ibid.
[68] Laing, *The Divided Self*, p. 28.

In the same book, Laing also made mention of two patients whose psychosis first manifests itself in religious terms. A 22-year-old man took a boat out to sea, saying that 'he had lost God, and had set out on the ocean to find him'.[69] A man in his fifties took all his clothes off at a family picnic, waded into the nearby river, and refused to come out, claiming 'he was baptizing himself for his sins'.[70] In a notebook entry Laing compared the work of the therapist to that of the Lord: 'Jesus Christ came to bring "life more abundantly". Such is the true task of all psychotherapy.'[71]

In later years, Laing was to expand on the connection between madness and spiritual problems, most notably and most notoriously in *The Politics of Experience and the Bird of Paradise*. While this book was denounced by many as romanticizing mental illness, it is clear that Laing had been exploring the relationship between madness and spirituality from an early age. For example, he read Bernard Hart's 1946 book, *The Psychology of Insanity* and marked the passage, which suggested that, in the Middle Ages, people who had visions or underwent trances were viewed as having an intimate communion with God, and were consequently revered, rather than being dismissed as lunatics.[72]

However, his old mentor, Karl Abenheimer, identified what he saw as the flaws in Laing's line of thought:[73]

> He argues that in this civilisation or even in every civilisation man is alienated from his childlike innocence, creativeness and at-one-ness with the whole of existence, and only madmen take this seriously and won't accept it. Thus they sometimes have 'transcendental' experiences which Laing regards as valid . . . When schizophrenics experience the presence of gods or spirits or when they claim to be aware of the migration of the soul then Laing suggests that this has to be accepted as literal revelations of metaphysical truth . . .
>
> It is old wisdom that man has been driven out of paradise and has to live in a state of conflict with others and with himself. It is equally old wisdom that any attempt to remain in a pre-natal state of unity with everything, or any attempt to return there by a shortcut, is madness. If one goes on complaining about the state of conflict in which one finds oneself, and about one's alienation, one ends up in spurious claims of superiority over everybody else and in destructive nihilism about everything human.

Abenheimer's critique highlighted what he regarded as the impossibility of Laing's position and his tendency to elitism and disdain for others. Again it is informative to look at William James's *The Varieties of Religious Experience*, in particular his chapter on mysticism. James mentions the Christian mystics to whom Laing was to make repeated reference: Dionysius the Areopagite, Meister Eckhart, and Jacob Boehme; but he also discussed Hindus, Buddhists, and Mohemmedans. James concluded that

---

[69] Ibid., p. 161.

[70] Ibid., pp. 161–2.

[71] MS Laing A713.

[72] Glasgow University Library Special Collections. Laing's personal library 1448. Hart, B. (1946). *The Psychology of Insanity*. Cambridge University Press, Cambridge, p. 4. Passage underlined by Laing.

[73] Quoted in Calder, R. (1988). 'Abenheimer and Laing—some notes'. *Edinburgh Review*, **78–9**, 108–16.

'the existence of mystical states absolutely overthrows the pretension of non-mystical states to be the sole and ultimate dictators of what we may believe'.[74] Mystical states, he suggested, may even provide a superior point of view, a window to a more extensive and inclusive world. Such sentiments would have found a sympathetic response from Laing.

This chapter has described Laing's early encounters with religious matters: his apologetic and furtive reading of the Bible when he was ten years old; his membership of Christian societies as a school boy; his adolescent protests against Christian authority; his recurrent doubts as a young adult about the existence of God; and his attempts during his training as a psychiatrist to reconcile scientific and spiritual explanations of madness. These encounters took place in the culture of mid-twentieth century Presbyterian Scotland, at a time when the legitimacy of religion was being questioned by science, psychoanalysis, politics, and philosophy. Laing felt compelled to immerse himself in this debate and to engage fully with the many arguments for and against religion. This debate was not simply a theoretical exercise. To Laing it concerned profound existential issues, and it was of the utmost importance to him as a psychiatrist to work out his own response to questions of faith. It determined how he conceived of 'the mental misery' of his patients.

Laing continued to wrestle with spiritual questions for the rest of his career. He seems to have found some kind of resolution to his agonized searching, if we are to judge by remarks he made during his last years. In an interesting article, entitled 'God and DSM III', which Laing wrote towards the end of his life, he said he was a 'negative theologian': he could define God by what he was not, but he did, nevertheless, believe in God.[75] In conversation with Bob Mullan,[76] Laing again described himself as a negative theologian and referred to Dionysius the Areopagite, a figure in whom Laing had an abiding interest, and who had defined God by what he was not. Laing had used a key passage by Dionysius the Areopagite in his 1979 book, *Sonnets*.[77] He declared that Dionysius had articulated, what was integral to all religious traditions:

> The truth of every myth is an ineffable mystery, which cannot reveal its secrets to the outsider and cannot be uttered by the insider, and cannot be known to any knower, outsider or insider.

[74] James, *The Varieties of Religious Experience*, p. 427.

[75] MS Laing A514/1. Annotated proof of 'God and DSM III', which appeared in the *Times Literary Supplement*.

[76] Mullan, *Mad to be Normal*, pp. 44–5.

[77] Laing, R.D. (1979). *Sonnets*. Michael Joseph, London, pp. 60.

Chapter 6

Laing and the arts

> The Greeks regarded medicine as primarily an Art. The God of Medicine was Apollo—
> also the God of Music, Poetry and the Fine Arts—the Sun-god. We are not accustomed to
> think of the Art which we hope to practice as having a close relationship to these things.
> That we do not so think is an artefact of our culture and education. The Greeks were
> nearer the truth of this matter than we are.[1]

Thus Laing as a medical student in 1949. One of Laing's most significant contributions
was his emphasis on the role of the arts in medicine and how they could provide
insights into human distress. As Laing's observation suggests, the link between the arts
and medicine has a venerable history, although historical eras have differed in
the importance they have accorded to the link.[2] Advocates claimed that exposure to
the humanities deepened the understanding of suffering and conferred wisdom on
clinical practice. There has long been a fruitful interaction between medicine and the
arts. Many clinicians wrote essays, novels, and poetry, and writers embraced medical
themes. In the eighteenth century, Tobias Smollett, a fellow-Glasgow medical graduate, achieved fame as a novelist with such books as *Roderick Random* and *The Expedition
of Humphry Clinker*. John Keats, the great English Romantic poet was a qualified doctor, while Laurence Sterne made frequent references to medicine, health, and sickness
in *The Life and Opinions of Tristram Shandy, Gentleman*. The nineteenth and early
twentieth century saw such medical authors as Anton Chekhov, Arthur Conan Doyle,
Mikhail Bulgakov, Arthur Schnitzler, William Carlos Williams, and the Scottish playwright, James Bridie, whose work Laing knew. Even Emil Kraepelin, viewed by Laing
and others as an incorrigible somaticist, was a published poet. The eminent French
neurologist, Jean-Martin Charcot, dubbed the 'Napoleon of the Nerves', held evening
soirées to which the leading writers, artists, and doctors of Paris flocked. The great
modernist writer, Marcel Proust was influenced by many physicians and psychologists, including Binet, Charcot, and Janet. His masterpiece, *In Search of Lost Time*,
deals with several medical and psychiatric topics, such as hypochondria, hysteria,
grief, and mental breakdown. Sigmund Freud was well versed in European and
Classical culture and his case reports were admired as much for their literary as for
their scientific merits.

At some point, however, there appears to have been a loosening in the link between
the arts and medicine. In an influential lecture delivered in the year before *The Divided*

[1] MS Laing A408. Laing, R.D. (1949). 'Philosophy and medicine'. *Surgo,* June, p. 135.
[2] Beveridge, A. (2009). 'The benefits of reading literature'. In Oyebode, F. (ed.) *Mindreadings.
Literature and Psychiatry*, RCPsych Publications, London, pp. 1–14.

Self was published, C.P. Snow,[3] the physicist and writer, contended that society was divided into 'two cultures', the scientific and the artistic. He maintained that this split was destructive and warned that 'Closing the gap between our cultures is a necessity in the most abstract intellectual sense, as well as the most practical.' The origins of the rift between the arts and the sciences are often traced to the Enlightenment, which held that reason would solve the problems of humanity. The Romantic Movement, which stressed spontaneity, the spiritual, and a sense of wonder, is seen as hastening the division between the arts and the sciences. However, this chronology has recently been challenged by the historian, Mark Micale,[4] who argues that the relationship between the humanities and medicine continued to enjoy a mutually rewarding relationship until at least the early part of the twentieth century. He maintains that the relationship only began to falter after the First World War with the ending of the liberal arts education to which doctors had previously been exposed. Micale is surely right to challenge the standard account by Snow, and his work receives support from Richard Holmes in his book *The Age of Wonder*,[5] which finds that scientific advances continued to exercise a fascination over artists and writers throughout the nineteenth century. In the case of Scotland, we can extend Micale's argument about liberal arts education even further. Would-be doctors continued to be exposed to an education which included the humanities throughout the twentieth century and, indeed, to the present day. Laing, it will be remembered, left school with a wide-ranging set of qualifications in the humanities. During this period in the 1940s, Scottish pupils were able to study both the arts and the sciences to pre-graduate level. Unlike the English system which aimed for narrowness but depth, the Scots curricula was based on width of experience. Laing's Scottish education, then, lent him certain advantages over his English-trained contemporaries. In addition, he was a talented musician and he was to compare writing prose to music: one should read out one's words to ensure that they had a suitable rhythm, he contended.[6]

The critic, Martin Esslin[7] who knew Laing expressed surprise that more psychiatrists had not made use of the vast body of creative literature which related to madness. However, he felt that Laing was an 'exhilarating exception', who combined psychological insight with great literary craft. Laing's immersion in literary culture influenced how he thought and wrote about mental disturbance. It is not just a matter of noting when he makes reference to literature, though that too is illuminating. Often there are allusions to other works without it being spelt out exactly what they are. For example, in *The Self and Others* in the discussion of 'The coldness of death', Laing writes: 'But none

[3] Snow, C.P. (1959). *The Two Cultures and the Scientific Revolution*. Cambridge University Press, Cambridge.

[4] Micale, M. (2007). 'Two cultures revisited: the case of the fin de siecle'. In Bivins, R. and Pickstone, J.V. (eds), *Medicine, Madness and Social History. Essays in Honour of Roy Porter*. Palgrave. London, pp. 210–33.

[5] Holmes, R. (2008). *The Age of Wonder. How the Romantic Generation Discovered the Beauty and Terror of Science*. Harper Press, London.

[6] Mullan, B. (1995). *Mad to be Normal. Conversations with R.D. Laing*. Free Association Books, London, p. 70.

[7] Mullan, B. (1997). *R.D. Laing. Creative Destroyer*. Cassell, London, pp.15–18.

of us wishes to bear too much reality: to wake up, for instance, at 3 a.m. and realize that we have been under the delusion of being alive.'[8] Here Laing is alluding to a line from T.S. Eliot's 'Four Quartets': 'human kind/cannot bear very much reality'. In fact Laing later revealed that *The Divided Self* had been influenced 'stylistically' by T.S. Eliot.[9] And of course there are specific literary references aplenty in Laing's work. To take just *The Divided Self*, mention is made of Beckett, Blake, Dante, Empson, Gorky, Holderlin, Kafka, Keats, Moore, Ophelia, Pascal, Rimbaud, Shakespeare, and Yeats. Laing was to claim that he saw himself in the tradition of Keats and his notion of 'negative capability'. Laing defined Keats's term as 'what he calls the capacity for uncertainty, mystery, and doubt, rather than certainty, objectification, and having arrived at the answers'.[10] Like Freud before him, Laing was able to bring a literary sensibility to the subject of madness, and this made his work accessible and appealing to a wide audience outside the psychiatric profession.

William Blake

As a young man Laing intended to write a study of William Blake, indeed at one stage he thought this would be his first book: it would be called *The New Man. An Existential Analysis/Study of William Blake*. Laing read the major biographies and made repeated notes on the nineteenth century poet and artist. Laing regarded Blake as 'one of the greatest prophets of our time' and felt that no Englishmen was comparable to him in the scope, depth, and clarity of his vision.[11] He maintained that Blake had a great insight into the workings of his imagination, and that unless 'we can do justice to Blake we cannot do justice to our patients'. Laing felt that Blake had a capacity for vision which he fiercely defended against destructive forces, both from within and without. Such a vision was the birthright of all men but it could become crushed or lost in our journey through life. Laing claimed that, if we studied Blake to discover the ways in which the vision could be destroyed, we could learn to see with greater clarity the processes in ourselves and in our patients that lead to mental disintegration.[12]

Blake rebelled against what he saw as the materialist philosophy of the Enlightenment, but also against those whom he felt promoted a repressive version of Christianity.[13] In his lifetime Blake achieved little success and on his death was regarded as talented but insane. His reputation slowly improved and by the 1950s he was being hailed by the Beat Generation and British poets of the underground movement as a liberator of humanity and as a prophet who had warned against the dangers of the mechanism of man. Blake's work was being triumphantly vindicated at around the same time that the young Laing was first exploring the world of culture, so it is not surprising that he

[8] Laing, *The Self and Others*, p, 66.

[9] Clay, *R.D. Laing*, p. 59.

[10] Evans, *R.D. Laing: The Man and his Ideas*, p. 90. Laing refers to 'negative *capacity*', though Keats's term was 'negative capability'.

[11] MS Laing A580 (ii).

[12] MS Laing A713. Drafts.

[13] Ackroyd, P. (1995). *Blake*. Sinclair-Stevenson, London; Drabble, M. (ed.) (2000). *The Oxford Companion to English Literature*. Oxford University Press, Oxford, pp. 107–09.

was aware of Blake, nor that he was so responsive to the message of the visionary poet, especially as it was being interpreted by the post-war generation.

In *The Divided Self*, Laing referred to Blake's notion of 'chaotic non-entity' to describe the schizoid's individual's dread of their self disintegrating.[14] In particular, he referred to Blake's Prophetic Books and maintained that, unlike the representations of the figures of Hell in Greek literature and that of Dante, Blake's characters no longer retained their inner cohesiveness but underwent divisions in themselves. Laing added, 'These books require prolonged study . . . in order to learn from him, what, somehow, he knew about in a most intimate fashion, while remaining sane'.[15] In the same book, Laing maintained that Blake did not fit in with conventional society and had to develop his own 'piercing vision': unlike many others, Blake possessed the ability to live by it. Those who were unable to live by their vision, Laing averred went mad.[16] In this, Laing is offering an essentially Romantic explanation of madness, and he is utilizing his particular picture of Blake to support his thesis. The mad are recruited from those sections of society that have visions: those who cannot retain their visions, either as a result of inner weakness or outside pressure, go insane.

In *The Self and Others*, Laing quotes with approval Blake's phrase 'the lineaments of gratified desire' in his discussion of sexuality.[17] The quotation is taken from these three lines by Blake:

In a wife I would desire
What in whores is always found—
The lineaments of Gratified desire.[18]

Laing writes that there are two basic intentions in sexuality: to obtain relief from tension, and to effect a change in the other. Laing takes Blake to mean that failure to witness the 'lineaments of Gratified desire' in one's sexual partner is a deeply frustrating experience.

Gerard Manley Hopkins

Early in his career Laing also planned to write a biography of the nineteenth century English poet, Gerard Manley Hopkins.[19] Characteristically, Laing hoped that it would be completed before he was 30, but as with the proposed book on Blake, he did not managed to write it. Laing was intrigued by Hopkins' recurrent bouts of depression and his struggles with his relation to God. Both were subjects in which Laing had a keen personal interest. As he wrote of his plan to write about Hopkins: 'Such a study might bring to sharp focus the problems which bother me.'[20]

---

[14] Laing, *The Divided Self*, p. 80 and p. 177, n. 1.

[15] Ibid.,p. 177.

[16] Ibid., p. 208.

[17] Laing, *The Self and Others*, p. 73.

[18] Bronowski, J. (1958). *William Blake. A Selection of Poems and Letters*. Penguin Books, London, p. 64.

[19] Drabble, M. (ed.) (2000). *The Oxford Companion to English Literature*. Oxford University Press, Oxford, pp. 494–5.

[20] MS Laing A410. Notes on Gerard Manley Hopkins.

Born into an Anglican family in Stratford, Hopkins went on to study at Oxford University where he attained a double first in Classics. In his final year he converted to Roman Catholicism and was subsequently ordained as a Jesuit priest. Hopkins worked in parishes around Britain, including Glasgow, but found the poverty and squalor of urban life overwhelming. He deemed Glasgow to be a 'wretched place' and 'repulsive to live in'.[21] He returned to academic life, taking up the chair of Greek and Latin at University College, Dublin. Hopkins was never able to reconcile writing poetry with his desire to serve God. When he joined the Jesuits, he symbolically burned his poems and stopped writing for eight years. However, he returned to poetry in 1875 with 'The Wreck of the Deutschland'. In this key poem, Hopkins developed what he called 'sprung rhythm', in which he sought to emulate the rhythm of common speech and written prose, rather than write in formal metre.

Hopkins' poetry embraced a nature mysticism, which explored the revelation of the divine in the physical world. The beauty of nature was the means through which humanity attained truth. Hopkins, like Laing, was interested in Duns Scotus, the medieval Scottish theologian, and his doctrine of the *haecceitas* or 'thisness', which refers to a principle of singular essence or individuating difference, the 'thisness' of a thing.[22] Martin Heidegger, as we have seen, was also interested in Duns Scotus and completed a post-doctoral dissertation on him.[23] Hopkins was inspired by his reading of the work of Duns Scotus to develop his notion of 'inscape', which was defined as the inner spirit of all things, animate and inanimate, as expressed in their outer form.[24] Hopkins felt that the poet's task was not merely to observe things, but to see *into* them in order to penetrate their souls. This, of course, has parallels with Laing's view of the task of the psychiatrist, who, he held, should look beyond the 'signs' and 'symptoms' of 'disease' to grasp the patient's particular mode of being in the world. Related to 'inscape' was Hopkins' concept of 'instress', which was defined as the force which sustained an 'inscape'. 'Instress' originated in the Creator and could be felt by a sufficiently responsive person. Hopkins derived this notion, too, from Duns Scotus.

Laing had a copy of the 1948 edition of Hopkins' poems by Helen M. Gardner, which provided an influential perspective on his work.[25] She had advised: 'Whoever would understand Hopkins must go not to Freudian psychology but rather to the "Spiritual Exercises" of St Ignatius Loyola, the founder of the Society of Jesus'.[26] Laing made numerous notes on the poet. He planned to study the place of poetry in Hopkins' life: how it emerged and for what purpose. He would draw on existentialism, the literature

[21] White, N. (2004). Hopkins, Gerard Manley (1844–1889), in *Oxford Dictionary of National Biography*. Oxford University Press, Oxford http://www.oxforddnb.com/view/article/37565.

[22] This is discussed in Brown, D. (2004). *Gerard Manley Hopkins*. Northcote House, Horndon.

[23] Dreyfus, H.L. and Wrathall, M.A. (eds) (2007). *A Companion to Heidegger*. Blackwell Publishing, London, p. 2.

[24] Van de Weyer, R. (1996). 'Introduction'. In Gerard Manley Hopkins (1996). *The Complete Poems with Selected Prose of Gerard Manley Hopkins*. Fount, London, pp. vii–x.

[25] Glasgow University Library Special Collections. Laing's personal library. 1902. Gardner, H.M. (ed.) (1948). *Poems of Gerard Manley Hopkins*. Oxford University Press, London.

[26] Ibid., p. xxi.

on the psychology of religion, and Duns Scotus. Despite Gardner's strictures, he would look at psychoanalytic approaches to creativity. Laing writes:

> When G.M.H. cries for his 'Comforter' he is indeed crying for his Saviour, and we do not intend to link . . . saviour with his mother's teat. [However] We do believe that there is a connection between this cry of the adult man in spiritual desolation and the cry of the baby abandoned by his mother, thirsty for milk.[27]

Laing was wary of psychoanalytical reductionism, but, nevertheless, he linked the spiritual yearnings of the poet to the plight of the abandoned infant. Laing was probably referring to these lines by Hopkins, which had been highlighted in the Gardner edition:[28]

> I cast for comfort I can no more get
> By groping round my comfortless, than blind
> Eyes in their dark can day or thirst can find
> Thirst's all-in-all in all a world of wet.

Although he never managed to write a biography of Hopkins, Laing was to refer to him in his published work. For example, in *The Divided Self*,[29] when discussing the case of James, he mentions Hopkins's contention that 'mortal beauty' was dangerous. Laing is alluding to a poem by Hopkins entitled 'To what serves mortal beauty?' The poem ends with theses lines:

> To man, that needs would worship block or barren stone,
> Our law says: Love what are love's worthiest, were all known;
> World's loveliest—men's selves. Self-flashes off frame and face.
> What do then? how meet beauty? Merely meet it; own,
> Home at heart, heaven's sweet gift; then leave, let that alone.
> Yea, wish that though, wish all, God's better beauty, grace.[30]

Laing writes that his patient, James, had been walking in the park when he had experienced a sense of oneness with nature. However, he had begun to panic and was terrified of losing his identity by this fusion of his self with the whole world. Hopkins had advised that if we met 'mortal beauty', we should then let it alone. Where more conventional psychiatrists might have depicted James's problems simply in terms of anxiety, Laing brought in poetry and religion to deepen the explanation.

In his 1961 book, *The Self and Others*,[31] Laing examined Hopkins in the context of the privacy of personal experience. Laing quoted a passage by Hopkins in which he

---

[27] MS Laing K16. R.D. Laing: Notebook, July 1953 to August 1962.

[28] Gardner, *Poems of Gerard Manley.* Poem no. 71, quoted in Introduction, p. xxv. There is another poem which Laing might also have had in mind. 'No worst, There is none': No worst, there is none. Pitched past pitch of grief/More pangs will, schooled at forepangs, wilder wring/Comforter, where, where is your comforting?/Mary, mother of us, where is your relief? Hopkins, G.M. (1996). *The Complete Poems with Selected Prose of Gerard Manley Hopkins.* Fount, London, p. 65.

[29] Laing, R.D. (1960). *The Divided Self.* Tavistock, London, p. 97.

[30] Hopkins, *The Complete Poems*, p. 61.

[31] Laing, R.D. (1961). *The Self and Others.* Tavistock, London, pp. 18–19.

described the absolutely unique and inaccessible world of what the poet called 'selfbeing'. Hopkins writes:

> . . . my selfbeing, my consciousness and feeling of myself, that taste of myself, of *I* and *me* above and in all things, which is more distinctive than the taste of ale or alum, more distinctive than the smell of walnutleaf or camphor, and is incommunicable by any means to another man . . .[32]

Laing drew on this observation to discuss what he considered to be one of the most difficult tasks of the psychiatrist: to understand the self-being of another person. What makes a psychiatrist decide that *their* perception of their patient's self-being is evidence of mental disturbance? Laing sounded a warning note: psychiatric intervention might do violence to an individual's experience of their self-being, and leave them estranged from themselves.

Dostoyevsky

> After D[ostoyevsky] one wonders whether philosophy is possible anymore.[33]

So observed Laing in one of his personal notebooks from the early 1950s. Laing was a passionate admirer of Dostoyevsky and, as a young man, had planned to write a biography of the great Russian novelist. He had read all his books, analysed the characters, and pondered their dilemmas. He read Dostoyevsky's letters and journalism, and also the major biographies. Laing made copious notes and considered writing an analysis of Dostoyevsky based on the object relations theories of Fairbairn and Klein. In his second book, *The Self and Others*, Laing made extensive reference to Dostoyevsky, and in later works, such as the *Politics of Experience and the Bird of Paradise* and *The Politics of the Family*, he again referred to the Russian writer.

Laing's first exposure to Dostoyevsky seems to have been when he was around four years old. Although he liked to advertise his intellectual precocity, even Laing did not claim he was actually *reading* the writings of the Russian novelist at this early age. Rather, as we have seen, he had access to a series of volumes entitled *The World's Library of Best Books*, which contained extracts from literature from different countries with pictures to illustrate the text. One such illustrated extract was of 'Raskolnikov being surprised in the street by "Murderer" hissed in his ear'.[34] The image obviously made an impact on Laing, as he remembered it into adulthood. As we have seen, Laing's student essay, 'Health and happiness' referred in admiring tones to Dostoyevsky.

Laing's private papers demonstrate that he continued to be very interested in Dostoyevsky. He felt there was a 'peculiarly passionate, turbulent quality' to Dostoyevsky's work and that it displayed an 'unreal realism'.[35] He went through *Crime and Punishment*

---

[32] Hopkins, *The Complete Poems*, p. 92.

[33] MS Laing K14. R.D. Laing: Notebook and partial diary covering Laing's stay at the military hospitals at Netley and Catterick, January 1952 to June 1953.

[34] MS Laing K1. Elements of an Autobiography by R.D. Laing, p. 25.

[35] MS Laing K16. R.D. Laing: Notebook, July 1953 to August 1962.

and made extensive notes; he wrote draft papers on Dostoyevsky in relation to love and nihilism; he devoured Andre Gide's biography of Dostoyevsky and copied numerous extracts into his notebook, for example:

> The intellect in D[ostoyevsky] is always demonically possessed, and its exercise leads to perdition of the self and the suffering of others . . . D[ostoyevsky] cannot be forced into a simple formula—not even 'the religion of suffering'.[36]

Elsewhere in his notebooks, Laing observed:

> Though Dostoyevsky is a rich mine for the psychologist, it would be a 'comic' error to call Dostoyevsky a psychologist. It is difficult to find the correct word. Berdyaev suggested pneumatologist, a symbolistic metaphysician, a mystical realist. . . .[37]

In this passage, Laing makes reference to Berdyaev, a Russian religious philosopher, whose writing he had also studied. By the time Laing began to publish his work, his continuing interest in Dostoyevsky remained apparent. He drew on his familiarity with the work of the Russian novelist to discuss Dostoyevsky at some length in his 1961 book, *The Self and Others* and later in *The Politics of Experience and the Bird of Paradise*, and *The Politics of the Family*. Why did the work of Dostoyevsky interest Laing?

As we have seen, Dostoyevsky can be seen as part of the tradition of existentialism. In *Existentialism from Dostoyevsky to Sartre*, Walter Kaufmann[38] portrays the Russian writer as occupying a seminal role in the development of existential thought. Laing was familiar with this book and cited it in the first edition of *The Divided Self*. Many of the writers who inspired Laing acknowledged their debt to Dostoyevsky. Nietzsche declared with characteristic modesty: 'Dostoyevsky was the only psychologist from whom I had anything to learn'.[39] Sartre was an admirer, while Camus drew on the insights of the Russian novelist in *The Rebel* and adapted *The Possessed* as a play. Many themes in the work of Dostoyevsky would have struck a chord with Laing.

Dostoyevsky is the novelist par excellence of mental disturbance. Even a cursory acquaintance with his work reveals that most if not all his characters seem to be verging on insanity. 'Is everyone mad?' asks the narrator of *A Raw Youth*.[40] In his novels, Dostoyevsky presents a many-stranded and complex account of mental derangement, which takes account of emotional, social, and spiritual aspects. Dostoyevsky read current medical writers and his novels contain numerous discussions of the contemporary theories of insanity.[41] In his *Diary of a Writer*, he commented on the court cases and the stories of human interest, described in the newspapers.[42] Dostoyevsky often took issue with

---

[36] MS Laing K14.

[37] MS Laing A 223, p. 3.

[38] Kaufmann, W. (1958). *Existentialism from Dostoyevsky to Sartre*. Meridian Books, Cleveland and New York.

[39] Gide, A. (1967). *Dostoyevsky*. Peregrine Books, London, title page.

[40] Dostoyevsky, F.M. (1947). *A Raw Youth* (trans. Garnett, C.). Dial Press, New York, p. 65.

[41] Rice, J.L. (1985). *Dostoyevsky and the Healing Art: An Essay in Literary and Medical History*. Ardis, Ann Arbor.

[42] Dostoyevsky, F.M. (1984). *The Diary of a Writer* (trans. Brasol, B.). Ianmead, Haslemere.

other commentators if he felt they had put forward fanciful psychological explanations of the reported events. Laing and Dostoyevsky shared a relish for mocking the pronouncements of the so-called experts on insanity. In the trial scene in *The Brothers Karamazov*, Dostoyevsky has fun presenting the conflicting psychological opinions about Dimitri, who stands accused of the murder of his father. Likewise, in the trial of Raskolnikov at the end of *Crime and Punishment*, Dostoyevsky portrays the psychological theorizing in a sceptical manner.

In the opening pages of his first book, *The Divided Self*, Laing examined the interview style of Emil Kraepelin, the eminent German professor of psychiatry. Like Dostoyevsky, Laing used the clinician's own words to damn him. In two of his later books, *The Politics of the Family* and *The Facts of Life*, Laing used the same technique to undermine the ideas of clinicians such as Morel, Bion, and Binswanger. Both Dostoyevsky and Laing were concerned that abstract theorizing often led to denial of the essential humanity of the other person—or as Laing put it, 'the power to bury them alive and screaming in their tomb of words'.[43]

Laing and Dostoyevsky are further linked by the work of Sigmund Freud, who wrote an essay on the Russian writer, 'Dostoyevsky and Parricide'.[44] Laing, as we have seen, had an ambivalent attitude towards Freud, sometimes hailing him as an intellectual hero, at others, damning him as a crude determinist. Freud considered Dostoyevsky to be a great artist and was impressed by his depiction of the workings of the unconscious mind. Freud stated that *he* had not discovered the unconscious: the poets had discovered it long before him. However, Freud's essay on Dostoyevsky, which has been heavily criticized,[45] displays the characteristics of analytical theory that so troubled Laing. Freud adopted a rigidly deterministic approach and saw in the work of the novelist evidence of a whole array of mental pathology. Freud maintained that Dostoyevsky harboured unresolved parricidal wishes, had criminal tendencies which were sublimated through his art, was a passive homosexual, and was given to excessive masturbation.

Laing disliked Freud's treatment of creativity, feeling that he was applying an inappropriately reductionist model to something which was spontaneous and which dealt in a profound way with the human condition. By claiming that the content of a work of art was the outward manifestation of unconscious forces, Laing felt that Freud was missing the point about the nature of creativity. As Laing's former analyst, Charles Rycroft wrote: 'Since the results of creative activity are by definition novel, unexpected, and therefore unpredictable, creativity is a concept hard to include within a causal determinist framework.'[46]

Freud had also been contemptuous of Dostoyevsky's belief in God, condemning it as the novelist's avoidance of harsh reality and his need to masochistically humble

[43] Laing, R.D. (1982). *The Voice of Experience*. Penguin Books, London, p. 62.

[44] Freud, S. (1961). 'Dostoevsky and parricide'. In *Complete Psychological Works*, Vol. 21. Hogarth Press, London, pp. 177–94.

[45] Frank, J. (1977). *Dostoyevsky: The Seeds of Revolt, 1821–1849*. Robson Books, London.

[46] Rycroft, C. (1995). *A Critical Dictionary of Psychoanalysis* (second edition). Penguin Books, London, p. 30.

himself before figures of authority. Laing disagreed with Freud's approach to religion, feeling that, once again, an inappropriate model was being applied to a subject that was, by its very nature, mysterious and inexplicable. Although Laing frequently referred to Freud, he does not seem to have made any specific reference to his essay, 'Dostoyevsky and parricide'. We know that Laing must have been familiar with it, because he had read the complete works of Freud. Perhaps Laing was too hostile to the thesis of the essay to find it useful. However, he did make a reference to the application of psychoanalytic theory to Dostoyevsky's work in *The Politics of Experience and the Bird of Paradise*. He wrote:

> When Ivan in *The Brothers Karamazov* says, 'If God does not exist, everything is permissible', he is *not* saying: 'If my super-ego, in projected form, can be abolished, I can do anything with a good conscience'. He *is* saying: 'If there is *only* my conscience, then there is no ultimate validity for my will'.[47]

Here Laing is emphasizing the folly of translating imaginative literature into Freudian terminology, and the passage reflects his scepticism as to the value of psychoanalytical approaches to art. In the course of his career, Laing entertained several and sometimes contradictory models of madness. However, he and Dostoyevsky often expressed similar views on the subject. Both saw madness as being on a spectrum, with sanity at one end and insanity at the other. Laing drew on the tenets of psychoanalysis to support this contention, while, in *Crime and Punishment*, we find Dostoyevsky has his character, Dr Zossimov, observe:

> We're all rather often almost like mad people, only with the slight difference that the 'sick' are somewhat madder than we are, so it's necessary to draw a line here. And the harmonious man, it's true almost doesn't exist.[48]

Laing was against categorising people, and his writing examines what he saw as the negative consequences of making a psychiatric diagnosis. In *Notes from the House of the Dead*, Dostoyevsky's fictional account of his time in a Siberian labour camp, the main character states:

> I am trying to classify all the prisoners into categories; that, however, is not really possible. Reality is infinitely various when compared to the deductions of abstract thought . . . and it will not tolerate, rigid, hard-and-fast distinctions. Reality strives for diversification. We, too, had our special form of life . . . and it was not merely some official existence but our own, inner, private life.[49]

One feels that Laing would have been sympathetic to these sentiments, and, in particular, the dichotomy that Dostoyevsky's character emphasizes between the institution's abstract perception of the inmate, and the individual's actual experience of the situation. Laing made much of the conflict between doctors and patients in their

[47] Laing, R.D. (1967). *The Politics of Experience and the Bird of Paradise*. Penguin Books, London, p. 114.

[48] Dostoyevsky, F.M. (1992). *Crime and Punishment* (trans. Pevear, R. and Volokhonsky, L.). Vintage, London, p. 226.

[49] Dostoyevsky, F.M. (1985). *The House of the Dead* (trans. McDuff, D.). Penguin, London, p. 305.

respective perceptions of the clinical interview. Doctors are guided by concepts of psychiatric illness, based on the general and the statistical, while patients view their experiences as particular and unique to themselves.

Laing was acutely aware that judgements about madness take place in a social context. His books, such as *The Self and Others, Sanity, Madness and the Family*, and *The Politics of the Family*, explored this in some detail. In the novels of Dostoyevsky, madness also takes place in a social context. It is perceived differently by each person and each person's judgement can also change over time. In *Problems of Dostoyevsky's Poetics,* the Russian literary scholar Mikhail Bakhtin highlighted this aspect of the novelist's art.[50] Dostoyevsky, he stated, offered a distinctive view, based on an awareness of the relativity of a given situation. Instead of a one-sided view-point, he offered a multidimensional perspective, where many independent voices are heard and interact. None is afforded priority. Dostoyevsky created what Bakhtin called a *polyphonic* novel. Laing was especially interested in this approach. He had been impressed by Dostoyevsky's juxtaposition of the voice of Raskolnikov alongside the voices of other characters. Laing stated that he had reflected on the structure of *Crime and Punishment* for the years leading up to his first books.

In *The Self and Others*, Laing gave his most extended commentary on Dostoyevsky, particularly the novelist's portrayal of the dynamics of the mind. Laing wrote: 'Dostoyevsky's genius is unmistakable in his handling of the merging of dreams, phantasy, imagination, and reality. All his novels explicitly reveal or openly imply his characters' simultaneous participation in the world of these modalities.'[51] Laing takes the depiction of the mental turmoil of Raskolnikov in *Crime and Punishment* as a good example of this aspect of Dostoyevsky's genius. He spends several pages analysing Raskolnikov's dream, which occurs on the day before he murders an old pawn-broker and her daughter with an axe. In his dream, Raskolnikov is a small boy and witnesses an old horse being beaten to death by a peasant, who eventually uses an axe to finish off the animal. Laing was impressed by the way Dostoyevsky showed the interplay of the different aspects of Raskolnikov's disturbed mind. In his imagination he sees himself as Napoleon; in his dream he is a little boy; and in his fantasy he is a beaten old horse and also the old woman he is about to kill. Laing returned to this theme in *The Politics of the Family* and observed that Raskolnikov had created a fantasy family.

In a later section of *The Self and Others*, Laing once again considers Raskolnikov, this time in relation to a letter he has received from his mother. For Laing, the requests expressed in the letter put Raskolnikov in an impossible position. They place several mutually contradictory injunctions on him, and Laing analyses them in some detail. This was a subject that enthralled Laing. He knew that social interaction could be understood on many different levels, and that individuals often sent out conflicting signals to each other. In *The Self and Others*, he had drawn on the 'double bind' thesis, as outlined by Bateson and colleagues, to examine the ambiguities of human interaction. In *Sanity, Madness and the Family*, he examined the communication patterns of

[50] Bakhtin, M. (1984). *Problems of Dostoyevsky's Poetics*. Manchester University Press, Manchester.

[51] Laing, *The Self and Others*, p. 50.

families, where one of the members had a diagnosis of schizophrenia.[52] He explored the subject further in *Interpersonal Perception*,[53] when he attempted to construct mathematical models of communication, and yet again in *Knots*,[54] when he set human dialogue to verse.

Laing was interested in Dostoyevsky's novel, *The Double*, which depicts the mental disintegration of Goladyakin, who believes he has a double.[55] For Laing, the origins of Goladyakin's problem lie with his own secret intention not to be himself, to oust himself from his place in the world. Goladykin attributes this intention to others, a mechanism which is one of paranoid delusion. In his attempts to resolve his situation, Goladykin tries another strategy: he will become a spectator. In *The Self and Others*, Laing quotes a passage which, in its description of the schizoid process, could have come from one of his patients:

> . . . This is what I'll do—I'll just be an outside observer, and nothing more. I'm an onlooker, an outsider, that's all, I'll say. And whatever happens it won't be me who's to blame.[56]

Another work of Dostoyevsky's that could have been a case study from *The Divided Self* is his short story, 'White Nights'. It describes a solitary young man who lives in his imagination but finds, as a consequence, that his inner world becomes progressively more atrophied. This is similar to the case of a youth described in *The Divided Self*. Laing writes:

> . . . he maintained himself in isolated detachment from the world for months, living alone in a single room, existing frugally on a few savings, day-dreaming. But in doing this, he began to feel he was dying inside; he was becoming more and more empty . . .[57]

Laing was intrigued by Prince Myshkin, the central character of *The Idiot*. In the novel, Dostoyevsky considers what happens when a Christ-like figure comes amongst society. Myshkin is the Christ-like figure who initially disarms people with his innocence and essential goodness, but who is eventually driven insane by a rapacious society. Laing was struck by the fact that Dostoyevsky's ideal of a perfect man was 'sexually harmless'. In a notebook entry he commented:

> When he [Dostoyevsky] set out to portray a perfect and good man in 'The Idiot' . . . he ended by portraying a man who pitied everyone but was incapable of fulfilling love. The most radical nihilist among Dostoevsky's characters is not Ivan Karamazov, Stavrogin, or Kirilov—it is Prince Myshkin.[58]

---

[52] Laing, R.D. and Esterson, A. (1964). *Sanity, Madness and the Family*. Penguin Books, London.

[53] Laing, R.D., Phillipson, H. and Lee, R.A. (1966). *Interpersonal Perception*. Tavistock, London.

[54] Laing, R.D. (1970). *Knots*. Tavistock, London.

[55] Dostoyevsky, F. (2003). *Notes from the Underground and the Double* (trans. Coulson, J.). Penguin Books, London.

[56] Laing, *The Self and Others*, p. 125.

[57] Laing, *The Divided Self*, p. 56.

[58] MS Laing A223, p. 9.

Dostoyevsky's underlying philosophy has resonances with that of Laing. He lived at a time when scientific materialism was in the ascendancy.[59] Many of Dostoyevsky's contemporaries believed that the evolution of society obeyed laws that the natural sciences were discovering. Not only that, but individual human beings were held to be subject to these laws. A fully defined science of man was considered to be just within reach. While many of his contemporaries welcomed this new materialist philosophy in the conviction that it would usher in a better world, Dostoyevsky looked upon such developments with horror. He did not believe that human beings could or should be approached in this deterministic fashion. He stressed the essential and irreducible uniqueness of each individual. Materialist philosophy turned people into objects, into automatons.

Laing was interested in Dostoyevsky's *Notes from the Underground*, which put forward a powerful critique of positivistic concepts of man. Dostoyevsky argued in favour of free will and felt that determinist accounts of man offered a deeply impoverished and essentially false description of what it was to be human. The main character observes:

> Science itself will teach man . . . that he really has neither free will nor caprice and never did, and that he himself is nothing more than a kind of piano key or organ peg . . . everything he does, he does not at all according to his wanting, but according to the laws of Nature. Consequently, one only has to discover these laws of Nature and then man will not answer for his acts . . . All human actions, of course, will then be calculated by these laws, like a table of logarithms . . .[60]

Such a perspective chimed with Laing's own views. He praised Dostoyevsky because, as he commented in one of his notebooks, he 'resolutely refused to petrify man, to turn him into stone, or even a piano'. As we know, Laing devoted much of his writing to exposing the reductionist, scientific models of *his* day. Dostoyevsky was concerned that the materialist conceptions of man promoted by nineteenth century thinkers left no room for God. Man was perceived as the summit of creation. While many of Dostoyevsky's peers saw the new materialist philosophies as triumphantly sweeping away the older religious views, Dostoyevsky was appalled. In his novels he contrasted the supposedly sophisticated intellectuals who were contemptuous of religion with the supposedly simple, common people who retained their faith. The intellectuals were influenced by fashionable ideas derived from the European Enlightenment and which were being discussed in the salons of Paris and Berlin. The common people still held to the older, and, for Dostoyevsky, more authentic, teachings of the Christian Church. This conflict troubled Laing throughout his life. Laing criticized mainstream psychiatry because it did not engage with the spiritual aspects of life. Indeed, Laing felt that psychiatry viewed religious experience as pathological in itself. In his openness to a divine account of human experience, Laing sided with Dostoyevsky's common people rather than with the intellectuals.

---

[59] Thompson, D.O. (2002). 'Dostoyevsky and science'. In Leatherbarrow, W.J. (ed.), *The Cambridge Companion to Dostoyevsky*. Cambridge University Press, Cambridge, pp. 191–211.

[60] Ibid., p. 196. Quoted by author.

Laing and Dostoyevsky shared certain similarities in their political outlook. In his opposition to the socialist and utilitarian ideas of his day and his support for the authority of religion, Dostoyevsky is usually regarded as being a conservative, Likewise, Laing referred to himself as a 'conservative anarchist'. Both were suspicious of socialism or indeed of any grand-encompassing system that emphasized the mass over the individual. Both rejected the idea that reorganizing society along rationalist lines would lead to universal happiness. Dostoyevsky objected to the idea that human beings were rational creatures who only needed to be shown their true rational interests to follow them. If a rational society was created, Dostoyevsky declared, people would bring it tumbling down. Laing believed that revolution sprang from within: from changes in the individual rather than in the wider society. Both were critical of any system which discarded God. In his classic work, *The Devils*, Dostoyevsky articulated his vision of the moral implications of a political theory that denied the existence of God. It was a novel that greatly interested Laing. As he wrote in one of his notebooks:

> Dostoyevsky is continually seeking to demonstrate that if man takes to the finite relative as a flight from the Absolute—and displaces on to the finite what properly belongs to the Absolute,—this is Nihilism. It leads not to progress, humanism, but to the negation of man. If man seeks to become the ground of his own existence, he makes himself God. Socialism, humanism, etc. are nihilistic—they lead to man's own self destruction.[61]

In this we see Laing's support of Dostoyevsky's view that a philosophy that denies the transcendent leads man to believing that he has replaced God. The character in *The Devils*, who is the philosophical embodiment of this line of thought, is Kirilov. Laing saw Kirilov's suicide as a 'ghastly, fantastic caricature of the crucifixion of God'.[62] In his notebook, he went on:

> It is atheistic humanism lived out to the ultimate absurdity. K[irilov] kills himself on behalf of all men. To demonstrate that everything is possible for man. That is his vision. History can now continue without God. K[irilov]'s sacrifice is the existential demonstration that man is now god [*sic*]. It is the final assertion of the self-sufficient self-will. It is necessary in order to render God's sacrifice unnecessary. It is the final rejection of Grace.[63]

Although Dostoyevsky is seen as conservative, he championed the common people. Unlike Tolstoy and Turgenev, whose novels are set amongst the upper classes, Dostoyevsky is the poet of the urban poor, of the 'insulted and injured'. In his writing, the voice of the downtrodden is heard and treated seriously. Likewise, a major aim of Laing's work was to allow the voice of the mentally ill to be heard and to be accorded respect. Indeed, Laing and Dostoyevsky had much in common. Both were troubled by matters of belief and wrestled with the subject throughout their lives. Both men were perceived by their peers as mentally imbalanced. In his early years, Dostoyevsky was ridiculed by his fellow writers for his excitable and nervous behaviour, while Laing was regarded as a madman by some of his medical colleagues. Both were interested in

---

[61] MS Laing A223, p. 9.
[62] MS Laing K 14.
[63] Ibid.

the extremities of the mind and shared many similar ideas about the nature of insanity. Both Laing and Dostoyevsky objected to the prevailing materialist philosophy of their day and stressed the irreducible uniqueness of the individual.

Chekhov

Laing remembered that he was very affected by Chekhov's *Ward No. 6* when he read it as a young man.[64] Anton Chekhov, the great Russian playwright and short-story writer, drew on his medical experience to tell a tale set in a grim provincial lunatic asylum.[65] The story charts the career of Dr Andrey Yefimych Ragin, who had originally intended to train as a priest but, as this was vigorously opposed by his father, became a doctor instead, despite having 'never felt any vocation for medicine or, come to that, for any specialized science'. When Ragin takes up his asylum post, his initial response to the hospital is that it is 'an immoral institution, highly injurious to the health of its patients' and that it should be closed down and the patients discharged. However he makes only half-hearted and ineffectual attempts to improve the place and rapidly comes to accept its abuses. Over the years his idealism and enthusiasm are ground down by the immense workload and by a sense of futility about clinical intervention. He stops his daily visits to the wards. Instead Ragin takes up reading, particularly books on history and philosophy, and quaffs continuously from a carafe of vodka, while dreaming of having erudite discussions with intellectuals. On a rare visit to Ward No. 6 he strikes up a conversation with Gromov, a young male patient who appears to be an intellectual and who challenges Ragin's quietist philosophy. Ragin considers that Gromov is the only intelligent man he has met in 20 years of living in the provinces and he takes to visiting him every day. This is perceived by a new member of the asylum staff, Dr Khobotov, and by others as evidence that Dr Ragin is becoming insane. Khotobov is a philistine and the only book he owns is *Latest Prescriptions of the Vienna Clinic 1881*, which 'he invariably takes with him when visiting patients'. This detail reflects Khotobov's exclusively somaticist approach to mental illness. Ragin is summoned before a committee, which includes Dr Khotobov, and asked various questions, such as what day of the week it is. Finally, he is asked if it was true that 'there was a remarkable prophet in Ward No. 6'. Ragin replies: 'Yes, he's a mental patient, but he's an interesting young man'. This seems to the committee to be unequivocal evidence of Ragin's insanity and he is asked no further questions. Ragin suddenly realizes that he has been subject to a psychiatric interview and 'for the first time in his life he felt bitterly sorry for medicine'. He thinks, 'They don't have a clue about psychiatry!' He is left feeling 'outraged and infuriated'. Later, Khotobov will repeatedly try to treat him with potassium bromide and rhubarb pills, much to Ragin's disgust. Eventually, Ragin is admitted to Ward No. 6 and, like all the other inmates, is beaten by the male attendant. In his pain he realizes that: 'it must be precisely this kind of pain that was suffered every day, year in year out, by those people who now appeared like black shadows in the moonlight. How could it be that for more than twenty years

[64] Mullan, *Mad to be Normal*, p. 268.
[65] Chekhov, A. (2002). *Ward No. 6 and Other Stories, 1892–1895*. Penguin Books, London.

he had not known and had not wanted to know this?' The next day he dies of a stroke.

One can see why the story interested Laing. The central character, Dr Ragin, bears some similarity to Laing. Both have spiritual yearnings and are unenthused by science. Both like drinking and are voracious readers. And while both are appalled by the state of the mental hospital, only Laing sought to do something about it. Ragin too easily succumbs to indifference and apathy. One of Chekhov's main points in the story is to stress that if individuals do nothing to alleviate the suffering of their fellow-men, then they deserve to suffer in the same fashion. The story also contains, in the character of Gromov, a portrait of a madman who speaks more sense than his psychiatrist. This is, of course, a typically Laingian trope. One is reminded of the female patient who became his 'mentor' when he first entered the long-stay wards of Gartnavel Hospital. One also thinks of Laing's account of his Army doctor days when he took to visiting a manic patient in his room each night and conversing with him for several hours. Like Ragin, Laing claimed that he found these conversations more illuminating than those he had with his medical colleagues.

In the character of Dr Khotobov, Chekhov describes a physician with a simplistic and crudely physicalist approach to mental suffering: pills are the answer to mental torment. Laing would have sympathized with Ragin's objection to Khotobov's regime of bromide and rhubarb, and he would also have had sympathized with Ragin's condemnation of the psychiatric interview to which he was subjected. Laing often portrayed the psychiatric interview as a means of invalidating the experience of the patient, and he would no doubt have been amused, if not aghast, at the idea that the main proof of Ragin's insanity was that he took an interest in one of his patients and talked to him! This short story by Chekhov dealt with many of the themes that were to preoccupy Laing in his subsequent career.

Kafka

In *The Divided Self*, Franz Kafka appears as the patron saint of the schizoid condition. He receives no less than six mentions, and early in the book Laing uses Kafka and his fictional world to illustrate what he calls the 'basic existential position of ontological insecurity', which, for Laing, characterizes the schizoid experience. In Kafka's work, characters have no firm sense of themselves as 'real' people, interacting with other 'real' people in a 'real' world. Laing draws on the views of the American literary critic, Lionel Trilling, to compare Kafka's world with the 'ontologically secure' world of Shakespeare, where no matter how grim life becomes, characters can at least hold on the their belief in themselves as *bona fide* people in a self-evidently tangible world.[66] Kafka's characters, like Laing's schizoid patients, have no such comfort.

Later in *The Divided Self*, Laing makes several references to a short story by Kafka, called 'Conversation with the suppliant', which, in the years leading up to his first

---

[66] Laing, *The Divided Self,* pp. 40–2.

book, he was to read and analyse.[67] For Laing, this story gives a stark account of the schizoid existence. Laing quotes the suppliant as saying, 'There has never been a time in which I have been convinced from within myself that I am alive.' This, as Laing sees it, is a clear expression of ontological insecurity. The suppliant's aim in life is to gain evidence of his own aliveness and of the realness of the world. As *his* world is not real, he must try to become the object in the world of other people. Hence his statement, which Laing quotes: 'it is the aim of my life to get people to look at me'.[68] Later in *The Divided Self*, Laing points to the similarities between the utterances of a number of his schizoid patients and that of the suppliant.[69]

Laing sees Kafka, himself, as 'schizoid',[70] and, as such, maintains that he had an uneasy relationship with the outside world. According to Laing, Kafka had the constant choice of remaining detached in order to preserve his inner world, or engaging with life but at the price of great anxiety. Laing states that Kafka knew this dilemma very well and had confessed that 'it was only through his anxiety that he could participate in life, and, for, this reason, he would not be without it'.[71] Laing takes a direct quotation from Kafka to further illustrate this schizoid dilemma:

> You can hold yourself back from the sufferings of the world, this is something you are free to do and is accord with your nature, but perhaps precisely this holding back is the only suffering that you might be able to avoid.[72]

Laing, however, had reservations about Kafka's work, as he conceded in a notebook entry:

> I cannot bring myself into the intricate complexity of Kafka's minute and tenacious scrutiny of the world—not an 'active' process, rather in his case, allowing or letting the world come to him.[73]

As a young man, Laing was more interested in engaging with the world, as the accounts of him in his student days attest.

Camus

Although he took the side of Sartre in his famous dispute with Camus, Laing was nevertheless interested in and influenced by the Algerian writer. As a student he had written an essay on the symbolism of the sea in the work of Camus and Kafka, but his mother had destroyed it.[74] Fortunately another student work which made reference to

---

[67] MS Laing K13. R.D. Laing: Notebook, 1951–1960, no page numbers. The story, 'Conversation with a suppliant' can be found in Kafka, F. (1953). W*edding Preparations in the Country and Other Stories*. Penguin Books, London, pp. 77–83.

[68] Laing, *The Divided Self*, p.116.

[69] Ibid., p. 128 and p. 159.

[70] Ibid., p. 95.

[71] Ibid., p. 95.

[72] Ibid., p. 82.

[73] MS Laing K14, p. 2.

[74] Mullan, *Mad to be Normal*, p. 269.

Camus has survived. This was Laing's essay, 'Health and happiness', in which he discussed Camus's novel, *The Plague*. Laing was struck by a comment by Tarron, one of the characters in the novel, that everyone carried the plague within themselves and that they had to be ever-watchful that they did not pass it on to others—'health, integrity, purity (if you like) is a product of the human will, of a vigilance that must to not falter'.[75] Laing continued to be interested in the novel, and he quoted an excerpt from it at the beginning of his autobiography *Wisdom, Madness and Folly*, in which the narrator, Dr Rieux concludes:

> None the less, he knew that the tale he had to tell could not be one of a final victory. It could only be a record of what had had to be done, and what assuredly would have to be done again in the never-ending fight against terror, and its restless onslaughts, despite their personal afflictions, by all who, while unable to be saints, but refusing to bow down to pestilences, strive their utmost to be healers.[76]

It is clear that Laing felt that this was an apt description of himself and of his aspirations as a doctor. In the story, Dr Rieux wrestles with questions which tormented Laing throughout his career. First, there was the question of one's response to human suffering. Earlier in the book, Rieux tells Tarron that he was still upset by the death of patients. He says of his first encounter with mortality:

> ... I saw that I could never get hardened to it. I was young then, and I was outraged by the whole scheme of things ... I've never managed to get used to seeing people die.[77]

Rieux's response anticipates that of Laing as a medical student. A sensitive young man, Laing was both moved but also angered by some of the terrible cases of human affliction he witnessed in the medical and surgical wards of Glasgow hospitals. Laing anguished over how such things were possible in a world created by God. Dr Rieux, however, is an atheist and is critical of those Christians who laud the 'excellence' of suffering, as the priest, Paneloux, does in a sermon to the beleaguered town, which we have considered in Chapter 5. Later, when Laing qualified and was working in psychiatric wards he continued to be 'outraged by the whole scheme of things'.

Laing was also interested in Camus's essay, 'The myth of Sisyphus' and the concept of the absurd. The absurd related to the indifference of the world to the hopes and aspirations of human beings. Man does not want to die but there is nothing more certain than he will. Laing felt that Camus's idea of the absurd had been 'grossly misunderstood' and observed:

> It states the paradox between the world of man, and the rest of the Universe. The rest of the world is not hostile to us, we are not integrated within a stupendous extra-human Destiny which is reaching fulfilment in some inscrutable fashion—the world is an alien place, where there is to be found no answer to our questions, or solace in our trouble ... We are strangers, outsiders.[78]

---

[75] Quoted in Laing, 'Health and happiness', MS Laing A64, pp. 6–7.

[76] Quoted by Laing at beginning of *Wisdom, Madness and Folly*.

[77] Camus, A. (1960). *The Plague* (trans. Gilbert, S.). Penguin Books, London, p. 107 (originally published in French, 1947).

[78] Undated letter by Laing to Marcelle Vincent during his time at Catterick. Quoted in Mullan, *R.D. Laing: Creative Destroyer*, pp. 86–8.

Laing went on to write that by refusing to accept religious explanations or any theory which justified the human condition, Camus held that we discover an essential identity with other human beings. He wondered though whether it was possible to live without hope, without illusions.[79]

Artaud

Antonin Artaud, the French actor and writer, who championed what he called 'the Theatre of Cruelty', occupies a suitably dramatic place in the story of Laing's early development. It was the reading of one of Artaud's essays when he was a 20-year-old medical student that was to have a profound effect on Laing's attitude to madness and psychiatry, or so he was later to claim. Laing recalled that it 'came as a revelation to him and played a decisive part in his development'.[80] The essay was entitled, 'Van Gogh, the man suicided by society', and Laing had read it when it appeared in the January 1948 edition of *Horizon*.[81] It was written in the aftermath of Artaud's discharge from Rodez asylum in Aveyron, where he had been admitted several years before, suffering from a severe psychotic breakdown. The essay represents Artaud's attack on conventional psychiatry and on the wider culture for its inability to cope with men of genius (like himself). The essay appealed to Laing's notion of the gifted individual being driven mad by an uncomprehending society. It is worth considering some of the sentiments that Artaud expressed in the piece. It began:

> You can say all you want about the mental health of Van Gogh who, during his lifetime, cooked only one of his hands, and other than that did no more than cut off his left ear . . .
>
> For it isn't man but the world that has become abnormal . . .
>
> So a sick society invented psychiatry to defend itself against the investigations of certain visionaries whose faculties of divination disturbed it . . .
>
> Faced with Van Gogh's lucidity, always active, psychiatry becomes nothing but a den of gorillas, so obsessed and persecuted that it can only use a ridiculous terminology to palliate the most frightful anxiety and human suffocation . . .
>
> And what is a genuine lunatic?
>
> He is a man who prefers to go mad, in the social sense of the word, rather than forfeit a certain higher idea of human honour.
>
> That's how society strangled all those it wanted to get rid of, or wanted to protect itself from, and put them in asylums, because they refused to be accomplices to a kind of lofty will.
>
> For a lunatic is a man that society does not wish to hear but wants to prevent from uttering certain unbearable truths . . .
>
> It is almost impossible to be a doctor and an honest man, but shamefully impossible to be a psychiatrist without bearing the stigma of the most indisputable insanity at the same time . . .

[79] Letter from Laing to Marcelle Vincent, undated. Quoted in Mullan, *R.D. Laing: Creative Destroyer*, pp. 68.

[80] Esslin, M. (1976). *Artaud*. Fontana/Collins, Glasgow, p. 61.

[81] Clay, *R.D. Laing*, p. 30; Hirschman, J. (1965). *Antonin Artaud Anthology*. City Lights Books, San Francisco, pp. 135–63.

Artaud goes on to blame Van Gogh's physician Dr Gachet for the artist's suicide. In his book on Artaud,[82] Martin Esslin, who sought Laing's psychiatric opinion of the writer, suggested that the Frenchman was, in part, writing about himself. He had spent nine years in asylums and was pleading his own cause as well as that of Van Gogh. Artaud claimed that psychiatrists were trying to kill men of genius, but he also thought that he had been the victim of a vast occult conspiracy which had put a spell on him. This spell affected other men of genius, such as Baudelaire, Kierkegaard, and Holderin. Esslin suggests that, from the beginning of his career, Artaud had taken a pride in being different from others, in having some kind of nervous debility. As Esslin writes:

> And as he never saw himself as, and never wanted to be, a run-of-mill, *normal* human being, as he was proud of his separateness, his claim to be exceptional, in fact a genius, the issue between Artaud and society never really amounted to a debate whether he was 'mad' or not ... but merely whether society was entitled to incarcerate him for nine years ... .[83]

There is much in Artaud's article, though expressed in an extreme fashion, which Laing was to articulate later in his own work. There is the notion that the talented and the visionary are not accepted by the dull, uncomprehending masses. There is also the idea that psychiatry has been set up by society as a kind of police force to shut-up and shut-away the original and the challenging. There is the time-old conceit that it is the world rather than the individual that is mad. On a personal basis, Laing seemed to share Artaud's desire to be different and non-conforming: it was evidence of one's authenticity. And what of Artaud's bleak assessment of the role of the psychiatrist—a shameful impossibility, as he put it? Records suggest that Artaud's own psychiatrist at the Rodez asylum, Dr Gaston Ferdiere, approached him with great humanity and respect. Dr Ferdiere treated Artaud as a friend, invited him round for lunch, gave him a small room of his own, encouraged him to draw and lent him books.[84] However, Ferdiere did prescribe several courses of ECT. Critics have seen this as an act of barbarity, while supporters have pointed out that Artaud actually improved after undergoing this treatment and was discharged following nine years in various asylums. This episode in the history of psychiatry does underline several dilemmas for Laing, and indeed, for anyone with an interest in the care of the mentally ill. Was a humane psychiatry possible? Could it be achieved within the framework of orthodox psychiatry? Were physical treatments necessarily barbaric? Or was blanket opposition to them a sign of personal prejudice which deprived patients such as Artaud of the chance to be released from hospital? Laing's subsequent career would see him changing his mind on these questions, working within and without the psychiatric system, inveighing against physical therapies and, latterly, in his BBC radio interview with Anthony Clare, accepting that medication might have a role to play.

---

[82] Esslin, *Artaud*. Chapter 5 has a discussion of Artaud's sanity.

[83] Ibid., pp. 97–8.

[84] Ibid., pp. 53–6.

The Unquiet Grave

One of Laing's favourite books was *The Unquiet Grave* by Palinurus, a pseudonym for Cyril Connolly, the editor of *Horizon*.[85] A former colleague, James Hood, suggests that Laing was drawn to the book in the wake of his grief over the death of his best friend, Douglas Hutchison.[86] The book, which appeared in 1944, became a classic and it is easy to see why it appealed to Laing. Dealing with angst, melancholia, suicide, and loss, Connolly sought to make sense of his own personal turmoil by wide-ranging references to the great writers, thinkers, and artists of Europe and beyond. The book consists of a series of fragments, containing extensive quotations from such luminaries as Adler, Aristotle, Baudelaire, Blake, Buddha, Chuang Tsu, Dali, Flaubert, Freud, Heidegger, Kierkegaard, Leopardi, Montaigne, Nietzsche, Pascal, Picasso, Rimbaud, and Voltaire. The names would all have been familiar to Laing and indeed they provide a sketch of the cultural preoccupations of intellectuals in mid-twentieth century Britain. Like Connolly, Laing was fond of crowding his texts with the names of intellectual heavyweights. They were both voracious readers and neither was shy of advertising their erudition. In his later works such as *The Facts of Life* and *The Politics of Experience and The Bird of Paradise*, Laing also emulated Connolly's fragmentary technique. Connolly begins the book by asserting that 'the true function of a writer is to produce a masterpiece'.[87] Needless to say, this was a sentiment to which Laing readily assented: it was his ambition that his first work would be one of greatness.

Connolly writes of the uncertainty of modern man, for whom neither religion nor politics holds the answer: 'when I consider what I believe, which I can do only by proceeding from what I do not, I seem in a minority of one, and yet I know that there are thousands like me: Liberals without a belief in progress, Democrats who despise their fellow-men, Pagans who must live by Christian morals, Intellectuals who cannot find the intellect sufficient—unsatisfied Materialists, we are as common as clay'.[88] Laing, as we have seen, expressed similar thoughts in his notebooks. Another passage by Connolly anticipates Laing's tormented battles with spiritual versus materialist explanations of humanity:

> We can either have a spiritual or a materialist view of life. If we believe in the spirit then we make an assumption which permits a whole chain down to a belief in fairies, witches, astrology, black magic, ghosts, and treasure-divining . . . On the other hand a completely materialist view leads to its own excesses, such as a belief in Behaviourism, in the economic basis of art, in the social foundation of ethics and the biological nature of psychology . . .[89]

[85] Palinurs (1944). *The Unquiet Grave*. First published by Horizon in 1944, Revised edition, 1945. Published in London by Penguin, 1967.

[86] Hood, J. (2001). 'The young R.D. Laing: a personal memoir and some hypotheses'. In Steiner R and Johns, J. (eds), *Within Time & Beyond Time. A Festschrift for Pearl King*. Karnac, London, pp. 39–53.

[87] Palinurs, *The Unquiet Grave*, p. 19.

[88] Ibid., p. 25.

[89] Ibid., pp. 53–4.

The book also makes mention of that characteristically Laingian concept, the 'false self', which Connolly saw in the context of retaining one's individuality. He writes:

> Birthday resolution: From now on specialize; never again make any concession to the ninety-nine parts of you which are like everybody else at the expense of the one which is unique. Never listen to the False Self talking.[90]

In the book, Connolly railed against those who would undermine the irreducibility of man.[91] To the physiologists, he said: 'I am not a cell, but myself'. To the sociologists he said: 'those who lack the herd-instinct are generally in advance of the herd which is conservative, stupid, intolerant and bourgeois'. And to the psychologists he said: 'those who have been all their lives used to intellectual isolation are the ones best fitted to remain isolated; they grow adjusted to their mal-adjustment'. In like fashion, for example in his student essay, 'Health and Happiness', Laing was to extol the superiority of the independent individual over the grey, unimaginative majority.

Another major parallel between the two writers occurred towards the end of the book, when Connolly argued that madness was sometimes the solution to an individual's life-long problems.[92] In fact, he asserted, the lives of the mad were often 'rich and crowded above the normal'. Connolly declared: 'Insanity beckons us to fulfil high destinies and to recognize our paraphrenic vocation'. Laing's later pronouncements that insanity represented an exalted state had many precedents.

Other writers

Laing read many other writers, but did not necessarily make extended notes about them. In *The Divided Self*, he compared a female patient to Tinkerbell from J.D. Barrie's *Peter Pan*, because, like the fairy creature, she needed someone else to believe in her existence. He was obviously intrigued with this character, and, in one of his notebooks, he recorded: '"If I did not exist, God would not exist". Tinker Bell in Peter Pan'.[93] Laing was interested in Thurber's short story, 'The Secret Life of Walter Mitty'. One can see the appeal: a character who lives in a world of fantasy to compensate for the drabness of his existence offered a comic version of the schizoid position. Laing was also intrigued by Thomas Mann's uncompleted novella, *The Confessions of Felix Krull, Confidence Man*.[94] The novella told the story of a con man who uses his ability to take on different personas in order to exploit others. Felix adopts a variety of masks to ease his way into society circles. He states: 'The real I could not be identified because it actually did not exist'.[95] Laing had a life-long interest in deception, and one of his first papers, as we have seen, was on 'On the Recognition of Simulated and

---

[90] Ibid., p. 123.

[91] Ibid., pp. 130–1.

[92] Ibid., pp. 150–1.

[93] MS Laing K12. R.D. Laing. Notebook, 1951–1952, p. 99.

[94] Mann, T. (1958). *Confessions of Felix Krull, Confidence Man* (trans. Lindley, D.). Penguin Books, London.

[95] Ibid., p. 205.

Functional Deafness'.[96] Krull describes how as a youth he had fooled his doctor that he was ill in order to be excused from school. Later he uses his skills to convince an army doctor that he suffers from epilepsy and, thus, should be exempted from military service. Laing referred to Felix Krull in *The Facts of the Life*, when he discussed a Glasgow surgeon he had encountered in his training. The surgeon, clad in pin-striped trousers, arrives at the hospital to do his Monday ward round and confers with his registrar. Laing writes:

> He reminded me of Felix Krull, Thomas Mann's confidence trickster, who makes his way around different countries of Europe, with two or three words of French, two or three words of Italian, and gets by wherever he goes without having to say practically anything.[97]

Laing obviously found the surgeon to be a phoney, going through a medical ritual without having anything meaningful to contribute. He was also interested in the ways an individual could deceive *themselves*. As we have seen, the existential notion of 'bad faith' held that individuals could lead 'inauthentic' lives by not being true to themselves.

Laing had read *Auto Da Fe* by the Nobel Prize winning novelist, Elias Canetti.[98] The book is interesting because it contains a portrait of a psychiatrist, Dr George Kein, who is strikingly similar to Laing in his approach to patients and in his rather romanticized view of madness. Unlike his predecessor at the Institute, who had 'embraced official psychiatry with the obstinacy of a madman',[99] Dr Kein 'treated his patients as if they were human beings'.[100] He listened to their stories. He laughed and cried with them. He claimed that he learnt an immense amount from the mentally ill. They 'enriched him with their unique experiences . . . their ideas were never reduced to paper, they flowed from a heart which beat outside realities, on which they fell like alien conquerors'.[101] Having immersed himself in the life of his patients, Kein comes to prefer their mad worlds to those of the 'sane', which he increasingly finds flat and colourless in comparison. He had become a psychiatrist 'out of admiration for the greatness of the distracted'[102] and he has a 'burning sympathy for those men who had so far separated themselves from others as to pass for mad'.[103] Dr Kein's assistants think that he relates so well to the mad because he is half-mad himself. This was a charge that was sometimes levelled at Laing too.

Another book that Laing read was H.G. Wells' *War of the World*, about which he observed, 'science fiction defines the form of the images of our terror'. These were

[96] MS Laing A518. Lieutenant Murray Brookes and Captain Ronald D. Laing, 'On the Recognition of Simulated and Functional Deafness'. Unpublished manuscript.

[97] Laing, R.D. (1976). *The Facts of Life*. Penguin, London, p. 106.

[98] Glasgow University Library Special Collection. Laing's personal library 621. Canetti, E. (1946). *Auto Da Fe* (trans. Wedgwood, C.V.). Jonathan Cape, London.

[99] Canetti, E. (1978). *Auto Da Fe* (trans. Wedgwood, C.V.). Pan Books, London, p. 363.

[100] Ibid., p. 364.

[101] Ibid., p. 365.

[102] Ibid., p. 370.

[103] Ibid., p.371.

alien creatures with whom human beings made unsuccessful attempts to communicate. They threatened unimaginable destruction. The only response was to destroy them, but this was impossible because against them, 'the cross, nor the Atom Bomb is of any avail'.[104]

There were writers that Laing did not care for. For example, in a commentary on *The Portrait of a Lady* by Henry James he wrote:

> I simply have not the sustained passionate interest in anyone—or at least in those aspects of people which are James' preoccupation—to write at such length . . . but there is too little of a sharpness, of an edge—it tails off to the stale, sterile, stuporose ennui . . . Isabel, as James sees her, does not seem to me of great importance . . .

Laing's choice of books reflects the preoccupations of the mid-twentieth culture in which he grew up. His relation to Scottish culture is more curious. His library shows that he certainly read works from his native land but his notebooks and early writings do not suggest that he was hugely influenced by them, at least, not overtly. A classic Scottish work that one might have expected to feature prominently in Laing's reading was James Hogg's *Private Memoirs and Confessions of a Justified Sinner*, dealing as it does with madness, religion, and divided selves. However, Hogg's 1824 work remained largely overlooked until it was re-discovered and hailed by the French writer, André Gide in 1947. Whether or not Laing was aware of Hogg's novel is difficult to determine, but he never seems to have made any reference to it. We will consider Laing's relation to Scottish culture in more detail in the final chapter.

Laing's relationship with the arts echoes that of Freud. Both were widely read in European literature and this shaped how they thought and wrote about mental disturbance. Both were lauded for their prose style, and while Freud was wary that such praise might detract from what he saw as his essentially scientific mission, Laing was pleased when his writing attracted the regard of the literary world. He was grateful to win the approval of Ted Hughes and William Burroughs, and was delighted when Christopher Isherwood told him that he would include the last two pages of *The Divided Self* in any anthology of English prose.[105] Laing's work was to inspire such authors as Doris Lessing, David Edgar, Peter Schaffer, J.G. Ballard, Will Self, and Allen Ginsberg, as well as a host of Scottish writers, and he, himself, was to go on to write poetry, and to appear as a character in a novel, *Zone of the Interior* by Clancy Sigal. It could be argued that the work of Laing, like Freud, has appealed more to those in the humanities than in the sciences.

The first part of this book has examined Laing's quest to master diverse but interconnected fields of knowledge in order to become an intellectual and make a contribution to the understanding mental disorder. In the second part we will look at how Laing drew on this knowledge when he entered the world of clinical psychiatry and how it shaped his therapeutic practice.

---

[104] MS Laing K16.
[105] Ibid., p. 360.

Part II

Laing and practice

Chapter 7

Laing in the Army

In the first half of the book we considered Laing's engagement with psychiatric theory, the humanities, and religion. In the second half, we will examine Laing's clinical practice, beginning with his days in the British Army, following him to his posts in Glasgow mental hospitals, and ending with his time in London and the Tavistock Clinic. Commentators have wondered what Laing actually *did* in therapy,[1] and some have speculated as to what he *might* have done. For example, Burston tells us:

> One of the hallmarks of Laing's approach was that he never demanded anything from patients, either silence or speech, and that he did not interrogate them as a conventional psychiatrist would have. On the contrary, he maintained a relaxed, nonthreatening posture in their presence and allowed them to open up their thoughts, feelings, and fantasies at their own pace.[2]

Kotowicz maintained that Laing had an 'effortless facility to engage in the barmiest of conversations . . . he had no trouble whatsoever in meeting a psychotic on his/her territory'.[3] Kirsner claimed: 'When Laing visited the back wards during his medical training in Glasgow, he simply could hear and understand what the schizophrenics were saying. He just had an uncanny ability to be able to hear the communications.'[4]

These rather idealized portraits of Laing at work appear to be based on what he *said* he did in therapy. In a classic paper on the history of medicine, Erwin Ackerknecht emphasized that we need to distinguish theory from practice: 'what a doctor thought and wrote' from 'what a doctor did'.[5] The medical historian, Akihito Suzuki, has suggested that the contrast between theory and practice is probably at its most extreme in psychiatry.[6]

In the case of Laing, we are fortunate that archival records shed considerable light on his practice. Thanks to his habit of assiduously retaining his medical notes, we have extensive primary source material that helps us to build up a picture of how Laing

1 Schneider, K.J. (2000). 'R.D. Laing's existential-humanistic practice: what was he actually *doing*?' *Psychoanalytic Review*, **87**, 591–99.
2 Burston, D. (1996). *The Wing of Madness*. Harvard University Press, Cambridge, Massachusetts, p. 33.
3 Kotowicz, Z. (1997). *R.D. Laing and the Paths of Anti-Psychiatry*. Routledge, London, p. 73.
4 Kirsner, D. (2005). 'Laing and philosophy'. In Raschid, S. (ed.), *R.D. Laing. Contemporary Perspectives*. Free Association Books, London, pp. 154–74.
5 Ackerknecht, E.H. (1967). 'A plea for a "Behaviourist" approach in writing the history of medicine'. *Journal of the History of Medicine and Allied Sciences*, **22**, 211–14.
6 Suzuki, A. (2006). *Madness at Home. The Psychiatrist, the Patient, and the Family in England, 1820–1860*. University of California Press, Berkeley and Los Angeles.

behaved in clinical encounters. We have access to case notes, court reports, and Laing's own contemporaneous observations and records. Of course these documents do not necessarily represent the 'truth' of the matter, as they were shaped by the circumstances and constraints under which they were written. However, they do have the advantage of immediacy in that they were composed at the time Laing saw the patient and they reveal his first impressions, undistorted by retrospective embellishment or editing. These documents can also be compared with the many individual case descriptions, which subsequently appeared in his books and which were based on these early clinical interviews. We see Laing in a variety of psychiatric settings as he tries to apply theory to clinical practice. We see him utilizing standard psychoanalytical methods, as well as recommending orthodox physical treatments, such as medication and ECT. We see him questioning these approaches, and experimenting with social therapies and existential analysis. In his personal notebooks, he puzzles over the patients he is seeing and draws on religion, philosophy, and literature to make sense of it all. It should be stressed that these clinical documents are taken from the early stages of Laing's career, when he was learning his craft. As he mastered the orthodox methods of interviewing patients, he felt free to be more spontaneous in clinical encounters and to question whether technique could sometimes hamper rather than aid therapy.

Laing felt that his experience in the Army heralded his first serious reservations about the nature of psychiatry. He wondered if his chosen discipline actually made patients worse, and he began to feel uncomfortable in his role as a psychiatrist. In an autobiographical passage written when he was about 40, Laing claimed that when he first started working with psychotic patients he found that, to some extent, he seemed to understand and see their point of view more than the psychiatric point of view he had been trained to adopt.[7] He admitted to being somewhat alarmed by this development. He also felt that such an attitude would be regarded as heretical by orthodox psychiatrists and that, at this early stage in his career, he would have to be careful to whom he expressed his views if he did not want to ruin his prospects. Of course this was a retrospective assessment and Laing may have exaggerated the differences in his attitude to that of others. However, it is clear he felt that there were serious problems in applying psychiatric theory to the patients he met. Elsewhere, Laing observed: 'Psychiatry, for me, quickly became primarily the study of the collapse of relatedness between human beings, for whatever reasons.'[8]

Army psychiatry

We are able to compose a picture of Laing as an Army psychiatrist because we have access to his hand-written notes and the many typed patient reports he filed during his period of office.[9] At Netley, Laing was a lieutenant in the Royal Army Medical Corps and his post was 'Medical Officer'. He was based on the Psychoneurotic Wing,

[7] MS Laing A662. Draft notes by R.D. Laing.
[8] Research Fellowship Application to Foundations' Fund for Research in Psychiatry by Laing, 15 March 1960.
[9] MS Laing DB85. Notes taken by R.D. Laing.

which had 200 beds, and for a period of 3 months he was in joint charge of the Deep Insulin Unit.[10] In addition he completed reports, in which he assessed whether soldiers were fit to continue in military service, or whether they should be discharged. On occasions, he also saw the wives of soldiers or staff. All Laing's reports were countersigned by his superior officer, a Lieutenant-Colonel J.F.D. Murphy, who was a 'Senior Specialist in Psychiatry'. Thus, even if Laing had concerns about the psychiatric approach at Netley, he would have been constrained by his junior position from objecting too vociferously. His diaries during this period certainly show him struggling with the dictates of military psychiatry, and in his autobiography he described his unease at his work. However, he did not adopt an attitude of outright rejection. As he recalled:

> From pretty well the very beginning, I *was* interested in learning the clinical method of a psychiatric medical examination. I felt that I had to internalise and make myself competent in what was going on. I never had any temptation to be swallowed up by it, but I also didn't have a simplistic contempt for everything that serious and intelligent people had brought to bear on this subject.[11]

However, the claim that Laing was practically the only Army psychiatrist who did not want mentally ill soldiers returned to active service is surely erroneous.[12] On a purely practical level, men with psychotic disorders would have been a liability, and the Army was keen that they did *not* return to the normal duties. From Laing's reports, it is clear that such men were sent to either military or civilian psychiatric hospitals. In these situations the decision was often clear-cut: the psychotic soldier was simply not capable of performing his duties. It was much more of a problem with soldiers who fell into the group exhibiting 'hysterical', 'psychopathic', or 'neurotic' symptoms, or who were simply 'malingerers'. It was often difficult to decide what was going on with such soldiers, and decisions had to be made whether to take a firm stance and send them back to active service, or whether they were so unstable that they should be discharged from the Army. Laing's reports suggest that he was quite able to make pragmatic decisions about such men. As he later observed, if it was felt that a soldier should be removed from active service, it was an easy matter to diagnose him as having a 'personality disorder'.[13]

When he transferred to Catterick, Laing was promoted to the rank of captain and had more clinical autonomy. He was in charge of a 16-bedded Neurosis Unit as well as a Detention Unit. He was involved in 'Intake Selection' at various centres in Carlisle, Newcastle, and Durham. He examined Army personnel who were in prison, wrote psychiatric reports on those awaiting court-martial, conducted outpatient clinics, and was an acting neurologist for the RAF.[14] In a letter to Marcelle Vincent written during

---

[10] Unarchived application by Laing for post of Registrar at Royal Mental Hospital, Glasgow, 23 September 1953.

[11] Mullan, *Mad to be Normal,* p. 316.

[12] Burston, *The Wing of Madness,* p. 34.

[13] Evans, *R.D. Laing. The Man,* pp. 38–9.

[14] Research Fellowship Application, p. 2.

his time at Catterick, Laing described his work.[15] He reported that he had to see a lot of the Army's 'bad boys', who tried to act 'daft' by cutting their wrists, tearing their clothes, or smashing up their environment. There was a detention ward for those that were deemed to need 'medical observation'. He was also asked to see any soldier who had a criminal history, in order to judge whether they were likely to continue their life of crime in the Army. If it was judged that they were, Laing discharged them. He wrote that his role was not to 'treat' such people, and, in any case, he did not think treatment was appropriate. These criminal types were the products of poverty, domestic abuse, and inadequate education. The appropriate response, he averred, was political: the reordering of society. However Laing had no faith that such a response would materialize, and he felt it was Utopian to think otherwise. In his autobiography, Laing wrote: 'The decisions I had been called upon to make . . . entailed all sorts of man management, administration, organisational institutional power and structure, that had nothing to do with medicine'.[16]

In an interview with Bob Mullan[17] about his military days, Laing stated that the Army was not interested in resolving the 'rather scholastic clinical niceties' as to whether a soldier was malingering. The Army had two considerations: the morale of the Army, which was affected if there were too many soldiers who did not want to be there; and ensuring that it was not too easy to get discharged on medical grounds, especially as it meant that the person would then be entitled to a pension for the rest of their lives.

The Army reports

Judging from his reports, the majority of men Laing saw suffered from neurotic disorders. He diagnosed numerous cases of 'hysteria' and 'anxiety', but there were also occasional cases of 'psychopathic personality' and 'paranoid schizophrenia'.

Of one soldier, Laing wrote: 'He is full of reasoned but idealistic critism [sic] of the Army, of society & people. He hardly accepts their consequences: or reflects on the practical means of amending affairs'.[18] He was given a diagnosis of 'hysterical amnesia' and returned to duty. There was another 'awkward' patient, whom the later Laing might have championed because he displayed a mixture of rebellion and religious preoccupation. However, in the context of the Army psychiatric report, Laing adopted a rather more orthodox perspective:

> Since the day of arrival at Unit he has refused to wear uniform or to obey orders. He was brought to the camp under escort as he refused to report for Military Service . . . He accounts for his own indifference by his confidence & trust in God. He says the Army has no authority over him, only God has authority . . . He never experienced a dramatic

---

[15] Letter by Laing to Marcelle Vincent from Catterick, undated, in Mullan, *Creative Destroyer*, pp. 86–9.

[16] Laing, R.D. (1985). *Wisdom, Madness and Folly*. Canongate, Edinburgh (1998 reprint), p. 120.

[17] Mullan, *Mad to be Normal*, p. 129.

[18] MS Laing DB85. Report on R., 5 November 1951.

conversion but for over a year in his early teens he found a 'change' was taking place in him. For some time he was puzzled and then he realised it was because he was becoming a Xian [Christian]. . .[19]

However, Laing was clearly intrigued by him and wrote: 'His cast of thought is unusual and eccentric. His "world" is structured differently from the statistically normal person.' Laing was to remain especially concerned about 'statistical' definitions of normality, seeing them merely as measures of conformity. Laing concluded that, although he would hesitate to diagnose the young man as psychotic, he felt enforced Army service would precipitate a major breakdown. He gave the official diagnosis as 'Psychopathic Personality/with Emotional Abnormality'.

Another observation in the reports anticipates the concerns of the later Laing. Of Corporal W., Laing wrote: 'This man is largely responsible for his actions, but he is in such bad faith with himself that acknowledges few of his desires, and actions as his own . . .'[20] Private C. was given a diagnosis of 'psychopathic personality', which seemed to be based on his 'heavy drinking & homosexual practices'.[21] Laing noted: 'After a number of drinks he always came round to looking for another homo'. He was discharged from the Army. Laing could be blunt in his assessments. Of one soldier, he concluded: '. . . it is evident that this man is a gross hysteric, and a psychopath. There is no prospect of him becoming a useful soldier'.[22]

Laing saw several soldiers with psychotic illnesses. Private H. had been transferred from Singapore and was very disturbed on the ship to England.[23] His talk was incoherent, he was violent, and he had started urinating and defecating in his cell. He constantly repeated the phrase, 'I am the King. I am the f . . . King', and stared vacantly. A diagnosis of 'schizophrenia complex' was made and he was discharged from the Army. Of one soldier, Laing wrote: 'His spoken language is not abnormal though his written production shows the classical stigmata of a schizophrenic & language disorder.'[24] Another patient was also suspected of suffering from schizophrenia. Laing wrote: 'There are many features to suggest that this man is an early schizophrenic—his apathy, his solitariness, his vague woolly philosophising, his propensity for nasty jokes and his distorted sense of humour.'[25]

Of another patient, Laing wrote: 'He believes himself to be "psychotically affected by the Free Masonic way of life" and by "ventric sound radiation attracting the lunar nerves" acting through "the free body field"'.[26] He was given a diagnosis of 'paranoid schizophrenia'. Laing was intrigued by a Corporal M., who had a short history of

---

[19] MS Laing DB85. Report on S., 15 July 1953.
[20] MS Laing DB85. Report on Corporal W., 15 June 1953.
[21] MS Laing DB85. Report on Private C., 26 February 1952.
[22] MS Laing DB85. Report on S., 23 June 1953.
[23] MS Laing DB85. Report on Private H., January 1952.
[24] MS Laing DB85. Report on H., March 1852.
[25] MS Laing DB85. Report on R., 21 May 1952.
[26] MS Laing DB85, Report on H., 11 September 1952.

disordered thinking, was hallucinating, and had ideas of reference.[27] Laing wrote that the underlying mechanism was projection and denial. Laing observed:

> He feels that in his head he has 'two minds'. Some sensations and impressions are registered by the one & some by the other. The result is that many impressions have no meaning for him because their meaning has been registered in one of his minds, and at the time of the impression, the other mind is working. This is really an ingenious theory to explain the fact that his thinking is retarded, memory is poor, he often does not understand what is said to him, or quickly forgets.

This is an early example of Laing trying to find meaning in the utterances of a psychotic patient. However, he made a diagnosis of 'paranoid schizophrenia', considered the corporal was in urgent need of treatment, and transferred him to P wing at Netley—P standing for 'Psychosis'. Of another patient, he commented: 'I feel that the schizoid features about this man are in danger of forming into a frank psychosis.'[28] In another clinical aside about a soldier suffering from schizophrenia, Laing made a comment, which again anticipated his later preoccupations, this time about the pretence of sanity. He wrote: 'This man can pass for normal over quite long periods, yet at other times his behaviour is quite phantastic. One has the impression that he can "play at being normal" when he wishes to.'[29] Laing was to recall: 'I developed an intense desire to be able to ferret out the differences between deception, malingering, self-deception (hysteria), neurosis and psychosis, functional and organic.'[30]

Laing also encountered a patient who was to appear as 'John' in *The Self and Others*[31] and who is also mentioned in his interview with Peter Mezan[32] and in *Wisdom, Madness and Folly*.[33] Laing recounted that he had looked in on 'John', who was manic and was confined to a padded cell. He found that by listening to him, the patient calmed down. Laing began spending time with him and joining him on his manic flights of fancy. 'John' could be anyone he wanted to be merely by snapping his fingers. Laing wrote notes about 'John',[34] and he also mentioned him in a letter to Marcelle Vincent on 10 January 1951:

> I have a patient—a young lad of 18. He has everything he wants—if he wants to be Caesar, or Christ, or Hamlet, or Keats he is—immediately, at will. If he wants to live in Roman times, or in a work of fiction he does so. In his life he has had virtually nothing of the things he had set his heart on; he is well aware that he is regarded as mad but he says why should he not be: now he is anyone he wants to be: has anything he wants: does everything he likes: why should he return to a world where he is unable to satisfy every one of his fundamental desires? Why indeed I find it very difficult to give him an answer.[35]

[27] MS Laing DB85, Report on Corporal M., 8 April 1953.

[28] MS Laing DB85, Report on S., 28 May 1953.

[29] MS Laing DB85, Report on D., 21 April 1953.

[30] Laing, *Wisdom, Madness and Folly*, p. 108.

[31] Laing, *The Self and Others*, pp. 85–7.

[32] Mezan, P. (1972). 'After Freud and Jung, now comes R.D. Laing'. *Esquire*, **77**, 92–7; 160–78.

[33] Laing, *Wisdom, Madness and Folly*, pp. 103–04.

[34] MS Laing A590/1. Draft by R.D. Laing, pp. 6–8.

[35] Letter from Laing to Marcelle Vincent, 10 January 1951, in Mullan, *Creative Destroyer*, pp. 84–5.

In this passage Laing presents the case for being mad, or, at least, its attractions. He goes on to cite Sartre and his notion that we are 'free' to choose insanity. However when he came to write up the case in *The Self and Others*, Laing found the patient's flight into madness unsatisfactory. He referred to Binswanger who called 'the manic life form' a 'swindle'. In this book Laing adopts an existential perspective and observes: 'By his delusional make-believe that he could be anyone he wanted, he swindled himself out of realizing the inauthentic grounds of his despair at this being genuinely possible.'[36] Laing returned to this patient again in the 1969 revised edition of the book, now titled *Self and Others*.[37] The explicit existential perspective is dropped, and Laing now writes: 'One has been tricked out of one's heritage by being told one is a beggar, so one tricks oneself back by pretending one is not really a beggar but really a prince'. In both versions, Laing considers that 'John's' solution is untenable. However, note Laing's theoretical position in the second version: madness is something that involves 'tricking' oneself and 'pretending' to be what one is not. When Laing recounted the story in 1972, he compared 'John's' penchant for living in imagined worlds with the aim of people who took LSD or hashish.[38] They, too, wanted to escape from suffering and from the constrictions imposed upon them by 'the system'. Laing judged that both were pursuing an inauthentic goal. Laing was later to reflect on his experiences in the padded cell:

> The issue of solidarity and camaraderie between me as a doctor and those patients did not arise for me, it did not occur to me until I was in the British Army, a psychiatrist and a lieutenant, sitting in padded cells in my own ward with completely psychotic patients . . . For the first time it dawned on me that it was almost impossible for a patient to be a pal or for a patient to have a snowball's chance in hell of finding a comrade in me.[39]

Dream analysis

At Catterick, Laing carried out dream analysis with several patients. He had extended sessions with a young soldier called C.[40] It is worth quoting one session in some detail, as it gives a good picture of what Laing was actually doing with patients. The session started with the patient telling Laing about a dream. It concerned two young boys, whom the dreamer had never seen before and who were playing at a piano or an organ. They looked at each other and the patient was watching for signs to show that they were embarrassed but could not see any evidence of this. Laing gives an account of the interview:

LAING: Two young boys?
PATIENT: Rather like choir boys—young.

---

[36] Laing, *The Self and Others*, p. 87.
[37] Laing, R.D. (1969). *Self and Others*. Penguin Books, Harmondsworth, p. 97.
[38] Mezan, *After Freud*.
[39] Laing, *Wisdom, Madness and Folly*, p. 31.
[40] MS Laing DB85. Dream Sessions with C. To facilitate comprehension, the speakers, 'Laing' and 'Patient' have been identified, whereas in the original, this was left blank. This method will be used in subsequent extracts of Laing's clinical interviews.

LAING: Never seen before?

PATIENT: No.

LAING: Suggest anything?

PATIENT: No.

LAING: Playing the organ.

PATIENT: Singing and playing.

LAING: Duet?

PATIENT: Sort of duet—same piano. Singing was the important thing.

LAING: What does that situation suggest?

PATIENT: Amazed that other people must enjoy doing certain things—singing for instance.

LAING: Why embarrassed?

PATIENT: Upbringing among boys at school. Taught singing & I didn't like it—in band—expected to sing—no good.

LAING: Playing the organ?

PATIENT: Used to like the organ—used to break into church—break it open, play it.

LAING: Break it open?

PATIENT: Locked—had to pull it.

LAING: Suggest anything?

PATIENT: At school . . . very attracted to girl in choir—don't know of any connection.

LAING: What about girl?

PATIENT: Nothing to tell—prayers—came in.

LAING: Speak to her?

PATIENT: No.

LAING: . . . Very friendly with any of the boys in the choir?

PATIENT: No.

LAING: Masturbate with any of them?

PATIENT: One of them.

LAING: Tell me about him . . .

PATIENT: Nothing to tell really. Someone told me that he did it—got talking. Steered conversation around.

LAING: Ever masturbate in the church.

PATIENT: No.

LAING: Playing piano together & masturbated?

PATIENT: Yes, probably.

In this interview, Laing is clearly following a Freudian line. He almost suggests to the patient that he see his dream in sexual terms. Despite his embarrassment as a medical student when he witnessed the word 'masturbation' being mentioned by a consultant psychiatrist in an interview with a young man, here Laing appears to have no qualms in using it.

An instance of the Ganser syndrome

Laing's paper on the Ganser syndrome is worth considering for the light it sheds on his clinical approach during his time in the Army.[41] In it, he described the case of a

---

[41] Laing, R.D. (1953). 'An instance of the Ganser Syndrome'. *Journal of the Royal Army Medical Corps*, **99**, 169–72.

29-year-old man who was referred to Netley for a psychiatric opinion of his fitness to face a court-martial. The soldier's marriage had collapsed owing to his wife's infidelity and he also been involved in a road traffic accident. He had gone absent without leave and had spent seven months wandering around fairgrounds doing odd jobs. The soldier surrendered himself on impulse to the authorities and, while awaiting court-martial for desertion, he was referred to the Area Psychiatrist at Chester. He was admitted to Netley, and Laing gives a good description of his presentation:

> On admission he was completely mute. He would blow out his cheeks and become blue in the face in prodigious efforts to utter even a whisper. He would then cry, beat his head and tear his hair. He would communicate freely in writing and could understand what was said to him. Under pentothal narcosis he spoke fluently and released a torrent of obscene abuse against his wife and the army. He yelled himself hoarse in a few minutes, and then burst out weeping, crying 'Mom, me Mom's good . . .' He then enacted his driving accident, crying out, 'It's not my fault, not my fault'.[42]

Over subsequent sessions, he behaved in the same way, but, at times, complained of going blind, feeling weak and dizzy, and having headaches. These symptoms disappeared and he was left in a 'confused state of anxious excitement'. He was given 'fairly heavy sedation' and started to behave like a 'little child'. He played with toys, and he had to be fed and toileted. It proved impossible to elicit a correct answer to the most simple questions. He said that two times two were two. He called an apple an orange. He gave the date, month, and year incorrectly. When pressed to give the right answer he would laugh or cry, or fly into a rage. His hands had to be bandaged because he stubbed cigarettes out on the backs of his hands. Laing tried hypnosis but the soldier still gave incorrect answers to questions. However after six weeks he improved and was his 'old self' again. Laing saw the case in psychoanalytic terms, writing: 'He regressed to the age of two or three, he incorporated orally his Good mother and projected his psychic reality to the external world.' In this clinical encounter, we see Laing making use of drug-induced narcosis and sedative medication, employing the hypnosis techniques he had practised as a medical student, and formulating his patient's problems in psychoanalytic terms.

Peter/'David'

There is one particular report in Laing's papers which is more detailed than the rest and which formed the basis of the description of 'David' in *The Divided Self*.[43] As well as the official report, Laing made his own notes and there is also a letter from the patient's father. The case concerned an 18-year-old man called Peter, who was admitted to Netley on 20 November 1951.[44] The official report revealed that he had joined the Army nine weeks previously but was displaying symptoms of anxiety and obsessional behaviour, such as stopping in the middle of an activity to pray.

---

[42] Ibid., p. 70.
[43] Laing, *The Divided Self*, pp. 72–81.
[44] MS Laing DJ27. Psychiatric Report on Peter, 20 November 1951.

He had attended a grammar school but had unexpectedly failed his higher English exam. He wanted to be an actor and Laing regarded his views on theatre as 'intelligent, sensitive, informed', although he noted that Peter preferred feminine roles such as Lady Macbeth. His mother had died when he was six or seven. As far as Peter remembered he was 'rather pleased', though he added 'perhaps I did feel some real sorrow I'd like to think so anyway'. This comment was reproduced verbatim in the case of 'David'. His father was a retired clerk with no interest in the theatre. Peter had a 'mentally defective' brother, and a sister who had died before he was born. Since early childhood he had to cope with a tendency to be awkward and shy. Laing wrote:

> Says he has deliberately schooled himself to act effectively in whatever situation he may be in. In fact he is always playing a part, always acting with a view to the calculated or expected effect. He now hardly knows what it might mean to 'be himself' to act naturally. He is never himself—he is always someone else, as it were. He is now unable to take off the 'persona'. As 'he' never risks revealing 'himself' 'he' need never feel shy, or awkward, or embarrassed. 'He', imagines, as he says of the actor, [that he] can be the skilled craftsman watching the impression he himself is making. His ideal is to be utterly frank and honest with himself, while never giving himself [away] to others.

This passage forms the basis of Laing's more extended treatment of 'David's' false-self system in the book.

Peter had realized three or four years ago that he was unpopular because 'he' had a 'nasty tongue'. In the book, 'David' says 'it' rather than 'he' had a nasty tongue, and Laing makes great play of the fact that he uses the impersonal pronoun. Like 'David', Peter took steps to remedy this. However, Peter had lost all genuine spontaneity. As a child he had dressed himself up in funny clothes or imagined himself gorgeously attired with an abundance of jewellery. He was worried about his compulsions and how ridiculous they were. He prayed as often as thirteen times in three minutes, and kept repeating 'sorry, Lord' over and over again. He worried that if he didn't pray some disaster would befall him. If he looked around when walking he would have to do it again and again, and if he touched something with one hand, he would have to touch it with his other hand as well.

Peter was described as a tall, pale, young man with facial tics. Laing considered he was 'schizoid', but that there was no evidence of schizophrenia. He gave the official diagnosis as an 'obsessional' state, but he added hand-written comments that he thought Peter was homosexual, 'extremely narcissistic', and might be in the early stages of schizophrenia. It is not entirely clear when Laing added these comments later, as he tended to go over his papers and make annotations.

In his own hand-written notes, Laing added more details. Peter heard 'an imaginary voice telling him what or what not to do'.[45] It was not located in space and it frequently gave him good advice. At times Peter tried to disobey the voice but this was extremely difficult. This detail was not mentioned in the report or the book. It is not clear why. Was Laing trying to simplify the clinical narrative? Did he think this aspect was not important? Or did he want to minimize the suggestion that Peter

---

[45] MS Laing DJ27. Hand-written notes on Peter by Laing, undated. Also typed notes, undated.

was psychotic? Laing also described Peter as having multiple facial tics and that his hands were constantly engaged in various magical gesticulations. These clinical details were not mentioned in the book.

Laing also noted that when he had lived with his father, Peter had taken over much of the running of the house, such as cooking, decorating, and going for messages. Laing had contacted Peter's old English teacher and reported:

> His English teacher told me that his performance was remarkable for its characterisation—the way he carried himself, played with a ring on his finger etc.—he wondered how a boy of 15 could so well have understood a woman.

After this performance his behaviour caused some concern to his teachers because he continued to play a feminine role in everyday life. He was forbidden to play female parts, and the following year he played Causius in *Julius Caesar*, but his performance was judged merely competent and not in the same league as his Lady Macbeth.

Laing noted that Peter gave his own private performances in front of a mirror at home and that he always played the part of a woman. He was rather frightened because the role of Lady Macbeth had, indeed, gained possession of him, and it was only with great difficulty that he was able to discard it. He was only able to do so by playing the part of an obnoxious character, which he did during his last years at school. His teachers were puzzled that he seemed to be going out of his way to make himself unpopular. Peter was aware of this, but could not help himself because it was the only way he could stop himself being effeminate in manner. Of Peter's sexuality, Laing wrote that he was attracted to men and was 'prepared to regard himself as a homosexual'. He'd had sexual intercourse with men, who picked him up on the street.

Laing also contacted Peter's father, who sent him a letter about his son.[46] He said that his son would have joined RADA if he had not been conscripted into the Army. He had acted in several plays at school and had taken up 'such unusual things for a boy as embroidery, sewing and in fact he designed and made the dresses for both male and female, for one of his stage productions'. Peter's father went on to write: 'He lost his mother when he was 7, so I have been both parents from that time and maybe that has reacted on him.'

Curiously, although the case of Peter formed the basis for the description of 'David' in *The Divided Self*, there are important differences. For example, 'David' was described as an only child and he was said to have gone to university to study philosophy. He attended classes in a cloak and carried a cane. David brought forth one of the most memorable images in the book. Laing writes: 'The boy was a most fantastic-looking character—an adolescent Kierkegaard played by Danny Kaye.' There was no mention of 'David' suffering from obsessional symptoms, having facial tics, hand gesticulations, or hearing a voice. Why the differences? Was Laing trying to protect the patient's anonymity by changing the details? Was he simplifying the case history by omitting some of the clinical symptoms? Was the description of the cloak and cane taken from another patient's history? Did Laing make any of it up? It is impossible to answer these

---

[46] MS Laing DJ27, Letter from father to Laing, 6 December 1951.

questions, but they do demonstrate how case histories can undergo substantial modifications in the passage from the clinic to the page.

In the book, the father's account, which Laing described as 'meagre', is also different. The father was said to be unable to see why his son needed to consult a psychiatrist, because there was nothing wrong with him. He claimed his son had always been perfectly normal and his current problems were just an adolescent phase. His son had always been 'a very good child, who did everything he was told and never caused any trouble'. Now Peter's father said none of these things in his letter to Laing. There may have been other letters from the father or Laing may have talked to him directly, but, if so, there is no record of this. One does have to consider the possibility that Laing attributed these statements to Peter's father. They do fit in with Laing's theories about the origins of schizophrenia, particularly the notion that children who went on to become psychotic were often perceived by their parents as consistently 'good'. Such parental descriptions were regarded by Laing as demonstrating that the child was being stifled and crushed; this might lead to madness in later life.

In the book, the father states that his son had been inseparable from his mother and that, when she died, he took over her role 'even to the extent of showing her flair for embroidery, tapestry, and interior decoration'. The father 'spoke highly' of Peter's newly acquired talents. Again, this account does not accord with the father's letter. In the letter he admits that his son's interest in sewing and so forth was a bit unusual. He also writes that it was *he* who took on the role of mother as well as father. Laing's original notes do not mention that Peter had a very close relationship with his mother; in fact, it was said that he 'remembered little of his mother'. Of course there might be missing documents that support this, but one does harbour the suspicion that Laing was distorting the clinical narrative to fit his theory. We also learn in the book that the son had simply been 'what his mother had wanted him to be'. Again this account is not to be found in the original clinical papers, but, of course, it fits with the theory that mothers can contribute to the development of psychosis in their offspring.

In the book, Laing states that 'David' first came to him when he was concerned that the female role he had been adopting was now taking him over: in fact he had reached crisis point. Laing writes that 'David's' fantastic get-up of cloak and cane was his attempt to prevent himself being 'entirely engulfed by the woman who was inside him, and always seemed to be coming out of him'. As we have seen, Peter in the original notes had experienced this problem at school and had tried to resolve it by adopting an obnoxious persona. So once gain we seem to have pretty substantial discrepancies between the published account and the clinical notes. In general, the published narrative offers a more dramatic picture, with the young man as a philosophy student in flamboyant attire, rather than an unwilling conscript to the British Army. Many of the original symptoms have been shorn to provide a more coherent narrative. In an interview with Peter Mezan in 1972, Laing claimed that in *The Divided Self*, he had tried 'to find a theory to fit the facts, rather than the other way round'.[47] In the case of 'David' it would seem that he selected and even changed the facts to fit his theory.

---

[47] Mezan, P. (1972). 'After Freud and Jung, now comes R.D. Laing'. *Esquire*, **77**, 92–7; 160–78.

There is an interesting footnote to the case of Peter. In April 1961, Laing received a letter from the principal of a drama school in England, in which she wrote that Peter was a student there and that they were wanting to take him on as member of staff.[48] Peter had asked her to write to Laing before they made the final decision. This indicates that not only was Peter doing well and had perhaps found his niche, but that he still remembered Laing and seemed to value his opinion. However, in *Wisdom, Madness and Folly*, Laing appears to attribute this *denouement* to another patient. He tells the story of another 'Peter', who was a patient he met when he was in the Army and whom he had taken home with him on leave in an effort to try and help him.[49] Laing advised 'Peter' to try and act in a normal manner so that he would be discharged from the Army in a few weeks. If he didn't manage this, a lengthy psychiatric career awaited him. 'Peter' successfully achieved his discharge and Laing writes that, years after this, he went on to become 'the director of a well-known college of dance and drama'. Laing congratulates himself that he had saved the patient from institutionalization. What is going on here? Were there two patients who went on to have successful careers in drama? This seems unlikely. Did Laing confuse the two patients? Or did he deliberately fabricate the ending to make a better story? It is difficult to reach a firm conclusion. Laing's biographers have accepted Laing's account of the story, and, for example, Clay commended Laing for his timely intervention.[50]

The anecdote about 'Peter' in *Wisdom, Madness and Folly* also illustrates a key aspect of Laing's approach to madness. For him, it was a condition that one could adopt or keep disguised. Just as he felt that patients could deliberately express 'mad' beliefs, so he also felt that they could hide their disturbed thoughts, especially from the unwelcome gaze of psychiatrists. In this anecdote Laing portrays himself as being on the side of the patient by telling him to cover up his problems. His account is seductive and the reader feels that 'Peter', thanks to the intervention of Laing, has escaped from the clutches of the evil empire of institutional psychiatry. However, although this might have been the case, there are alternative readings. If Peter was suffering from a psychotic illness, might he have benefited from some kind of psychiatric intervention? Because Laing has painted such a bleak picture of mainstream psychiatry during this period, many readers, including some of his biographers, would scoff at such a suggestion. Laing provides a happy ending to his story of 'Peter', which seems to clinch the case for non-intervention, but, as we have seen, there must be some doubt as to whether Laing accurately reported what eventually happened to his patient.

There is yet another aspect to the case of Peter, which raises more doubts about the veracity of the published version in Laing's autobiography. On 10 January 1951, Laing wrote to Marcelle Vincent about taking an ex-patient home with him to Glasgow.[51] Laing had discharged him from the Army and thought he might fix the man up with an analyst in Glasgow. He wanted to help his ex-patient escape admission to a mental

[48] MS Laing DJ27. Note by Laing.

[49] Laing, *Wisdom, Madness and Folly*, pp. 106–08.

[50] Clay, *R.D. Laing*, p. 49.

[51] Letter by Laing to Marcelle Vincent, 10 January 1951. Quoted in Mullan, *Creative Destroyer*, p. 83.

hospital, where he would be subjected to physical treatments that Laing was 'not very happy about'. He took him to see a psychoanalyst, who was most probably Karl Abenheimer. He agreed with Laing that analysis was a good idea. Laing writes: 'Things seemed to be working out well when he went quite "off" and the whole project had to be abandoned.'

This letter gives a quite different account to that in Laing's autobiography. In the letter we learn that the patient was *already* discharged from the Army before Laing took him home. In *Wisdom, Madness and Folly*, Laing claimed he had taken him home because, otherwise, the patient would have been subjected to physical treatments in Laing's absence. There was nothing in the letter about coaching the man to put on a normal façade to avoid hospitalization. And in the letter it ends badly for the former patient, who appears to have suffered some kind of breakdown. Again we have to ask: why the discrepancy? Since the letter was written contemporaneously, it is likely to be nearer the truth than Laing's autobiography, written some thirty years after the event. The kindest explanation is that Laing misremembered what had happened. However the tale has been refashioned to portray Laing as the sensitive hero and the fate of the patient, after his narrow escape from institutionalization, a happy one. Whether Laing deliberately changed the plot of the narrative or whether it was done subconsciously is impossible to say. Certainly Appignanesi takes Laing's account at face value and praises him for his treatment of 'Peter, whom he took home with him, despite the diagnosis of schizophrenia, so as to save him from ECT'.[52]

During Laing's time in the Army, he employed physical treatments, such as insulin coma therapy, pentothal-induced narcosis, sedative medication, and ECT, but he also had the opportunity to develop his analytic skills in the Psychoneurotic Wing, where he saw patients individually and in groups. He assessed the mental fitness of soldiers for military service, and adopted a business-like and unsentimental manner in rejecting the unsuitable. In his notebooks he expressed his unease and unhappiness about the nature of psychiatry, but he also encountered at least two patients who were to feature in his early books and one who formed the basis of his first professional publication.

---

[52] Appignanesi, L. (2008). *Mad, Bad and Sad. A History of Women and the Mind Doctors from 1800 to the Present.* Virago, London, p. 360.

Chapter 8

Gartnavel Hospital and the 'Rumpus Room'

R.D. Laing's time at Gartnavel Hospital in Glasgow was arguably the most crucial experience of his clinical training. It was here that he encountered patients with severe mental illness, many of whom were to appear in his first two books, *The Divided Self* and *The Self and Others*. It was at Gartnavel that he conducted with others the famous 'Rumpus Room' experiment, which he was to discuss repeatedly throughout his career and which was to assume such mythological proportions in the re-telling. Here Laing first experienced working in a large and over-crowded mental hospital, and, although he was later to say that he was appalled by much of what he saw, he also spoke warmly about many aspects of the institution: the sense of camaraderie amongst staff; the essential decency and humanity of the older psychiatrists, such as the superintendent, Angus MacNiven; and, above all, the patients, whose often strange and seemingly inaccessible worlds, he attempted to penetrate and understand. He spent hours with individual patients, making notes—over and above the official records—in which he tried to fathom their disturbed mental conditions. In his endeavours, Laing drew on psychoanalysis, as well as sociology, existentialism, and religion. He spent time in the long-stay wards, observing the behaviour of the patients and their interaction or, more commonly, lack of interaction with others. He read voraciously, and, although he was later to give scant mention to his Gartnavel colleagues, they were well-versed in the latest psychiatric theories and were able to provide Laing with a forum in which to discuss his emerging ideas. The hospital that Laing was joining had a venerable history, particularly in the early part of the twentieth century, when David Henderson brought his experience of working in Europe and America to bear on practice in the Glasgow asylum. Henderson also co-authored with his Gartnavel colleague, R.D. Gillespie, the most important and enduring British psychiatric textbook of its era.

The historical background to Gartnavel Hospital

Gartnavel Hospital opened in 1814 and was originally called the Glasgow Asylum for Lunatics. It moved to the Gartnavel site in 1843 and in 1931 it changed its name to the Glasgow Royal Mental Hospital.[1] The hospital catered for private patients, who were housed in the West wing, and non-fee-paying patients, who were housed in the East wing. In 1948, it was incorporated into the National Health Service, but still retained

---

[1] Andrews, J. and Smith, I. (1993). *'Let there be light again.' A History of Gartnavel Royal Hospital from its beginnings to the present day*. Gartnavel Royal Hospital Press, Glasgow.

the West and East nomenclature. It was in the latter wing of the hospital that Laing was to work and where he was to study long-stay patients. The hospital had links with Europe and America. Dr David Henderson was Superintendent of the hospital from 1921 to 1932, and, prior to taking up his post at Glasgow, had spent several months in Munich at the clinic of Emil Kraepelin, whose approach to psychiatry Laing was later to challenge. Henderson, himself, although expressing great admiration for the German clinician, felt that his clinical manner was marred by his lack of sensitivity to the feelings of his patients.[2] Henderson had also worked in New York with Adolf Meyer, who championed the 'psychobiological' school of psychiatry. Meyer exercised a profound influence over Henderson and British psychiatry generally.[3] By psycho-biology, Meyer meant attending to the whole person and considering a wide range of factors in the aetiology of mental illness. Meyer opposed the prevailing idea that insanity was hereditary and that it ran a predetermined and usually unfavourable course. Instead, Meyer contended that each person was a product of social forces and life experiences, and that heredity played only a small part. Clinicians should study the biographies of their patients, rather than just assign them to diagnostic categories. Meyer saw psychiatric disorders as the reactions of a person to the cumulative events in his or her life.

According to Dr Isobel Hunter-Brown, who worked at Gartnavel at around the same time as Laing, the key to the Glasgow approach to mental illness is to be found in the pages of Henderson and Gillespie's *Textbook of Psychiatry*.[4] The first edition came out in 1927 and it was this edition that Laing referred to in his autobiography, though the textbook went through several successive editions and it was more likely that it was the 1944 one that Laing consulted when he was training.[5] We know Laing made notes from the book, in particular its references to Bleuler and Kretschmer.[6] The authors of the *Textbook of Psychiatry* were heavily influenced by Meyer and wished to bring his work to a British audience. In the Preface, they declared:

> Most of all the biological viewpoint of Adolf Meyer and his followers of the American school has seemed to us to shed fresh light on the nature of mental illness, and to offer new hope in its prevention and treatment. This biological hypothesis regards mental illness as the cumulative result of unhealthy reactions of the individual mind to its environment, and seeks to trace in a given case all the factors that go to the production of these reactions.[7]

[2] Henderson, D.K. (1964). *The Evolution of Psychiatry in Scotland*. E. & S. Livingstone, Edinburgh, p. 173.

[3] Gelder, M. (1991). 'Adolf Meyer and his influence on British psychiatry'. In Berrios, G.E. and Freeman, H. (eds), *150 Years of British Psychiatry 1841–1991*. Gaskell, London, pp. 419–35.

[4] Hunter-Brown, I. (2007). *R.D. Laing and Psychodynamic Psychiatry in 1950s Glasgow: A Reappraisal*. Free Association Books, London, p. 98.

[5] Hunter-Brown discusses a 1949 edition but the 6th edition was 1944 and the 7th was 1950.

[6] MS Laing A694.

[7] Preface to the 1st Edition, 1927, Reprinted in Henderson, D.K. and Gillespie, R.D. (1940). *A Textbook of Psychiatry for Students and Practitioners* (5th edn). Oxford University Press, London, p. ix.

Henderson and Gillespie saw mental illness in terms of the social problems of everyday life. Disturbed relations or family discord could contribute to psychological disturbance. Further, it was held that mental illness should be understood in terms of the individual, and that symptoms had little meaning if considered apart from the specific context in which the patient experienced them. The patient's own view of themselves and their world was to be taken into account. The psychiatrist should make use of the patient's own words in describing the clinical problem. The *Textbook of Psychiatry* maintained that ordinary rather than technical language was to be preferred when describing the patient. The authors stated:

> We have made a point of quoting at length clinical records of cases in our own practice. Mental illness is an individual affair . . . general descriptions of clinical syndromes, while interesting, are not of the first importance. What is wanted always is an understanding of the patient as a human being, and of the problems which he is meeting in a morbid way with his 'symptoms'.[8]

This passage could have been written by Laing, especially the use of inverted commas around 'symptoms', with its implication that medical terminology was inappropriate or inadequate when applied to problems of living. Lengthy individual case accounts were to be preferred to abstract and anonymous descriptions of syndromes. This, of course, was the approach that Laing adopted when he came to write his own books.

Hunter-Brown, with some justice, observes that Henderson and Gillespie's *Textbook of Psychiatry* expressed many of the ideas that Laing was to advance later in his career. If we consider Henderson and Gillespie's account of schizophrenia, where they favour a Meyerian rather than Kraepelinian line, we see further parallels with Laing. They write:

> . . . schizophrenia is the outcome of progressive maladaptation of the individual to his background. Schizophrenia is not a 'disease', but a congeries of individual types of reaction having certain general similarities . . . The individual may be loaded in various ways— by inheritance, by physical defects of an endocrine disorder or some grosser kind, by intellectual deficiency, or what not—but none of them is in itself a sufficient cause of schizophrenia. It is only when the subject, whether handicapped or not, has to face the usual concrete problems in his life that reactions can appear which cumulatively lead to one of the numerous conditions which have been included under the designation of 'dementia praecox' or 'schizophrenia'.[9]

Laing would have agreed with the notion of seeing schizophrenia in terms of the individual's response to the particularities of his or her social environment, but he laid much less emphasis than Henderson and Gillespie on physical factors. In *The Divided Self*, Laing adopted a neutral position as to whether there was a physical aetiology to schizophrenia, but in later work he tended to dismiss such a possibility altogether.

---

[8] Ibid., p. x.
[9] Henderson, D.K. and Gillespie, R.D. (1940). *A Textbook of Psychiatry for Students and Practitioners* (5th edn). Oxford University Press, London, p. 204.

Henderson and Gillespie's account of Meyer's approach to schizophrenia also anticipates Laing's:

> It was from a careful study of patients, and especially of their history before any breakdown was recognised by friends or relatives—a line of investigation commonly neglected—that Meyer concluded that 'schizophrenia' is the end result of an accumulation of faulty habits of reaction.[10]

Again we note the use of inverted commas, this time around 'schizophrenia', a polemical strategy that Laing was later to adopt. Like Meyer, Laing was to trace the origins of schizophrenia to a time well before the onset of symptoms, in fact, in the case of Julie from *The Divided Self*, as far back as infancy.

Henderson brought the 'case conference' to Gartnavel, a concept which had its origins in the work of Meyer. The case conference involved the clinical presentation of a patient's history to a group of psychiatrists. The patient was brought in and interviewed, and this was followed by a discussion about diagnosis and treatment. This tradition continued at Glasgow and Laing, as we will see, also participated in such events when he was a senior registrar at the Southern General Hospital under Professor Rodger.

Henderson's successor was Dr Angus MacNiven, who was still in post when Laing arrived at Glasgow in the 1950s. From the Island of Mull, MacNiven was a Glasgow graduate, who had also trained with Meyer, and had a signed portrait of Sigmund Freud on his wall. MacNiven believed that there was no sharp dividing line between normal and abnormal functioning. He was instrumental in finding work for refugee Jewish psychiatrists and psychoanalysts before and during the Second World War. Smith and Swann detect considerable scepticism about physical methods of treatment during the Henderson/MacNiven years: both men were very influenced by psychoanalysis.[11] Under MacNiven, physical treatments, such as insulin coma treatment, leucotomy, and ECT, were used at a later date than in other institutions and with greater caution.

Laing at Gartnavel

Laing took up his post as registrar at Gartnavel Royal Mental Hospital in October 1953.[12] Patient numbers at Gartnavel were mounting throughout the 1950s and topped the 900 mark for the first time in its history by the end of 1953, just after Laing's arrival.[13] There was also a shortage of medical staff, which, combined with

---

[10] Ibid., pp. 204–05.

[11] Andrews and Smith, *A History of Gartnavel*, pp. 75–6.

[12] Laing gives this date in his Research Fellowship Application. Hunter-Brown gives the date as a month later, *R.D. Laing*, p. 147.

[13] Andrews, J. (1998). 'R.D. Laing in Scotland: facts and fictions of the 'Rumpus Room' and interpersonal psychiatry'. In Gijswijt-Hofstra, M. and Porter, R. (eds), *Culture of Psychiatry and Mental Health Care in Postwar Britain and the Netherlands*. Rodopi, Amsterdam, pp. 121–50.

rising inmate numbers, meant that doctors were unable to spend as much time with their patients. Looking back in 1972 at Gartnavel, Laing recalled:[14]

It wasn't such a bad place in many ways—it was full of eccentrics, and the patients were allowed to be far more eccentric than you'll find nowadays in modern hospitals, where they won't put up with it.

In *Wisdom, Madness and Folly*, Laing described his early experiences as a psychiatrist:

As a young psychiatrist in general hospitals and psychiatric hospitals, I administered locked wards and ordered drugs, injections, padded cells and straitjackets, electric shocks, deep insulin comas and the rest. I was uneasy about lobotomies but not sure why. Usually all this treatment was against the will of its recipients. I went around in a white coat, with stethoscope, tendon hammer and opthalmoscope sticking out of my pockets, like any other doctor. Like them, I examined patients clinically. I had samples of blood, urine, spinal fluid sent for laboratory analysis, ordered electroencephalograms and so on.

It looked the same as the rest of medicine, but it was different. I was puzzled and uneasy. Hardly any of my psychiatric colleagues seemed puzzled or uneasy. This made me even more puzzled and uneasy.[15]

In this chapter we look at Laing's involvement in a social psychiatry project that came to be known as the 'Rumpus Room' experiment, while the subsequent chapter will examine his treatment of individual patients at Gartnavel.

Background to the 'Rumpus Room' experiment

The 'Rumpus Room' experiment occupies a crucial stage in Laing's development and he was repeatedly to return to it throughout his career, culminating in his last thoughts on the subject in *Wisdom, Madness and Folly* and *Mad to be Normal*. The experiment was set up to see if changing the social environment of long-stay patients improved their mental condition. This should be seen in the context of the time when such ideas were in vogue. The World Health Organization had pointed to the dangers of institutionalization and many psychiatric hospitals in Britain, such as in Yorkshire, Cambridge, and London introduced measures to improve the experience of long-term inmates.[16] There has been debate as to Laing's exact role in the experiment, given that others were also involved.

Jonathan Andrews has studied Laing's involvement in 'The Rumpus Room' experiment. He emphasized that Laing's approach was shared by a number of psychiatrists in Glasgow and the proposed project received the backing of Ferguson Rodger, the Professor of Psychiatry in Glasgow, and Dr Angus MacNiven of Gartnavel. Work on schizophrenia and group therapy pre-dated Laing's arrival and continued for some time after he left. Psychotherapeutic approaches to schizophrenia and an interest in the social environment of the mental hospital were features of contemporary psychiatric thinking both in Glasgow and beyond. The idea that disturbing symptoms in

---

[14] Mezan, P. (1972). 'After Freud and Jung, now comes R.D. Laing'. *Esquire*, **77**, 92–7; 160–78.

[15] Laing, *Wisdom, Madness and Folly*, p. xvi.

[16] Hunter-Brown, *R.D. Laing*, pp. 122–3.

patients with chronic psychosis might be more to do with the nature of custodial care than with any underlying illness was familiar to psychiatrists during this period.

Andrews points to the importance of Thomas Freeman who was a consultant at Gartnavel during Laing's time there.[17] Freeman, who was a Belfast medical graduate, combined his Gartnavel work with being a Lecturer in Psychotherapy at the Department of Psychological Medicine at the Southern General.[18] He had previously worked as a senior registrar with Maxwell Jones at Belmont Hospital in Surrey and was a contributor to Jones' book, *Therapeutic Communities*, which outlined the group approach at Belmont.[19] In it Freeman emphasized the importance of the nurse–patient relationship and the need for it to become a therapeutic one.

Another significant presence at Gartnavel was John Cameron, who was a Glasgow graduate, and, like Laing, had begun his career at the Killearn Neurosurgical Unit. Laing had known Cameron as a medical student. Cameron was a war veteran and was six or seven years older than Laing. He apparently had taken Laing under his wing because he had been impressed by his intellectual precocity.[20] Laing was to fill his vacancy when he started at Gartnavel, and their past friendship may have inspired Laing to participate in the schizophrenia research project that Cameron was now pursuing full-time as a research assistant. According to Andrews, despite the impression conveyed by Laing's writings, it was Cameron not Laing who had initiated the practice of the therapist sitting in the midst of patients in the refractory ward. Burston[21] follows Laing's lead in this, claiming that his wish to spend time with patients was exceptional amongst Gartnavel psychiatrists, who generally preferred to avoid visiting such wards. Cameron was a registrar at Gartnavel between 1952 and 1953, before leaving his post to become a research assistant at the Department of Psychological Medicine. He was to leave Glasgow to go and work at the Chestnut Lodge Sanatorium in Rockville, USA.

Laing's other research colleague was Andrew McGhie, who was a Glasgow graduate in the arts and was initially a research psychologist at the Department of Psychological Medicine, before becoming Senior Clinical Psychologist at Gartnavel in 1955. Freeman, Cameron, and McGhie went on to publish a book, entitled *Chronic Schizophrenia*[22] in 1958, a development which upset Laing as he felt he did not receive sufficient acknowledgement for his contribution. Laing is only mentioned once. The book details the authors' perspective on psychosis. They favoured a psychological approach, which drew on Kraepelin's nosology, but also 'the dynamic theories of Bleuler and Meyer'.[23] They saw the symptomatology of mental illness as a reaction to an adverse environment

[17] Andrews, *R.D. Laing,* 130–2.

[18] Ibid., pp. 136–7.

[19] Jones, M. (ed.) (1952). *Social Psychiatry: A Study of Therapeutic Communities.* Tavistock, London.

[20] Andrews, *R.D. Laing*, p. 140.

[21] Burston, *The Wing of Madness*, p. 36.

[22] Freeman, T., Cameron, J.L. and McGhie, A. (1958). *Chronic Schizophrenia.* Tavistock, London.

[23] Ibid., p. 2.

or psychological stress. The authors felt it was important to make a longitudinal study of a patient's life and to uncover the significant events.

Group psychotherapy was being employed by Cameron and Freeman at Gartnavel in the 1950s before Laing arrived. Indeed they had begun their first project around 1952.[24] At the time of the 'Rumpus Room' experiment, there was also a project investigating the effects of group analytic psychotherapy on chronic schizophrenic patients.[25] The grant for research into schizophrenia had already been obtained by the time Laing arrived at Gartnavel and had been awarded to Cameron, Freeman, and McGhie. The 'Rumpus Room' project was funded from this grant. Freeman told Andrews that Laing's contribution was far from the original, instigating one that he later claimed, and that it was, in fact, rather brief and fleeting.[26]

Dr MacNiven had long been interested in psychological approaches to mental disorder, and in 1938, along with Dr David Yellowlees, had established the Lansdowne Clinic for Functional Nervous Disorders near the hospital.[27] MacNiven was cautious about the introduction of chlorpromazine, and, while acknowledging its benefits, felt that the improvement in the patients was not purely down to chemicals. Andrews feels that Laing, in his retrospective accounts of the 'Rumpus Room', unfairly minimizes the contribution of MacNiven in supporting the project and persuading the Hospital's Board of Management to agree to it. In his reports to the Board, MacNiven gave the new 'Rumpus Room' experiment his approval and described the initial results as 'very interesting'. He identified Laing as the principal researcher and suggested that the Board invite him to their meeting to describe the project. Although Andrews states that Laing's oral account was not transcribed in the minutes, there is an unpublished paper which probably formed the basis of his talk to the Board. Entitled 'Proposals for Active Treatment Unit for Deteriorating Psychotics',[28] in it Laing set out his plan. The aim was to re-socialize a group of patients who were very isolated. Laing wrote:

> A completely permissive atmosphere would of course be the aim, in the centre. Whether, as it is hoped, the feeling of security engendered by membership of the group would eventually help individual patients to resist the exhibition of their anti-social tendencies remains to be seen.[29]

Laing proposed that the nurses should not wear uniform because it acted as an armour behind which they could shelter and was a symbol of authority to the patients, as well as a barrier to communication. Laing contended that nurses participating in the therapy would have their morale increased. The project would stimulate discussion amongst staff, which would help to resolve tension. Thus Laing's pitch concentrated on the social benefits that such a project might bring. The Board, like MacNiven,

---

[24] Andrews, *R.D. Laing*, p. 133.

[25] MS Laing A501/1. Chronic Schizophrenic Patients and their Nurses: A Study in the Essentials of Environment.

[26] Andrews, *R.D. Laing*, p.135.

[27] Ibid., p 126.

[28] MS Laing A617. Proposal for Active Treatment Unit for Deteriorating Psychotics. This appears to have been written by Laing, although there is no name on it.

[29] Ibid., p. 3.

judged the project to be 'very interesting', and asked Laing to report back later.[30] However, he was soon to leave the hospital and did not return to the Board. Andrews talked to doctors who had worked under MacNiven and formed the impression that his 'liberal and encouraging attitude created a welcome climate of innovation'.[31] MacNiven let the junior doctors pursue their inclinations as to treatment.

Laing and his colleagues drew on the experience of Dingleton Hospital in the Scottish Borders, which Laing had visited on a fact-finding mission. Laing later recalled that Maxwell Jones was developing his ideas about the therapeutic community around this time.[32] Laing claims that he went to visit Jones at Dingleton but he wasn't there. Jones did not actually take up his post at Dingleton until 2 December 1962,[33] so it appears that Laing's memory is faulty on this point. However, Laing must have been exposed to Jones' published writings which had been available for some years.

The project doctors also looked to American researchers who were carrying out similar types of work. In particular, they drew on the work of Staunton and Schwartz and their 1954 book, *The Mental Hospital*.[34] The book was based on their research at the privately owned Chestnut Lodge Sanatorium, near Washington, which provided psychotherapy for psychotic patients. One of the authors, Morris Schwartz, was a sociologist and he provided a sociological analysis of the institution. Laing conducted a seminar[35] at Gartnavel in which he presented his comments on *The Mental Hospital*. Laing was impressed with the finding that communication difficulties in staff could lead to disturbance amongst the patients: psychiatric symptoms were dependent on the social milieu. He noted that even in schizophrenic patients with 'autistic' features, their disturbance was not simply a result of some internal problem, but was also influenced by what was going on in their environment. Laing drew on the work of another American psychiatrist, Harry Stack Sullivan, who had underlined the importance of the nursing staff in a ward environment. Sullivan had set up a ward, in which he had devoted most of his time to talking with the nursing staff about their interactions with patients. Laing also turned to history and referred to John Conolly's 1856 work, *The Treatment of the Insane without Mechanical Restraint*, whose title reflected the author's therapeutic philosophy.

Whether or not Laing was quite the lone innovator that he presented himself to be, it is clear from his private papers that he spent a considerable amount of time and energy thinking and writing about the 'Rumpus Room', as well as observing the patients in the wards. Laing made extensive notes on the various aspects of the project,

[30] Andrews, *R.D. Laing*, pp. 128–9.

[31] Andrews, *R.D. Laing*, p. 129.

[32] Millard, D.W. (1996). 'Maxwell Jones and the therapeutic community'. In Freeman, H. and Berrios, G.E. (eds), *150 Years of British Psychiatry. Volume II: the Aftermath*. Athlone, London, pp. 581–604.

[33] Anon (2000). *The Story of a Community. Dingleton Hospital Melrose*. Chiefswood Publications, Melrose.

[34] Staunton, A.H. and Schwartz, H.S. (1954). *The Mental Hospital*. Basic Books, New York.

[35] MS Laing DG57. Some comments on 'The Mental Hospital'.

such as the behaviour of patients, the role of nurses, and his own reactions to the long-stay wards of Gartnavel.

The refractory ward

As a preliminary to the 'Rumpus Room' experiment, Laing spent time in a 'refractory' ward, observing the social world of the patients. He chose a ward known as F.E.6. 'F' stood for female and 'E' for East, indicating it was in the part of the hospital that had originally catered for the poorer patients. The ward had padded cells and was reserved for the very 'worst' patients. Laing sat in the dayroom of the ward for one or two hours each day for several months. There were 40–50 patients in the ward. Most of them were huddled in chairs and did not converse with each other. As his contemporaneous notes indicate, Laing clearly found it a shocking experience and was appalled and frightened by the behaviour of the residents, at least initially. In the 1950s, long-stay psychiatric wards were, indeed, grim places. Overcrowded and understaffed, the wards contained individuals who were very disturbed and disturbing. Psychiatric staff throughout Britain and the United States were beginning to conclude that the quality of institutional environment could exercise a profound effect on an inmate's mental condition. But the nature of the patient's psychiatric condition also played a part. Healy has described the transformation that chlorpromazine wrought in people suffering from schizophrenia, when it was first introduced in the 1950s in France.[36] Thus, a combination of a toxic institutional environment and the severe psychiatric illnesses of the inmates rendered these 'refractory' wards unsettling places to inhabit for both staff and patients. It is not surprising, then, that Laing expressed his unease, though he has been criticized for his negative remarks about the patients he encountered there.[37] As we will see, despite his apprehension and distaste, Laing continued to spend time in the long-stay ward and soon discerned the humanity beneath the seeming chaos of its inhabitants.

Laing began recording his experiences on 2 April 1954:

> At first bedlam. The patients are crowded seat to seat, round dayroom. I feel rather scared. I'm afraid my clothes will be ripped off, or that I'll lose my balls. Several women are running about, shouting, singing, laughing, swearing. Several approach me. One swears. One pulls up her dress and exhibits her fannie . . .
>
> It takes some time before I can settle down to see more clearly what is going on . . . The noisy people who are setting the 'tone' of the ward are only 3 or 4 out of perhaps 40 people.[38]

Laing noted that the majority of patients sat in the foetal position on the chair, and occasionally one would look up, shout something or suddenly run, take the chair and throw it at the wire netting covering the windows. He concluded: 'It is incomprehensible, frightening, repulsive, horrible'. He spent the next five days trying to individuate' the

---

[36] Healy, D. (2002). *The Creation of Psychopharmacology*. Harvard University Press, Cambridge MA.

[37] Abrahamson, D. (2007). 'R.D. Laing and long-stay patients: discrepant accounts of the refractory ward and "rumpus room" at Gartnavel Royal Hospital'. *History of Psychiatry*, **18**, 203–15.

[38] MS Laing DG64. L.E.6 Dayroom, p. 1.

patients in his own mind. He jotted down his initial impressions.[39] He saw no unprovoked attacks on nurses. Some patients were friendly to him, but hostile to other patients. There were definite 'cliques', but some patients had no friends at all. Laing was constantly being given scraps of paper and orange peel by patients and being importuned for cigarettes or sweets. Some patients acted as his 'bodyguard'. He observed that there was a 'remarkable amount of miming and caricaturing going on'. He felt there was basically nothing for the patients to do on the ward and it was impossible to even read a book. The nurses only interacted with the patients if they were misbehaving, and Laing reasoned that patients were sometimes deliberately provocative to draw attention to themselves.

In an entry on 5 April 1954, Laing admitted his fear of one of the patients:

> Mrs W.—one of them I'm really afraid of. Large, wears her jacket like one of Napoleon's generals. Struts about in like manner. Foul teeth. Scowls. Expresses the highest disdain & contempt by inarticulated tones. She came up and forced my mouth open, puts her filthy face right up to mine & peers in.[40]

Laing described another patient that he found unappealing:

> A.F. is a grotesque stick of a woman, waddling around in shoes 2 times too large for her—underpants about her ankles. They are always falling down & she stops to pick them up. She bubbles saliva out of tightly pursed lips continually. From time to time she wipes some off her hand to smear over a table cover . . .[41]

Laing found that some of the patients tried to monopolize his time and he admitted he found their 'advances' repellent. On 9 April 1954, he witnessed another patient attack another but did not intervene. He was upset with himself at this reaction, and the next day he upbraided himself:

> I can't act the part of George McLeod's 'sociological observer from Wisconsin'. I have to defend myself and I have to protect the weak against vicious attacks from the strong. My presence incites intense jealousy, and there is no equivocating in its expression.[42]

However, two weeks into the venture, Laing was noting that the ward seemed less depressing and repulsive, and that he was starting to see the patients as individuals. He felt that, though the social processes were strange and unfamiliar, the patients lived *together*. He tried to puzzle out what went on between the patients. On one occasion, a patient led one section of the ward in singing 'Bonnie Charlie's noo awa' and a hearty chorus developed from the other side. Laing also noted that, despite their lack of personal attention to their appearance, the patients liked being dressed and complimented.

Laing wished to find out about: the eating and sleeping arrangements of the patients; who went out of the ward; and who had visitors. He wanted to know what correlation there was, if any, between clinical, psychoanalytic, and sociometric assessments of patients.

---

[39] MS Laing DG64, p. 4.

[40] Ibid., p. 7.

[41] Ibid., pp. 7–8.

[42] Ibid., p. 10.

What was the process whereby patients, 'rejected' by families and the more congenial wards, found themselves in F.E.6? He mused that the longer the patients had been in the ward, the longer they were likely to remain. He speculated as to why they were unable to be moved on, and considered that the most important factors were: dirtiness, obscenity, shouting, and, above all, violence.[43]

In an unpublished paper, written between 1955 and 1956, Laing reflected on his experiences in the refractory ward. This offers a more considered response than that revealed in his contemporaneous notes:[44]

> I think the first thing that happened to me when I had sat myself in a chair was that I got my trouser buttons ripped open, my hair ruffled, and my tie pulled. Several patients fought each other to hug me, or kiss me. The intensity of their reactions hardly abated during the whole time I spent in this ward. At first I tried to remain unperturbed—to defend myself without hitting back, and to reject the sexual advances of the patients without rejecting them. But this was not easy.[45]

He admitted that at times he was so shaken that he had to leave after half an hour. Initially Laing tried to understand what was going on in psychoanalytic terms. However he felt this was unproductive and concluded that the best approach was 'not through the head but through the navel'. He observed:

> When I gave up intellectualizing, I felt that occasionally I got a glimpse behind the veil of some of these mad creatures. And such a glimpse I still recoil from of complete and utter hopelessness; of nothing; of non-being. Each patient was a vacuum, filled only with hopeless terror for the beings all around who threatened by their abhorrence to obliterate her.[46]

Laing referred to an analogy a colleague, Dr Roy, had made to him about the refractory ward:

> He said that at first the ward sounded like an orchestra tuning up, each instrument unrelated to others, the total sound chaotic. Later, however, the actions and speech of each patient, although autistic, yet seemed to be interwoven with that of others . . . [as] when the jumble of sound of a difficult piece of music all suddenly makes sense. It did not make much sense to me but I had glimpses when I felt I could. Certainly it was [the] sense that the patients though isolated were *not* exclusively self-absorbed.[47]

Laing was evidently taken by this analogy: the reference to music and the notion that madness was potentially understandable would have appealed to him. In fact, Laing repeated the analogy in his autobiography, *Wisdom, Madness and Folly*, but this time attributed it to himself rather than his colleague.[48] Laing felt he was able to communicate with certain patients whom he called the 'ward philosophers'. In particular he mentioned

[43] Ibid., p. 4.
[44] MS Laing A153. R.D. Laing: The Rumpus Room, 1954–1955, Glasgow, 1956, p.1.
[45] Ibid., p. 2.
[46] Ibid., pp. 3–4.
[47] Ibid., pp. 4–5.
[48] Laing, *Wisdom, Madness and Folly*, p. 123.

one patient a Miss M., about whom he wrote individual notes,[49] and who was to reappear in his autobiography as his 'mentor'.[50] In his unpublished paper, Laing writes:

> For what I think I have learned about psychosis, I am indebted to a remitted manic patient, as much as to anyone. She sat by me often, and explained to me a great deal of what went one. One patient for instance, sitting in the far corner of the ward, gazing out a window, she told me was furious that I had not looked at her when I had entered the ward. Another patient who was curled up under a table, and emerged only to collect food . . . had been playing at being a snake for years . . .[51]

In this paper, Laing concluded that the ward was terribly overcrowded, the nurses were far too harassed and overworked, and the patients had nothing to do.

The 'Rumpus Room' as seen by Laing

Laing wanted to see what would happen if a small group of patients from the refractory ward were allowed to spend time in a more congenial environment and with the same nurses, day after day. A room was selected and it came to be called 'The Rumpus Room' by the nurses, although they also called it 'The Class' or 'The School'.[52] Laing called it by its official name, the 'Free Activity Centre', and, from the outset he kept detailed notes of his observations and experiences of the new unit.[53] On 8 June 1954 the experiment began. Eleven patients, all suffering from schizophrenia, had been selected from F.E.6 and at 9.00 am they were taken to the Free Activity Centre. They were to stay there until midday when they would return to the ward, before spending the afternoon between 2.00 pm and 5.00 pm in the Centre. Two nurses were to be permanently present. Initially the room was sparsely decorated, but facilities for sewing, knitting, rug and wool making, drawing, and playing with coloured wooden chips were available. The patients were also observed by one of the project's doctors in F.E.6 for one to three hours a day for the first six weeks.

Laing spent short periods at the beginning and end of the first morning observing and making notes. He recorded what each patient was doing and their relationship to other people and objects in the room. He was to continue this practice throughout his time at Gartnavel until he left in February of the following year. Altogether he was involved with the Rumpus Room for eight months, although he spent several weeks in the refractory ward before this.

In his notes Laing set out his ambitions for the project: There should be a detailed biographical study of each patient and information about their families and how often they visited. Special reference should be made to 'any previous attempt that broke down, to achieve "sublimation"—symbolic realisation, or in other ways to "live thro" their "problem"'.[54] Conversation with the patients should be encouraged, and whilst

---

[49] MS Laing DG53. Clinical notes by R.D. Laing, 1953–1954.

[50] Laing, *Wisdom, Madness and Folly*, pp. 121–2.

[51] MS Laing A153, p. 4.

[52] MS Laing DG64. Laing's notes, 25 September 1954.

[53] Ibid.

[54] Ibid., p. 3.

there would be no formal sessions of psychoanalysis, Rosen's concept of 'direct analysis' would guide the interactions. Laing wanted to improve the quality of the 'Rumpus Room' environment, especially the blank walls. He suggested that there should be clay modelling, adequate drawing facilities, dancing, and singing. He explained that he was following the concept of the 'total push' or 'throw in everything'. He was keen to see how the 'social process' in F.E.6 was affected by the project, for example if the number of violent incidents or the use of sedatives was reduced.

Laing began his record of the first day by making a diagram of where each patient stood or sat in the room and the position of the furniture. He then describes the behaviour of the patients, whom he identifies by their initials:

> L.C. sat in corner, muttering to herself—I heard her reciting a nursery rhyme—later joined group at Table A.
>
> M. McM. sitting, isolate.
>
> P.H. wandering back and forward. Smiles at nurses—kisses my hand, accepts a cigarette— 'I don't think my husband would like me to take that'—gives it back a little smoked later with thanks and a smile.
>
> M.W. shouting (esp at A.B.) objects to nurses having uniform & stockings, bangs chair repeatedly on floor. Is cautioned by Nurse McM. & stopped—goes to Table A, picks up chips, throws them on the floor—goes back to seat—Nurse McM. takes her off chair by arm & 'makes' her pick them up.
>
> I sit beside her for a little. She is talking about a girl's school—the Inspector, school doctor, teachers: objects to eating chemistry. Tells me to stop 'shoving twins up her guts'—spits repeatedly—'or to stop shoving an electric red-hot poker up her lily'—King Ed. & King John also come into it—a lot more too.[55]

Laing adds that at Table A. sits B.P., J.P., and D.L., one arranging coloured strips, two, doing nothing. C.S. is knitting something green 'for a baby'. Mrs D. 'mutters away unintelligibly' and A.B. 'occasionally struts around' upset by taunts of M.W., while Mrs E. sits, knitting at Table B.

By 14 June Laing recorded that he considered the patients behaved differently in the ward than in the activity room.[56] In the ward they reverted to the 'same stereotypes' and reacted to each other in a dull, uniform way. In the 'Rumpus Room' they were more likely to be involved in some activity and they were more emotionally responsive to each other. Laing felt that the behaviour of the patients was a function of their social setting. He also noted that when the patients returned to F.E.6, they did not stick together as a group. Nurses observed that the patients were more disturbed when they returned, possibly because they resented going back there. However, the ward was generally less rowdy. On 23 June three new patients were added and two removed, although Laing did not document the reason for this.[57]

Laing expended considerable energy trying to make sense of the patients' behaviour and utterances. After the first two weeks he commented with disappointment: 'I have

---

[55] Ibid., p.1.

[56] Ibid., p. 5.

[57] Ibid., p. 6.

not succeeded in finding my bearings in the psychotic worlds of any of the patients yet.' He made an attempt to understand a particular episode:

> M.W . . . shouts at me not to put my electric poker up her tulip. When I sat beside B.P. today she kept picking up the skeins of wool that lay in front of B.P. on a table and throwing them at her—apparently an expression of jealousy. [This would seem to indicate that there is libidinal transference as well as aggressive transference.] *brackets added by Laing.*[58]

Here he used orthodox Freudian theory, but he obviously had second thoughts about this interpretation, because some time later, he added the comment: 'Balls!' He recorded that Mrs U. shouted to him about penises and observed: 'I cannot catch the drift of what she is saying.'[59] Laing tried to make sense of another patient, called 'the Princess':

> Calls me her cousin. It seems that her mother is Queen of Scotland. Slander, defamatory to her character to the effect that she is a prostitute of the streets is circulated about her in hospital. Streetwalking plays a large part in her ideas and this may tie up with her perpetual perambulations. I think she regards herself as the Lord Provost's wife. The Canadian Mounties, & 'the Argyll & Cameron Highlanders' enter into it too, but I do not see how.[60]

On 1 July Laing recorded that little progress had been made that week. The patients did not talk to each other. He noted that some patients were being given sedatives before coming to the activity centre. However, by 25 September the situation had improved with 'no outbursts, no breakages, no running away, no need of sedation'.[61] The doctors had taken the decision to withdraw from participating on an interpersonal level and the place was being 'allowed' to run itself.

Laing continued to document the activities in the 'Rumpus Room', noting the fluctuating fortunes of the patients. Some he felt were definitely improving, but there were still occasional episodes of violence. For example, on 18 January 1955 Laing recorded of M.McM.:

> She is usually friendly to me. However, on one occasion she started shouting at me as soon as I came in. It was all jumbled but she constantly reiterated 'I'm not a pishy body, I'm not a pishy body'—she dashed across the room and attacked me as I sat on a chair—the force of the attack took me a bit by surprise. She almost toppled me onto the floor and she got in a few lefts and rights to the head. The Princess was very upset by this—she was flushed and trembling. L.C. adopted her stylistic gesture of abhorrence. P.H. ran out. All the others watched intently. The nurses dragged her away and she went back to her corner still shouting.[62]

---

58 Ibid., p. 7.
59 Ibid., p. 8.
60 Ibid., p. 7.
61 Ibid., p.10.
62 Ibid., p. 15.

On 6 February 1955, Laing was gratified to note that there had been 'a dramatic change in the social presence of M.W. and P.H'.[63] M.W. no longer always sat on the one spot, she was speaking sensibly and politely, and was controlling her jealousy. It was felt by the staff that the change was related to a strong bond she had recently developed with another patient. She was also pleased when Laing had called her by her Christian name, as she had previously complained that he did not even know who she was. It was observed that P.H. was much smarter in her dress. She managed to make clear statements, such as 'I'm very well thank you' and 'Goodbye', but the rest of her talk was a 'complete jumble'. Laing felt that there was now more interaction between the patients and with the nurses. He felt that a particular nurse, by virtue of her 'aura of emotional warmth', had played a major part in bringing about the improvement.

In his notes, Laing outlined his interpersonal approach to psychosis.[64] He maintained that the patient should not be considered in isolation, but, rather, one should consider the effects the patient had on others, and, in turn, how the patient was affected by those in her environment. He also brought in a psychoanalytic perspective:

> One could perhaps define 'illness' in terms of what *they do to others* i.e. in terms of what others do to them—*have done. Patients tend to regress not to their past but to what others have done to them.* [A schizophrenic] does not regress only to *her* infancy but to her *mother's* 'unconscious' (unacknowledged) attitudes to her in infancy. Her 'illness' is a persisting response to this, or, otherwise put:—What has been repressed is 'the bad mother'— it is she who returns, overwhelms the 'ego'.

Laing notes end in February 1955, because at that point he left Gartnavel to go to the Southern General.

Staff meetings

There were two types of staff meetings, a small one with Laing and the nurses from the 'Rumpus Room', and a larger one involving the other doctors involved in the project and nurses from the long-stay wards. Laing kept a record of the small meeting, which was held for the first time on 10 June 1954, two days after the 'Rumpus Room' experiment began.[65] At the meeting the purpose of the experiment was discussed. Laing explained his theoretical approach.[66] We all have an inner world and an outer world, he said: for staff, the inner world was related to dreams, while for patients it related to phantasy. Staff were incorporated into the patients' fantasies, appearing as mothers, fathers, or other significant figures. Later meetings revealed that one of the sisters was instructing nursing staff to give some of the patients sedatives, such as paraldehyde, before they came to the 'Rumpus Room'. This had been done without consulting medical staff. Laing suggested that if a sedative had to be given, it should be given just before the patient returned to the ward.

---

63 Ibid., p. 16.
64 Ibid. Laing's notes.
65 Ibid. Staff meetings.
66 Ibid. Staff meeting, 31 January 1954.

Laing felt that he had a very important role to play in meeting with the nurses every week and listening sympathetically to their account of the previous seven days. He described how, over time, nurses started to discuss the patients as people rather than in a formulaic way. By the last month of his time there, he observed that they never asked for an 'explanation' of patients' symptoms, as this had somehow become irrelevant.

In other notes, Laing made further comments about the nursing staff.[67] He described an episode when one of the patients had hit a nurse, but this was not reported. Laing felt that there were several reasons for this. First, the nurses took pride in the patients and identified with them in some way. Also they did not want one of the ward sisters who was critical of the 'Rumpus Room' to find out and have ammunition for her attacks. Perhaps, Laing speculated, they saw the doctor as a 'punitive father'.

The larger staff discussion meetings

Throughout the period of the 'Rumpus Room' experiment, there was a weekly support meeting for the staff involved in the study. Minutes[68] were kept and they provide a remarkable insight into the emotional and practical difficulties that the research created, as well as reflecting the climate of a 1950s psychiatric hospital, a period when new psychotropic medication was being introduced. There was great debate as to the comparative efficacy of chlorpromazine, social environmental approaches, and psychoanalytical therapy. Laing and his co-researchers, Dr Cameron and Mr McGhie, attended the meetings, as did the nursing staff.

At the first meeting[69] a large number of nurses attended and 'sat stiffly round the walls'. Dr Laing set out the aim of the project: it was to try and assess the chronic patients who were gradually increasing in number throughout the hospital. Dr Cameron said that the 'environment' of the hospital was 'other people', so that if one improved the chronic patients it would create a better environment for newcomers. Questions were then 'fired' at Dr Laing about Dingleton Mental Hospital, which was pursuing a similar project in social psychiatry. Laing replied that Dingleton had no more staff than Gartnavel, but nurses objected that with the present state of overcrowding it would be impossible for them to get to know the patients better. They said they had to spend part of their time cleaning up the wards, clearing up messes made by 'refractory' patients, and sewing torn clothes. Dr Laing remarked that at Dingleton, patients were sometimes enlisted to help with such chores, but nurses replied that because Gartnavel had been a private hospital this culture did not exist. However, as the meeting went on there was a marked change in the attitude of the nurses and the discussion became 'friendly and lively'. It was felt that the exchange of ideas had been useful.

---

67 Ibid. Laing's notes, 2 December 1954.

68 MS Laing DG63, Staff Discussion Group at Gartnavel.

69 Ibid. Unfortunately the report of this meeting was not dated but it seems from the content that it was the first one.

In a hand-written commentary which Laing added to his copy of the report of the meeting, he admitted that the initial stages of the meeting had been very inhibiting, but that two members of staff had managed to 'break the ice' by introducing humour. Laing observed: 'Neither Ian [Dr Cameron] nor I have that "natural" ease & warmth which makes this sort of thing very easy.'[70]

Future meetings discussed a variety of topics relating to the impact of the research project and patient care generally. Staff discussed treatments, including ECT, leucotomy, and also tube-feeding. On one occasion, Laing advised that a patient was not well enough to go home.[71] At another meeting, nursing staff reported that the patients not selected for the 'Rumpus Room' daily groups felt jealous of those who had been. They felt that they were being neglected by the doctors and that they were receiving no treatment. Dr Laing was reported as observing that group treatment was perhaps the only practical method of giving several patients the benefits of psychotherapy, rather than one.[72] However, at the meeting of 7 September 1954, a nurse reported that the disturbance amongst patients had reduced since Dr Laing had taken to wandering around the refractory ward, talking to the patients. She remarked that the most useful thing a doctor could do when visiting the ward was to talk to every patient so no one felt neglected.[73]

The meeting of 14 September was dominated by the reaction of the staff to the suicide of a female patient, Lydia A. and to their feelings of guilt and responsibility.[74] It was mentioned that another female patient, Miss McA., had also been threatening to kill herself. Dr Laing suggested that an attempt should be made to 'institute a tribunal within the scope of the patient's delusional system in the hope that this might give her a prop by feeling that powerful figures were at her side against the persecutors'. Laing's somewhat unusual suggestion was in the tradition of Philippe Pinel, the pioneering eighteenth century French alienist, who had tried many novel ways to help his patients. These included setting up a mock court for a man who thought he was going to be executed, and granting him a 'reprieve'.[75] Laing was well-versed in the history of psychiatry and may have been influenced by Pinel. The staff members thought Laing's idea would be 'an interesting experiment' and it was to be discussed with McNiven. However, it does not seem to have been enacted. Another rather curious therapeutic suggestion was that a patient, called Miss L., might translate some portion of Sartre's *L'Etre et Le Neant*.[76]

As the head doctor of Gartnavel, Dr Angus McNiven was often the object of criticism by staff. Laing, however, defended him and pointed out how supportive he had

---

[70] Ibid., Laing's written comments on undated report.

[71] Ibid., 17 August 1954.

[72] Ibid., 17 August 1954.

[73] Ibid., 7 September 1954.

[74] Ibid., 14 September 1954.

[75] Goldstein, J. (2001). *Console and Classify. The French Psychiatric Profession in the Nineteenth Century*. University of Chicago Press, Chicago and London, p. 83. See the case of 'the guilt-ridden tailor'.

[76] MS Laing DG63. Staff Discussion Group at Gartnavel, undated meeting.

been of the research project.[77] At times nurses complained about other medical staff, for example, that they had allowed a patient who was obviously a 'psychopath' to be admitted to the ward. The nurses also said that they were worried that the doors of the wards were left unlocked, as the 'open door' policy made the management of patients difficult. There was a feeling that the type of patient being admitted to the hospital had changed as a result of the introduction of the National Health Service. Prior to this staff had more say in who came in. In addition, overcrowding was getting worse but there had been no accompanying increase in staff numbers.[78]

Sometimes physical treatments were discussed but from a psychological point of view. For example, the group discussed insulin coma therapy which was still employed at Gartnavel during this period. The group agreed that an important aspect of the treatment was the amount of attention that was given to each patient undergoing such therapy. If one compared this type of treatment with that of the 'Rumpus Room', where patients received a similar amount of attention, then there was 'reasonable doubt as to the efficacy of insulin as a drug as when divorced from the setting in which it was given'.[79]

At the 11 January meeting in 1955, Dr Cameron asked one of the nurses if the newly developed tranquillity in the ward was related to the introduction of Largactil, the trade name for chlorpromazine. The nurse replied that she thought 'this drug was of value to the chronic patients' and that the ward had 'never been so quiet and quite a few patients were showing marked improvement'.[80] Another nurse agreed with this view. An unpublished paper[81] on the 'Rumpus Room' experiment by Cameron, Laing, and McGhie commented in more detail about chlorpromazine. They noted that three of the patients were on Largactil. Prior to its introduction to the hospital, there had been 'considerable strain and tension throughout the hospital'. The ward from which the research patients were drawn was described as having reached 'a crescendo of disturbance'. After Largactil was prescribed, patients improved 'remarkably' and some were 'completely changed'. Improvements in the 'Rumpus Room' were attributed to the drug. However, the authors noted that fluctuations in the patient occurred despite the use of the drug.

A psychodynamic perspective still dominated the staff approach to patients. For example, at the 1 February meeting we find Laing discussing a patient:

> He emphasised, in particular, Betty's sibling rivalry problems and showed how they might lead to difficulty in the ward. Betty's problems with her mother often led her to speak in a biting way to older women.[82]

This was to be Laing's last meeting as he left to take up his new post as senior registrar at the Southern General Hospital. The meetings still continued and Laing took an

---

[77] Ibid., 21 September 1954.

[78] Ibid., 28 September 1954 and 19 October 1954.

[79] Ibid., 8 March 1955.

[80] Ibid., 11 January 1955.

[81] MS Laing A150/1-2. Cameron, J.L., Laing, R.D. and McGhie, A. Chronic Schizophrenic Patients and their Nurses: A Study in the Essentials of Environment.

[82] MS Laing DG63, 15 February 1955.

interest in the reported minutes. Staff felt that the project had been a success, and, as it had progressed, there was a feeling that people were becoming more encouraged to try and understand the patients.[83] In the report of the meeting of 15 March 1955,[84] Laing would have read that Nurse Madden felt it would be ideal to have all patients in small wards similar to the 'Rumpus Room'. She went on:

> She felt that having seen how important little everyday happenings were to these patients it was now more clear that there must now be hundreds of things which happen in a crowded ward which must annoy the patients. She felt, for instance, that one great advantage in the 'Rumpus Room' was the fact that the nurses were never changed and a patient was allowed to make friends with the nurses . . .

In an unpublished manuscript entitled, 'Doctor–Nurse–Patient Relations',[85] written between 1954 and 1955, Laing made further observations about the 'Rumpus Room' experiment. He noted that, as time went by, the nurses were increasingly able to decode the apparently bizarre statements of the patients. As an example he described the patient who, every time Laing entered the room, accused him of 'trying to stick a red hot poker up her tulip'. Initially, the nurses thought that the patient was very angry, but later they began to see that she was frightened. Laing felt that the nurses were becoming adept at applying Freudian principles to their patients' utterances. This psychodynamic approach to psychosis reflected the ethos of the research staff's approach, and, for example, in the staff meetings, Dr Cameron talked about the Oedipus Complex and about delusions being a form of 'defence'.

The 'Rumpus Room' results

The results of the experiment were written up and published in the *Lancet* in 1955 under the title, 'Patient and nurse. Effects of environmental changes in the care of chronic schizophrenics'.[86] The order of authors was: John Cameron, Ronald Laing, and Andrew McGhie. The researchers stated that the environment exercised a powerful effect on a patient's mental well-being and that the most important therapeutic element in it was the people. They had set up an experiment in which patients and nurses were given the chance to develop sustained relationships with one another.

The authors reported that for six weeks one of them spent one to two hours each day in the female refractory ward, which housed 65 patients and was supervised by only four and sometimes only two nurses. In the later book, *Chronic Schizophrenia* by Freeman, Cameron, and McGhie, Laing was identified as the person who spent time in the refractory ward.[87] The noisy and violent patients tended to absorb the energies of the nurses and the quieter ones were neglected. They sat around the walls or lay on the floor, in the same place every day. From this ward, eleven patients were selected by

[83] Ibid., 29 June 1954.

[84] Ibid., 15 March 1955.

[85] MS Laing DG57. Doctor–Nurse–Patient Relations, 1954–1955.

[86] Cameron, J.L., Laing, R.D. and McGhie, A. (1955). 'Patient and nurse. Effects of environmental changes in the care of chronic schizophrenics'. *The Lancet,* **266**, 1384–6.

[87] Freeman *et al.*, *Chronic Schizophrenia*, p. 6.

Laing to spend time in an attractively decorated ward. The only criterion for selection was the patient's social isolation. Their ages ranged from 22 to 63 years and they had all been in the ward for at least four years. They all suffered from schizophrenia.

Two nurses were also selected to be with the patients. After the second day the patients were waiting at the ward door to be taken across to the room. Initially the nurses tried to mould the patients' behaviour by exhortation or disapproval. The nurses were anxious about the experiment, worrying that the patients would run away or become violent. They felt that the patients were more settled in the room but it was reported that they were extremely unsettled on return to the ward.

Gradually an improvement in the patients was noticed. They paid more attention to their appearance and were more active, sewing, drawing, or making tea. Some patients began to behave to the other patients in a more individuated way. The nurses became less worried and they also thought that the patients were becoming more comprehensible. In an earlier draft of the published paper the authors gave more details. They referred to Elizabeth T., who greeted one of the authors as her brother, the Duke.[88] The authors felt the patients were not making more sense; it was just that the nurses were beginning to understand them better and were more sensitive to their feelings. The nurses became less concerned with the prohibition of antisocial behaviour by direct action, and became more interested in anticipating the unsatisfied needs that had produced them. The patients did more and more of the work in the room. Violence diminished. Trips into town were organised and went well. In the draft version of the paper, the authors reported that three patients went home at weekends. One patient appeared to have improved considerably but after she returned from her third weekend away, she did not seem so well:

> She was depressed, and told the nurses that someone had been interfering with her and that she was now pregnant. Nurse B. pointed out that the patient had visited her mother's grave for the first time at the week-end, and that she had been talking for a long time to a ward nurse whom she had thought was a man while she was very ill.[89]

Laing would have supported this effort to find meaning in madness, and he was pleased that nurses were adopting this approach to their patients. In the *Lancet* paper, the authors described an incident which would have appealed to Laing's view that madness could be turned off and on:

> . . . Mrs Smith said to one of us at tea-time: 'Would you care for a cup of tea?' He accepted and she began to pour him a cup. Nurse asked her if the doctor took sugar and milk. 'Of course he does. One spoonful of sugar. Don't you remember. He always does.' This ordinary conversation, was quite startling both to the nurse and the doctor. Not only was the patient talking sense in sound syntax (this she had done before); but suddenly she had abandoned the stilted intoning of words which had characterised her speech for years, which is so characteristic to psychotics and so elusive to written description.[90]

---

[88] MS Laing A151/1. Cameron, J.L., Laing, R.D. and McGhie, A. Chronic Schizophrenic Patients and their Nurses: A Study in the Essentials of Environment, p. 9.

[89] Ibid., p.11.

[90] Cameron *et al.*, 'Patient and nurse', p. 1386.

After twelve months the authors felt that there had been many improvements in the appearance and behaviour of the patients. They were no longer social isolates and they took greater interest in themselves. They were less violent and their language ceased to be obscene. The authors felt that the main factor in the improvement was not the change to a more pleasant environment, but that the nurses and patients had been able to get to know each other and formed a bond. They concluded that the barrier between patients and staff was not erected solely by the patients but was a mutual construction.

Reflections

Laing continued to be preoccupied with the 'Rumpus Room' experiment for the rest of his career. He wrote notes and discussed it in interviews and in books. As he retold the story, he emphasized the centrality of his role and he exaggerated the benefits the experiment had brought to the patients. In an unpublished paper on the 'Rumpus Room', written in the wake of the completion of the research, Laing stated that he had been inspired by the nineteenth century English alienist, Henry Maudsley, who contended that what he called 'chemical restraint' to the brain cells was equivalent to physical restraint to the body. Laing remarked that the inscription on the foundation stone of Gartnavel Hospital promised that physical restraints would never be used, and he interpreted this to include medication and physical methods of treatment. Rather than physical methods of treatment, Laing felt that the human relationship between staff and patient was crucial. He observed that the nurses in the 'Rumpus Room' became fond of their patients and that it was important that they did not feel there was anything wrong with this. He wrote:

> The nurses I worked with had an ordinary aptitude and disposition for their job. Like their patients they were 'simply human'. If simple humanity is given an opportunity to display ordinary devotion, I believe with Conolly that 'the consequences may not be that a much greater number of perfect recoveries are affected . . . but the actual number of the insane thus kept in the living and intellectual world, enjoying a share of happiness, is immensely increased'.[91]

In an early draft of *The Divided Self*,[92] under the heading of 'Confirmation', Laing outlined how a psychiatric hospital could seriously undermine a patient's sense of their own identity. People's sense of identity was normally based on the clothes they wore, the place they stayed, and where they worked. But this was different for a psychiatric patient. First, they did not have their own clothes but were issued with institutional ones. Often they did not have a place to put them. Although they might sleep in the same bed for years they might suddenly be moved to another bed or another ward. They had no money. Although there was a sameness about the daily routine, there was no time of the day that was their own. They had to get up, eat, and go to bed when they were told. Laing concluded:

> Many patients feel very often, therefore, that the words they use are not their own. They are everyone's property. They may even feel that the words are strangers to them and

---

[91] MS Laing A153, p.12.
[92] MS Laing A590/1. Draft outline of *The Divided Self.*

therefore that they are in a sense persecuted by words, so they attack their own words by splitting them up and so on, or they invent words which come as far as possible to have meaning which they alone can understand, and in that sense achieve in language something private . . . They are using words to convey to others that their words have a private, secret meaning, rather than to communicate in terms of shared sounds and meanings of sounds.

On a reprint of the *Lancet* paper, Laing scrawled some comments, which he left undated:

After all that, I could just about stand to be an unbelieving psychiatrist even if it meant I was psychotic. But I was not in a minority of one. There were others, who did not believe that all these 'chronic deteriorated schizophrenics' in refractory wards were all suffering from some irreversible deteriorative degenerative process . . .[93]

In 1972, in an interview with Peter Mezan, Laing revisited the 'Rumpus Room' experiment.[94] He described the impact his visits to the refractory ward had on the patients, who would 'all start going through their schizophrenic numbers—muttering and walking up and down, or crouching in a corner, or whatever their number happened to be'.[95] Here Laing is talking his characteristic view that madness is something of an act, something the patient adopts in particular situations. Of his proposal to set a room aside for selected patients, he commented that the nurses were disconcerted he should want to see the patients alone, because it 'went against all the rules', although, as have seen, Laing received support from the hospital authorities for the project. He spoke dismissively of his research colleagues, whom he claimed to have 'brought' in with him because he was about to go to another job at the Southern General. Laing spoke contemptuously of their narrow psychoanalytic approach, which he felt prevented them from fully engaging with their patients as people. He claimed that Freeman, Cameron, and McGhie's book, *Chronic Schizophrenia* showed: 'after eighteen months all my patients had been released back to their families—because they seemed a lot better. And a year later they were all back again'.[96] He added: 'Naturally! Nobody in those days thought about the *family* in relation to schizophrenia.'

In 1976, Laing again discussed the 'Rumpus Room' experiment, this time in his book, *The Facts of Life*.[97] He conceded that 'Gart Navel [sic] wasn't too bad as a genuine refuge' and that quite a few people would admit themselves there of their own accord. He claimed that he had 'persuaded the hospital authorities to try an experiment of taking everyone off every drug that they didn't want'. He recounted that thirty windows in the ward were broken in the first week, but, he averred, the cost of replacement was still cheaper than the drugs. There is no evidence to support this account and it does seem to be one of Laing's fanciful re-tellings of events. Laing went on to write that he was the only doctor who ventured into the refractory wards. Other doctors

---

[93] MS Laing A535.

[94] Mezan, *After Freud.*

[95] Ibid., p. 168.

[96] Ibid., p. 171.

[97] Laing, R.D. (1976). *The Facts of Life.* Penguin Books, London, pp. 111–16.

might come in to perform the mandatory six-monthly physical examinations of the patients, but they left as soon as they could. Consequently they were unaware of what 'really' happened in the ward, which only, he, Laing, was privy to as a result of his more extended visits. He claimed that a nurse would warn the patients that the examining doctor was coming and that they would then 'take up their appropriate positions and start up their usual numbers'. Once again Laing has set himself up as the lone hero and friend to the lowly patients and nurses. He is accepted by them and is able to penetrate the reality of their world. And again Laing uses the trope that madness is a 'number' that patients perform when it suits them.

In *The Facts of Life*, Laing declared himself to be 'in full sympathy' with the patients and those nurses who wanted change, and, as a result, he wrote a report, recommending the 'Rumpus Room' project. He maintained that relationships formed amongst patients and staff were more important than medication. Typically, Laing claimed that he was only 25 at the time of the project when he was actually nearer 28. In the book, Laing recounts:

> On the first day, the twelve 'completely withdrawn' patients had to be shepherded from the ward across to the day room. The second day, at half past eight in the morning, I had one of the most moving experiences of my life on that ward. There they all were clustered around the locked door, just waiting to get out and get over there with the two nurses and me . . . So much for being 'completely withdrawn'.[98]

Once again he repeated the story that all the patients were discharged in eighteen months but re-admitted within a year.

In 1987, Laing again told the story of the 'Rumpus Room', on this occasion in his autobiography, *Wisdom, Madness and Folly*[99] and his account followed that of *The Facts of Life*. He claimed that there was 'no sense of threat or real physical danger' in the 'Rumpus Room', though the contemporaneous notes suggest it was rather more turbulent that Laing made out. He observed that:

> In that room, it became ever more clear to me that these patients were exquisitely sensitive to nuances that some people never notice, or dismiss as petty. Most of us walk over them but some people drown in them, patients or not.[100]

Laing was repeating a common belief of American psychoanalysts, such as Freida Fromm-Reichmann, that individuals who suffered from schizophrenia were in possession of an acute sensitivity that rendered them supremely vulnerable to social interaction. Laing reiterated the story that all the patients were discharged but were all re-admitted at a later date. This time he asked if they had found more 'companionship' inside the 'Rumpus Room', than outside, in the community.

In 1988 Laing was interviewed by Bob Mullan for the book that would become *Mad to be Normal*. He once again discussed the 'Rumpus Room' experiment, and claimed of the patient group that: 'The change in them was immediate and dramatic and was sustained over a period of about 18 months or so until all of the group left the hospital . . . by

---

[98] Ibid., pp. 115–16.
[99] Laing, *Wisdom, Madness and Folly*, pp. 120–6.
[100] Ibid., p. 125.

another year or so they were all back'.[101] As we have seen, the changes were more modest than Laing claims in this interview.

In a recent paper Abrahamson[102] has re-examined the 'Rumpus Room' experiment. Although the original *Lancet* paper made no mention of the patients being discharged, Laing, as we have documented, went on to claim that all the patients in the study had been discharged home but that eighteen months later they were all back in hospital. Abrahamson traced six of the original study patients and found that *none* of them were ever discharged. His findings raise questions as to whether Laing's memory was at fault or whether he deliberately fabricated the story. However, Dr Hunter-Brown, who was at Gartnavel at the time recalls:

> In 1956/57 when I was working in the hospital we heard that all Laing's therapeutic community patients had been so improved as to be able to leave the hospital, and after a year or so at home had all volunteered to return.[103]

It is difficult to be sure exactly what happened to the 'Rumpus Room' patients. Was it part of the hospital folklore that they had been discharged, or were some of them, whom Abrahamson was unable to trace, discharged?

Abrahamson maintains that Laing and his colleagues presented a very restricted view of the refractory ward and its inmates. He criticizes the authors for not mentioning the effect of the experiment on the patients who were not chosen for the 'Rumpus Room' and were left behind in the refractory ward, though this issue was discussed at staff meetings as we have seen. Abrahamson points out that, although Laing observed that it was a good development that nurses and patients began to enjoy each other's company, he, himself, did not participate in such a close relationship with the patients. The implication seems to be that Laing had only minimal involvement with these patients, though Laing's own contemporaneous notes suggest that he did spend a significant period of time on the ward.

Abrahamson criticizes the project for dissuading nurses from attempting to mould the patients' behaviour by using approval or disapproval. The medical staff were imbued with psychodynamic thinking and may have been hostile to behavioural methods. He also criticizes the doctors for interpreting the nurses' concern for patient safety as evidence of their own anxiety. Abrahamson comments that medical staff did not appreciate the extent to which patients sought out activities to structure their day and that they also underestimated the impact the greatly improved environment of the 'Rumpus Room' would have had on the patients' well-being. However, as we have seen from his notes, Laing put a lot of thought into how the environment of the 'Rumpus Room' could be improved.

In his review of the Gartnavel period, Jonathan Andrews concluded that Laing, in his retrospective accounts of his Glasgow days, had been less than generous to his colleagues in acknowledging their work, although he did concede that Laing' ex-colleagues had their own agendas, too, and may have minimized Laing's contribution. Biographers have

---

[101] Mullan, *Mad to be Normal*, p. 133.
[102] Abrahamson, *R.D. Laing and Long-Stay Patients*.
[103] Hunter-Brown, *R.D. Laing*, p. 82.

generally followed Laing's lead and paid little attention to his co-workers or the contemporary psychiatric interest in social approaches to mental illness. For example, Kotowicz[104] claims that, even as early as the 1950s at Gartnavel, Laing's 'distinctly different' approach was evident.

The 'Rumpus Room' experiment occupies a key place in Laing's narrative of the Psychiatrist's Progress, and his account of it has frequently been repeated uncritically by others. In Laing's version, he boldly enters the foreboding and forbidden territory of the refractory ward. His entry is fraught with danger, but our hero conquers his fears and his repugnance, to remain with the excluded ones. His reward is that he is accepted by this estranged community and begins to see behind their veil of obfuscation and learn their language. He plans to rescue his new companions, or at least some of them, and sets up an expedition to a kinder, happier land. Despite hostility and indifference from those in power, the expedition is a success, but when our hero departs, his companions falter and are returned to their former misery. To be fair to Laing, there is quite a lot of truth in this mythological account. He *did* show initiative, courage, and perseverance in spending time in the refractory ward. He *was* afforded a perspective on the institutional world of the long-stay patient that few had sought to investigate. He *did* try hard to understand this often intimidating and perplexing world. He *did* invest a lot of time and energy in setting up and following through the 'Rumpus Room' experiment. However, in later years he did rather exaggerate what the experiment had achieved and he did tend to downplay the contributions of others. The 'Rumpus Room' was to form the template for Laing's more radical experiment in the 1960s with Kingsley Hall, where mentally disturbed people could seek sanctuary without psychiatric intervention.[105]

---

[104] Kotowicz, *Laing and the Paths of Anti-Psychiatry*, p. 71.

[105] Abrahamson judges that Kingsley Hall came to resemble the refractory ward rather than the 'Rumpus Room'. He states that there was a deteriorated physical environment, inactivity, and the more vulnerable residents were not properly protected.

Chapter 9

Individual patients at Gartnavel

In March 1960, in the same year as *The Divided Self* was published, Laing reflected on his interest in psychotic patients:

> I think I found myself "drawn into" psychotherapy with psychotics because I seemed to under-stand them enough not to able to forget what they told me of their persecution and despair.[1]

During his placement at Gartnavel, Laing devoted a considerable amount of time to psychotic patients: talking to them, listening to them, and making efforts to understand their worlds. These were amongst the most disturbed and disturbing patients that Laing ever saw in his career, and their stories formed the basis of his early theorizing about madness. Several of them, such as 'Julie', 'Peter', and 'Mrs A.', were to make memorable appearances in *The Divided Self* and *The Self and Others*. We are fortunate that Laing made such extensive notes about his clinical work, because they provide an invaluable glimpse into his day-to-day encounters with patients and how his thinking about them evolved.

During this period Laing drew on fairly orthodox Freudian concepts. He asked patients to tell him what came into their mind and to remember what they had been feeling and doing; and he examined their past memories and dreams.[2] Laing made orthodox psychoanalytical comments, for example, he said of one female patient: 'She has withdrawn libidinal cathexis from love-objects (husband, son) . . . this relationship to self (under her own lash) reflected in transference—"I feel as tho' I've been whipped"'.[3] Laing was also influenced by those clinicians such as Frieda Fromm-Reichmann and John Rosen, who held, despite Freud's scepticism, that psychoanalysis was applicable to psychotic patients. He was inspired by *The Mental Hospital* by Staunton and Schwartz, who advised that, if the patient talked long enough to some-one, there was bound to be a favourable change. The authors maintained that it was ethically wrong to give up on 'chronic' patients. In his clinical notes, we also see Laing drawing on existential and spiritual perspectives on madness.

Mrs C.

Laing's encounter with Mrs C. illustrates how disturbed some of the patients at Gartnavel were during this time. It also shows Laing attempting to use Freudian notions, such as 'penis envy'. Laing saw Mrs C. several times in the summer of 1954.[4]

---

[1] Research Fellowship Application by Laing to the Foundations' Fund for Research in Psychiatry, 15 March 1960, p. 5.

[2] MS Laing DG53, Gartnavel Cases. Mrs M. Interview, 19 December 1953.

[3] Ibid. Interview, 18 September 1953.

[4] MS Laing DS92, Notes on Mrs C.

She proved to be violent and abusive. Initially he saw her on his own, but during an early interview, she attacked him. She put her arms round him and attempted to drag him to the floor. She then tried to kick him in the groin and to scratch his face. Laing decided that in the future he would only see her with a nurse.

Mrs C. believed that she was a white slave who had been bought and placed in Gartnavel by Dr MacHarg, whom she described as a 'stinking bastard'. In the hospital she believed she was being 'sexed up' by the doctors and that filthy, stenchy injections were administered to her through her vagina. She was going to complain to the Law Courts in Edinburgh and ruin not only all the doctors, but the whole country.

When Laing saw her with a nurse, Mrs C. began by asking them if they were sexually intimate and she also enquired about their sex life. Neither Laing nor the nurse replied, and Mrs C. commented, 'Well haven't you tongues in your heads, can't you answer!' Laing answered that her questions were intended to embarrass and provoke himself and the nurse. In further interviews, Mrs C. continued to be abusive towards Laing. On one occasion she again tried to kick him in the groin, but he side-stepped it and she was restrained by nurses, all the while scratching, biting, and spitting.

In one interview Laing said to her that she couldn't get over the fact that *she* didn't possess a penis. She replied: 'O if I had a penis, then there wouldn't be a woman in Glasgow who wouldn't have a baby by me.' She proceeded to express the most intense envy of males, before going into details about artificial insemination of cattle. Mrs C. then made remarks about the size of Laing's penis. The next day she was described as 'going round naked', and was locked in her room. Laing went to see her, but she attacked him again and drew some blood. She said to him: 'If it satisfies you I was shouting about penises all morning.' Laing commented in his notes: 'I think the next step is to extend the "penis envy" to the interpersonal context.'

Miss M.

Laing was interested in Miss M., who was an inpatient at Gartnavel and whom he described in *Wisdom, Madness and Folly*.[5] In his contemporary notes[6] of 1953, he wrote that she had a manic-depressive illness. He mused that a manic patient was said to deny or refuse to mention their 'secret sorrow', but Miss M. did neither. Instead she dwelt on what had been denied her: children and the loss of loved ones through death. The patient told him to read Psalm 32, verses 3 and 4, which she said described her situation. It read:

> When I kept silence, my bones waxed old through my roaring all day long.
> For day and night thy hand was heavy upon me: my moisture is turned into the drought of summer.

Laing tried to see her situation in existential terms and he referred to the work of Paul Tillich. He felt that because she saw her life as an existential failure, she had liter-ally 'gone to pieces'. In his autobiography Laing was to claim that Miss M. was able to

---

[5] Laing, R.D. (1985). *Wisdom, Madness and Folly*. Canongate, Edinburgh (1998 reprint). pp. 121–2.
[6] MS Laing DG53, notes on Miss M., 14 November 1953.

have lucid conversations with him and that she explained to him what was happening with the other patients in the ward. She became, he says, his 'mentor'.

Miss L.

Laing described sessions he had with a Miss L., an inpatient at Gartnavel with an agitated depressive illness.[7] Laing captured her distraught state well:

> She enters the room in great agitation, usually saying 'I don't want to see you, Dr. Laing. Dr. Laing please let me go. Oh, you're just torturing me. You can't do anything for me. You can't see into my mind. You've never had a case like mine before. Dr. Laing, why can't I get well . . . will you give me something. Some day . . . why not . . . Oh I can't sit down, I've got to walk about all the time and my feet are so sore'.

Laing said to her:

> You have thoughts that disturb you, that you've . . . you're ashamed of. They horrify you. You feel that you couldn't have such thoughts if you were yourself—in your right mind. Besides, you feel you deserve nothing more or better than this—to walk up and down in a Mental Hospital for the rest of your life.

Miss L. replied:

> I'm ashamed of walking up and down—there's nothing else for it.

At one interview Laing interpreted her behaviour as a consequence of guilt over her death wish for her mother, but admitted that it did not have any noticeable effect. On the next occasion she walked about as usual and Laing said nothing.

Miss A.

In *The Divided Self*, Laing described the case of Rose, who was trying to deal with painful memories by forgetting herself.[8] She felt that she was gradually killing herself, in fact later she claimed that she *had* killed herself. This case was based on a Miss A., a 23-year-old woman that Laing had encountered at Gartnavel in 1954. He made lengthy notes of what she said in interviews with him and he also summarized the clinical details of her case.[9] She was one of four children and had several office jobs. She became ill at the age of 18 and had four previous admissions to hospital. She had been treated with several courses of ECT and also insulin.

Laing felt that she had a 'borderline psychotic state'. Miss A. told him:

> Real self is away down: used to be just in my throat but now it's gone further down. Losing myself . . . Don't know what I'm trying to do all I know I'm killing myself slowly. I can't look forward. Can't plan time.
>
> Get scared. World of my own. They cannot get in and I cannot get out.[10]

---

[7] MS Laing DL3, notes on Miss L.

[8] Laing, R.D. (1960). *The Divided Self. A Study of Sanity and Madness*. Tavistock Publications, London, pp. 150–3.

[9] MS Laing DA23, Miss A., 1954.

[10] Ibid., p.3.

Laing considered that Miss A. had problems with ego boundaries: that she had difficulty in deciding between 'me and not-me'. He felt that the outlook was not good unless she was seen consistently by one therapist—by that point she had already been seen by eleven psychiatrists. Unless this happened, Miss A. was going to be ill indefinitely and probably end up having a leucotomy, Laing judged.

Betty

Laing made extensive notes on his psychotherapy sessions with Betty, who was an inpatient at Gartnavel and suffered from a manic-depressive illness.[11] She was to become 'Cathy' in *The Self and Others*.[12] Laing saw her on a regular basis and adopted a psychodynamic approach. It is clear that Betty was intermittently very disturbed during the period that Laing was seeing her.

Laing observed that, for a period Betty construed his every gesture as an attempt to annoy her. She repeatedly said that staff, too, wanted to annoy her, either by sending her to another hospital or by keeping her at Gartnavel. At one session, Betty greeted him: 'Why do you come here? Why don't you take another patient? I know what you will say; that I am testing out your feelings to see whether you are fond of me.'[13] We see how patients quickly became familiar with Laing's psychotherapeutic approach, particularly his strategy of turning their statements back on them. Laing responded by reminding her of a dream she had a few days previously. In the dream, she was running away, but 'as hard as she ran she could not get further away as she was being held here by a magnet'.[14] He told her that the feelings which held her here came from inside herself. Laing quoted this dream in *The Self and Others*, but changed her account so that it now read: 'I am running as hard as I can away from the hospital, but the hospital, and you in it, is a gigantic magnet.'[15]

At the next session Betty spoke about getting all her teeth out and wondered if her gums would be ripped. Laing suggested that 'such fantasies had to do with a need she experienced to suffer pain and punishment in consequence of the fantasies' she had about him. Two hours after this interview, the patient came into the room where Laing was sitting and poured a pail of water over him. She went out immediately but came back five minutes later and said, 'Do you think you will get pneumonia?' Laing replied that he didn't think so. She went back to the ward but was very agitated and had to be given a sedative. Later she half-heartedly apologized and said she had been annoyed because Laing had cut the interview short by five minutes. She was also annoyed that Laing had previously said to her that she was afraid of what his feelings towards her might be. She said, 'You don't feel anything for anybody'.

In the next few interviews Laing considered that Betty's sexual fantasies were becoming more conscious and were 'evoking an almost unmanageable super ego reaction'. She compared Laing to Dr Jekyll and Mr Hyde, saying: 'You are really very kind, but

---

[11] MS Laing DB87, Further notes on psychotherapy, October 1954.

[12] Laing, R.D. (1961). *The Self and Others*. Tavistock Publications, London, p. 142; also in Laing, R.D. (1969). *Self and Others* (2nd edn). Pelican, London, pp. 149–50.

[13] MS Laing DB87, Further notes on psychotherapy, p. 1.

[14] Ibid., p. 1.

[15] Laing, *The Self and Others*, p. 142.

at times you are horrible'. She described what might be construed as a prophetic dream that Laing was on trial for taking drugs. As we know, in later years Laing was to take drugs and was compelled to surrender his medical licence after facing accusations of alcohol abuse. In her dream, Betty reported, she had intervened in Laing's 'trial' to say it was her fault. She admitted that she was worried that she would drive him to drugs. She asked him why he smoked so much.

Sometime later she went on an overnight pass to her family home, but did not tell her parents she was allowed out. When they asked her to return to the hospital, she became convinced that her parents did not want her. She went to Glasgow Central Station and broke windows in a train. On being returned to the hospital by the police she broke 22 panes of glass in 'a frenzy of anger'. She absconded from the ward several times again, on one occasion she was found in Great Western Road in her dressing-gown.

A subsequent session is interesting because it reveals Laing's belief in the importance of early childhood experiences and their influence on later adult behaviour. This was, of course, a commonly held view amongst psychoanalytically-minded psychiatrists, but in this exchange we see how Laing introduced the concept to the patient. Laing commented that when Betty felt upset she often had difficulty putting her feelings into words and, instead, acted out her difficulties. He suggested that the way she felt now must bear some relation to the way she felt as a very young child, when she had 'incomplete mastery of language and when what words she did have seemed to her extremely powerful and dangerous weapons, that is when she was 18 months to 2 (and a half) years of age, just after one sister had been born and during the period when her second sister was born'. This provoked a heated response from Betty, who replied, 'You think I am upset by the birth of my sisters, see! I hate them, I hate the lot of them. I hate everybody, they are all the same'.

Some days later she took an overdose of sedative medication after a visit from her sister. Betty had said to her, 'What would you do if you knew I was going to kill myself in a quarter of an hour?—nothing?' When Laing saw her the next day he told her the story of the Chinese who, when they kill themselves, do so on their enemies' doorstep. Betty was by now in a state of 'manic excitement', and, at a subsequent interview, she paced up and down and talked in a most disjointed fashion. She was sent to the secure ward. When seen again by Laing, she remembered the Chinese proverb and said: 'That's a good idea. You remember that you said, "Just go ahead".' She threatened Laing that she would not go back to the ward when the interview finished. Laing went to phone nursing staff to bring her back and she promptly barricaded herself in the room and broke six windows. When she was taken out, she returned to the ward laughing, jumping, and skipping, evidently in high spirits.

Laing's notes reveal that he was dedicated in his attempts to help Betty and that he had to withstand considerable aggression from his patient. His employment of psychodynamic psychotherapy to treat a patient with a manic-depressive psychosis was in keeping with the Gartnavel tradition and, indeed, with other psychiatric hospitals during this period. In a revealing passage, headed 'Notes on Counter-Transference' he described his feelings about Betty:

I want to 'cure' her.

I want her to respect me.

I find her praise of me more difficult to interpret as transference than criticism.

I find I am . . . too ready to discount the 'real' intensity of her criticisms.

I tend to identify myself with her (my problems with my parents—I see parallels).

I want her to be concerned—I want to play a significant role in her life.

However at present, I am reasonably settled (secure & satisfied) in my own relationship.[16]

At times Laing was capable of great frankness and was able to acknowledge negative aspects of himself. After he left Gartnavel and had taken up his post at the Southern General, Laing kept in touch with Betty by letter for a short period.[17]

In *The Self and Others*, Laing wrote that Betty, whom he christened 'Cathy', was engrossed in a struggle to leave her parents. She could not do so in a real way, but 'developed a manic psychosis in which she "left" her parents in a psychotic sense by denying that her parents were her real parents'.[18] From Laing's perspective, psychosis did not arise by chance; rather it was a person's reaction to their life-situation. It was a way of dealing, albeit in an often maladaptive and destructive manner, with a personal crisis. In the case of Betty, her manic symptoms and behaviour were occasioned by what Laing perceived as her troubled relationship with her parents. Laing wrote that she was constantly running home, but when she arrived, she would berate her parents for not letting her lead her own life. In *The Self and Others*, Laing described 'Cathy'/Betty as having a 'transference psychosis', by which he meant that her reactions to him were re-enactments of past relationships and that they made themselves manifest in the symptoms of her psychosis. For Laing, insanity was potentially understandable, and Freudian techniques offered a key to unlock the secrets of psychosis, at least in this case. Laing's view of Freudian psychoanalysis was not uncritical, but in the clinical situation, especially early in his career, he drew heavily on it.

In the revised 1969 edition, Laing added that the only reason that 'Cathy'/Betty was in hospital was the disturbance she made when she got home. This is somewhat disingenuous, because, as we have seen, Betty was also very disturbed in hospital and public places. There were occasions when she was so unsettled that she was given sedative medication and sent to a more secure ward. Laing tended to play down just how disturbed some of the patients were that he described in his books. In tandem, he tended to exaggerate how easy it was to make sense of their psychosis.

Magda

Laing made notes on Magda, a long-term patient at Gartnavel who was one of the patients involved in the 'Rumpus Room' experiment.[19] His notes are of interest because they illustrate his clinical approach to severely disturbed patients and they

---

[16] MS Laing DB87. Notes on Betty.

[17] Ibid. Letters between Laing and Betty.

[18] Laing, *The Self and Others*, p. 142.

[19] MS Laing DF69. Notes on Magda, 1954–1955.

also reflect his belief, common at the time, that the mother played an important role in the genesis of schizophrenia.

When Laing first encountered Magda in 1954, she was 33 years old. She came from a large Roman Catholic family. Her parents had a strained relationship and her father, who was rather distant, had left it to the mother to bring up the children. Magda had a twin brother, three older brothers, and one older sister. Her mother remembered that she was not allowed to breast feed the twins in case it gave them 'rheumatism'.[20] The twins also had 'delicate stomachs' and, in the first few months, they lost weight. As we will see, Laing was to make much of the mother's breast-feeding difficulties in his interviews with Magda. The mother reported that Magda was easily toilet-trained.

Magda was devoted to her twin brother, and tended to hang around with him and his companions, rather than making friends of her own. Her mother told Laing that as a child Magda had been a 'delightful character' who was fond of dancing. She attended a fee-paying school and later went to work at the Post Office, which she found draining. Sometime later she enrolled at teacher-training school. She worried a lot about her work and her studies.

Her twin brother told Laing that their mother did not like Magda having boyfriends and generally thought that men were 'not much good'.[21] She actively broke up one of Magda's relationship because she thought the man was unsuitable. Her twin felt that their mother still treated Magda as a little girl, rather than as a woman of 33. He had escaped from the controlling nature of the mother by joining the Navy and becoming independent. When he married at the age of 27, he felt Magda had been upset and his mother was also unhappy because he had married a non-Catholic.

Laing first met Magda in August 1954. At that point she was very disturbed. She believed she was being tortured and that she was in hospital to be hypnotized. 'Town parole' or trips outside the hospital had been stopped because she had been noisy and drew 'unwelcome attention to herself'. She was annoyed about this and had increased her attacks on fellow-patients. Her mother had found her with a male patient in the hospital grounds and there was a suspicion that they had been having sexual intercourse. As a result of this, 'ground parole' or freedom to walk in the hospital grounds was curtailed and she became even more aggressive. She pleaded to get out and eventually took to her bed, saying 'I'm not well'. She spent her time lying bundled up under the bedclothes. She smeared food all over herself and urinated and defecated on the floor. She refused to get out of bed. At meal times she would however sit and allow herself to be fed by a nurse, albeit, keeping her eyes shut.

Laing writes that it was 'decided to do something about her as she had regressed possibly to a foetal stage'.[22] On his first visit Laing simply watched her being fed. On the second visit, Laing said to her: 'You feel you're a little baby. You're to be fed and nursed, and given every attention'. She replied: 'I get no attention in this place'. Laing assured her that he would see that she did. In a subsequent interview,

---

[20] Ibid. Interview with Magda's mother, 1955.
[21] Ibid. Interview with twin brother of Magda.
[22] Ibid. Notes on Magda, p. 1.

Magda began talking about the number 10. She said she was not 10. The exchange continued:[23]

> LAING You feel you weren't made perfect—10 is a perfect number—you've been born mutilated so you feel.
> MAGDA I get nothing in here.
> LAING It's not the nurses' fault. It's your mother's fault.
> MAGDA That's nonsense. I got on very well with my mother.
> LAING She's an old witch.
> MAGDA (pause, no comment). I get no tea in here.
> LAING If only your mother had some good milk to give you.
> MAGDA You talk a lot of nonsense.
> LAING I'll see you get tea.

Laing found that by keeping Magda supplied with tea and cigarettes she would agree to see him. A few interviews later, Magda again complained that the nurses tortured her and that the ward sister treated her 'like dirt'. Laing recorded:[24]

> LAING Sister's a good mother to you. She's very fond of you. I know that. She doesn't want to stand between us. Your mother's the bad one.
> MAGDA As a matter of fact I got on very well with my mother
> —long pause while she smoked her cigarette.

In a subsequent interview, Magda complained she was being kept in hospital in chains and that it was Laing's fault.[25] Laing asked her about her brother but she replied: 'It's none of your business . . . I don't attempt to be evolutionised—your psychoanalysis is all wrong.'[26] With this patient Laing seems to be following the example of John Rosen, who told patients that their mother was the problem, and that it was the task of the therapist to compensate by being a 'good mother'. Rosen also talked about 'good' and 'bad' milk. Thanks to Laing's honesty in reporting Magda's responses, we can see that she was not very impressed with this approach and continued to assert that she had a good relationship with her mother.

The coldness of death

Laing made extensive notes about Mrs McL., a 34-year-old patient who was suffering from a puerperal psychosis.[27] He completed 45 pages, detailing his psychotherapy sessions with her and he typed out her own hand-written account of her illness. He also typed out his formulation of her problems. Mrs McL.'s case formed the basis of Chapter 6, 'The Coldness of Death' in *The Self and Others*,[28] which was later revised and retitled, *Self and Others*.[29] In these books, she appeared as 'Mrs A.'.

---

[23] Ibid., p. 2.
[24] Ibid., pp. 3–4.
[25] Ibid., p. 5.
[26] Ibid., p. 6.
[27] MS Laing DM103. Typed and handwritten notes on Mrs McL., 1953–1954. Hand-written account by patient, typed up by Laing.
[28] Laing, *The Self and Others*, pp. 57–66.
[29] Laing, *Self and Others*, pp. 68–77.

Mrs McL. was a Roman Catholic from Barra. She was married to a ship's officer and they had four children. For three weeks after the birth of her fourth child in October 1953, she had felt unable to get up from bed, though her doctor could find nothing physically wrong with her. She felt a 'terrible storm in her head'.[30] One night her husband came back from a party at four in the morning and was a bit drunk. In the book Laing writes that he came back from a 'business trip' and makes no reference to drunkenness. The baby had been crying all night and she was angry with her husband. She accused him of having ruined her with repeated pregnancies, and said he was callous and cruel.

The next night she did not sleep but had sensations of sails flapping in her head, a violent storm going on inside her, and a strange sense of her thoughts running down and coming to a standstill. She fell asleep for three hours and felt better. She took the baby out of the cot and put him on the side of her bed to feed him but the baby fell on the floor. She was deeply upset but then came the realization that all this had nothing to do with her. She was no longer 'in the world'. The room and the baby in the cot now suddenly appeared as if seen through the wrong end of a telescope. She was 'absolutely and completely emotionless'.[31]

She developed a peculiar sensation in her tongue, and felt it was paralysed and twisted. She thought that she had been poisoned and that the poison had come from a germ in her bladder. Laing, in his typed notes, wrote that she thought of her illness and experiences in Gaelic. She said that *ollphiast*,[32] the Gaelic word for intestinal worm, also meant 'beast', and that the English word 'worm' did not capture her feeling of there being a beast inside her wreaking destruction. In *The Self and Others*, Laing dropped the Gaelic details and wrote that 'There was no one word that served to convey entirely to her satisfaction what she felt she had inside her.'[33] This is curious as the Gaelic context adds colour to the picture and helps us to understand the patient better. Also Laing's avowed intention in the book was to try and understand individuals in their social context. By divorcing the patient's narrative from her cultural background, Laing rendered her story less meaningful. Was he trying to protect her anonymity by changing the details, or was he keen to disguise the Scottish and Gaelic aspects of the narrative? As a Scot abroad in London, was he, during this period in his career, suffering from a 'cultural cringe' about his native background?

Laing made extensive notes of his psychotherapy sessions with Mrs McL. and estimated that he saw her on sixty occasions between November 1953 and April 1954.[34] His working diagnosis was 'depression' but he admitted he was not sure. He spent a large part of the sessions interpreting her dreams and what he saw as the 'transference' reaction in his patient towards him. He invoked such concepts as 'female castration fear'

---

[30] MS Laing DM103. Typed notes by Laing.

[31] MS Laing DM103, Typed notes by Laing.

[32] Laing left the Gaelic word for intestinal worm blank, possibly because he was unsure how it was spelt. Thanks to Chrisma Bould for giving me information about this word. Olliphiast is from the Irish Gaelic, which was spoken on Barra.

[33] Laing, *The Self and Others*, pp. 58–9.

[34] MS Laing DM103, Hand-written notes by Laing.

and 'negative narcissism', which was a term he took from the analytical writer, Karl Abraham. Laing felt Mrs McL. had delusions that she was suffering from a serious bodily illness. She would repeatedly ask him to examine her for physical symptoms, and he would repeatedly refuse.

At one session Mrs McL. blushed and said to Laing: 'Well I suppose I have to face the music and ask you to feel my pulse.'[35] Laing concluded that she was trying to force him into the role of 'seducer' or 'lover', and noted that there was a 'strong erotic transference'. At another session Mrs McL. said to Laing: 'I know what you're thinking. You think that I'm ill like this because I'm running away from my life in Barra—that I dislike my husband.' Laing thought that this was 'quite a succinct, masterly summary of her case'. But she added that this was not how she saw her situation: she felt that she was physically ill. She then repeated her requests to be examined. She also continued her pattern of wanting to be told by medical staff that she needed to remain in hospital. On this occasion Laing refused to do so. The following morning she left the hospital. Laing felt she was playing him off against her husband, and he was again being put in the role of 'seducer'. The patient returned soon after and the sessions continued.

At one stage, Laing felt that Mrs McL. was now beginning to drop her delusions, but always returned to them, albeit, half-heartedly. She would say: 'I suppose I have to ask you to feel my pulse.' However this did not last and an interview some weeks later was entirely taken up with Mrs McL. talking at length about her symptoms. Laing tried a new tact as he explained in his notes:

> This time I told her that they were plainly fantastic & didn't merit consideration. That her judgement, just what she took to be perfect, was hopelessly impaired in this aspect. That I was surprised that so intelligent a person could hold such fantastic views etc. I knew she held such views. She derived satisfaction from talking about them. But she reiterated them to bring all else to a stop. That it was obstructive tactics. That I had said all there was to be said about them etc.[36]

Laing was clearly trying a direct approach. He was certainly capable of being forceful in interviews and, in another session, he recorded that he 'insisted fairly strongly' about his point of view. Perhaps Laing was frustrated with his patient, but he may have been deliberately adopting a somewhat brutal approach in the hope of bringing about a change in her. Whatever his motivation had been, Laing wrote that the following interview seemed to be more constructive, and that Mrs McL. made no mention of her physical symptoms.

About a week later, Mrs McL. asked to see Laing because she had experienced three 'flashes of inspiration' about her condition.[37] First, it had occurred to her that she would not have been able to have been so physically active in attending to her baby, if she was as seriously medically ill as she had imagined. She was now beginning to think that she had been wrong. She also said that for the last seven years she had been preoccupied with death, disease, and disaster, and that she had been concentrating for so

[35] Ibid. Notes on Mrs. McL., 1953–1954.
[36] Ibid., 11 March 1954.
[37] Ibid., 20 March 1954.

long that her mind had brought about what she most feared, at least in her imagination. She had tried to connect her symptoms with past events in her life. She had suddenly realized that her perception of her hands as blue was related to her experience with her baby daughter, Marie, who had suffered a fit and lay with 'blue-black' hands for two hours afterwards. Mrs McL. had never felt so distressed and she feared her daughter was going to die. When her daughter's hands returned to their normal colour, Mrs McL. began concentrating on her *own* hands. Another flash of inspiration occurred when she asked herself why she had felt that splashing her hands with water made them blue. She realized that this was connected to her splashing water over Marie's hands when they were blue.

Her third flash of inspiration came when she considered why she was repeatedly asking doctors to examine her to see whether she was dying or not. She connected this with the illness of Marie, when she waited for the doctor's verdict as to whether her daughter was going to die or not. She said that she seemed to have been re-living that day for the last six months. She discussed the coldness over her body. She remembered her mother used to talk about *fuachd a' bhias*, the Gaelic phrase for 'coldness of death'. She also remembered at school touching a boy's head, which felt cold, and that he later died. Laing used the English translation as the title of the chapter about her. He made no reference to the Gaelic origins. In his original typed notes, Laing observed that, for a Roman Catholic from Barra, it was a condition to call in a priest to administer the last rites.

Laing said to Mrs McL. that he thought that the connections she had made were important. He thought she was exhibiting what Freud had called 'repetition-compulsion', defined as an innate tendency to revert to earlier conditions. Laing said to her that other events from the past might come to her. When she asked for reassurance about her physical health, Laing told her the story of Atalanta from Greek mythology. She was a virgin huntress and all suitors who could not outrun her were put to death. Atalanta was eventually beaten when one suitor dropped three golden apples which she stopped to pick up. Laing felt Mrs McL.'s recurrent requests for reassurance were perhaps designed to throw others off the scent and to disguise a deeper problem. Mrs McL. stated that she was now glad that Laing had ignored her appeals for reassurance and was considering the possibility that he was right when he said there was nothing medically wrong with her. If he had reassured her, she might not have had her 'flashes of inspiration'. However, the interview ended with Mrs McL. yet again asking for reassurance.

At other sessions, Laing discussed Gaelic culture with Mrs McL., talking about such topics as second sight and literature. Laing recorded that he and she had examined Mrs Mcl.'s fears in 'the cultural context of the islands', and that it was 'instructive and helpful background that she had to cover sooner or later'.[38] As we have seen, Laing entirely dropped the Gaelic background to the story in *The Self and Others*.

Towards the end of her time in hospital, Laing recorded this exchange:

> MRS. MC.L Do you think I'm in a metaphoric state? I have woven a beautiful tapestry of symbols and am living in it.
> LAING It may be that you are saying this, not so much because you feel such to be the case, but because you feel that I would like you to say something like this etc.

---

[38] Ibid., 10 March 1954.

MRS. MCL. Yes, that is partly so but that has occurred to me. Get flashes when that is how it appears.[39]

Laing used these evocative remarks of his patient in the account of her in *The Self and Others*, but he omitted his own sceptical observations. Laing was seemingly aware that patients often adopt the theoretical outlook of their therapists, but in the book he did not want to give the impression that he had, somehow, influenced Mrs McL.

By 13 April 1954 Mrs McL. was feeling much better. However, Laing still pursued dream analysis. He interpreted one of her dreams as showing her jealousy of her brother. He recorded himself as saying to her: 'Just because he has a little appendix, this little extra equipment when you were so better equipped in every respect'.[40] She recollected that as a child she had a male doll, which she threw into the sea after tearing off all its clothes. Shortly after this Laing decided that her recovery had gone far enough and that the 'limited aim' of therapy had been reached. Her psychosis had subsided, but she was now in the 'neo-neurosis described by Rosen', for which, he wrote, there were no treatment facilities. Treatment ended on 30 April 1954 and Mrs McL. returned to Barra. In his two published accounts, Laing did not mention that he thought the patient needed further, specialized therapy. In the second edition of his book, he added that she had kept well for five years after leaving hospital.

In his typed notes Laing provided more details about Mrs McL. and how he perceived her problems. These notes are undated, though it would seem that they were completed some time after the handwritten notes, which were composed during Laing's actual clinical contact with Mrs McL. In his typed notes Laing placed less emphasis on Mrs McL.'s own belief that the episode, when her baby, Marie, turned blue, had disturbed her and that it had subsequently influenced the nature of her symptoms. He did state that one of her children was 'subject for a while to what appears to have been breath holding attacks' and that Mrs McL. was 'quite distracted' by this. He went on to describe her perception of the event in a rather different manner from the way he had described it in his hand-written notes. In the typed notes, he wrote that she had been splashing water over hands and 'suddenly had a flash of insight that her left hand was the head of her second baby and that she was splashing water over his head as she had done on one occasion when he had either a fit or a breath holding attack and she was convinced that he was going to die'. The gender of the baby was changed and Mrs McL.'s explanation was more symbolic. Laing went on to write that she had a second flash of insight when she equated her heart with her baby and had anxiously listened to it beating, afraid it might stop, which would signify the death of her baby. This explanation did not appear in the original notes.

In the typed notes, Laing wrote that she felt her skin had a dying pallor, her hands had an unnatural blueness, her heart might stop beating, her bones were twisted, and her flesh was perishing. Laing observed that her parents and brother were all dead, and he was struck that all her complaints seemed to be drawn from the final illnesses of her family. He claimed that she, herself, had likened the sallowness of her complexion to

[39] Ibid., undated but near the end of Laing's notes.
[40] Ibid., 13 April 1954.

that of her brother before he died of tuberculosis. She had felt the coldness of death creep over her father before he died. The paralysis of her tongue seemed to be derived from the experience of her dying father, who had suffered a series of strokes; also, her mother had died from cancer of the mouth. These connections between past events and current bodily symptoms were to form the core of Laing's account of Mrs McL. in the two editions of his book. In *Self and Others*, Laing writes of these connections:

> She made them herself. They were as complete a surprise to me as they were to her. No interpretations remotely resembling them had come from anyone.[41]

We have seen that there are some discrepancies and changes of emphasis in the different versions of the case of Mrs McL. How do we explain the differences? There are certain comparatively trivial differences. For example, Laing shifted the family up the social scale so that the husband was now a business man rather than a ship's officer. He also reduced the size of their family so that there were three children instead of four. This might be explained by the need to make the patient's case anonymous, and one could possibly defend the decision to drop the Gaelic context along these lines. However, the difference in the accounts of Mrs McL.'s own understanding of her symptoms is potentially more problematic. The most generous explanation is that the typed and book versions represent a fuller account of what the patient said, and that the hand-written notes were merely an abbreviated record, composed hastily without the opportunity for in-depth analysis. However, another possibility is that Laing amended the material to fit with his theoretical perspective on the case. The connections the patient is said to have made appear less complex and less symbolic in the original contemporaneous notes. One has to be a little sceptical that the patient made these connections spontaneously and entirely free from the influence of Laing, if indeed she made them at all. The original notes demonstrate that she was aware of Laing's perception of her case, and that he, in his turn, was aware that she might make interpretations of her problems in order to please him. As narrative-based medicine contends, the doctor and patient are both involved in constructing a story of the illness, and influence each other as to what kind of 'narrative' emerges.

In his discussion of Mrs McL. in *The Self and Others*, Laing wrote: 'Jung has, of course, more than anyone else, succeeded in linking such modern psychotic experience with human experiences in other time and places'.[42] When he came to revise the book in 1969, Laing dropped this reference to Jung. By this stage he was much more critical of Jung and disenchanted with his views on madness. Laing was evidently fascinated by the case of Mrs McL. and was to provide alternative explanations of her breakdown. In *The Self and Others*, Laing compared Mrs McL.'s account to Blake's poem, which reads:

> O Rose, thou art sick!
> The invisible worm.
> That flies in the night,
> In the howling storm,

---

[41] Laing, *Self and Others*, p. 76.
[42] Laing, *The Self and Others*, p. 65.

Has found out thy bed
Of crimson joy,
And his dark secret love
Does thy life destroy.

Laing contended that Blake was saying that a single vision or having only one modality of experience was akin to death. He went on:

> This is what most people regard as sanity. At least a two-fold vision is necessary before the full world of delight can be glimpsed. Mrs. A.'s psychosis was a single vision. For practical purposes she was insane, but from an ultimate point of view, she was no more subsane, no more moribund than we are most of the time *without* realizing it. Her sanity returned with a two-fold vision that frightened her because it was too much, but which she finally sustained. But none of us wishes to bear too much reality: to wake up, for instance, at 3 a.m. and realize that we have been under the delusion of being alive.[43]

Laing is comparing what he regarded as Blake's superior perception of reality with that of the normal run of humanity, whom he considered lived an impoverished existence and were not even aware they were doing so. For Laing, Blake was a visionary who was able to access other realms of experience—'the world of delight'—whilst the majority of unenlightened plodders were condemned to 'only one modality of experience'. They were, to use Laing's term, 'subsane'. His patient recovered when she was able to withstand the experience of a 'two-fold vision' of the world. By implication, she had achieved a more exalted state than most of us, who—and here Laing alludes to T.S. Eliot—cannot 'bear too much reality'. From his early student essay onwards, Laing held there was a division in society between the superior individual and the dull uncomprehending masses.

In 1969 when he was re-writing *The Self and Others*, Laing dropped this passage and relegated Blake to a foot-note. He now observed: 'what we call psychosis may be some times a natural process of healing (a view for which I claim no priority)'.[44] Madness, Laing claimed, contained the seeds of its own recovery. Laing was to later comment that this observation did not create any controversy when he initially expressed it, but that when he repeated the notion, albeit in a more dramatic style and using the term 'metanoia' in *The Politics of Experience and the Bird of Paradise*, it provoked heated condemnation.[45] However, the revised version of *The Self and Others* appeared two years after *The Politics of Experience*.

Laing felt that orthodox psychiatry was quite unable to understand or explain Mrs McL.'s experience. In the 1961 edition of *The Self and Others*, he stated: 'While one may find much of psychiatric and psycho-analytic theory unsatisfactory, any criticism of theory can only be made on behalf of experience, not in order to deny the experience with which the theory attempts to come to terms'.[46] In the 1969 edition, Laing

---

[43] Ibid., p. 66.

[44] Laing, *Self and Others*, p. 74.

[45] Mullan, B. (1995). *Mad to be Normal. Conversations with R.D. Laing.* London: Free Association Books, p. 357.

[46] Laing, *The Self and Others*, p. 63.

was more emphatic: 'Theory can only legitimately be made on behalf of experience, not in order to deny experience which the theory ignores out of embarrassment'.[47] Laing portrayed himself as amongst those who did not deny what they could not explain, but it is arguable that he, too, was prone to let his theoretical perspective shape and even distort the experience of his patient.

The ghost of the weed garden

Edith E. was a young patient who became 'Julie' in the chapter entitled 'The ghost of the weed garden', which ends *The Divided Self*.[48] She suffered from schizophrenia, and in 1954 Laing spent a great deal of time with her, attempting to enter her world and to engage her in psychotherapy. His notes indicate that he had 180 interviews with her, amounting to 250 hours.[49] Family members were interviewed by Laing and by his colleague, the clinical psychologist, Mr McGhie who was also involved in Edith's care.[50] Laing stated that Edith was one of the patients included in the 'Rumpus Room' experiment, even though she was not from the refractory ward but from an adjoining one. Laing described her as a 'favourite' patient.[51]

Prior to her admission, Edith stayed with her parents and had an elder married sister. Her father was a police sergeant who had been having affairs with women for many years. Edith had worked as a receptionist at a hairdresser's but had to leave because she could not cope. She had originally been seen by Dr Angus MacNiven in the late 1940s when she was 17. He described her as a tall, flat-chested woman with a large head of straw-coloured hair.[52] She admitted to hearing voices. One voice had told her to take her clothes off while another had told her to go and stand in the subway in Hillhead where she would see at a window a person being beaten to a pulp. She was also told that a child's life was in danger. On another occasion a voice told her about a murder that had been committed. A girl who was wearing her clothes had been killed. Edith felt that she had been changed in some way and that there was something 'powerful' in her mind. She also felt that there was an invisible barrier between herself and others, and she found this upsetting. She felt that she had lost something essential in her life. Dr MacNiven wrote: 'She wants love and affection. It is an indefinable thing, but it is something that is missing. She is definite about that.'[53]

Her mother told Dr MacNiven that for the previous year Edith had been very difficult to live with. She constantly accused her mother of not bringing her up properly. She said that her mother had ruined her chances of marriage and a happy life.

---

[47] Laing, *Self and Others*, p. 75.

[48] Laing, *The Divided Self*, Chapter 11, 'The ghost of the weed garden: a study of a chronic schizophrenic', pp. 178–205.

[49] MS Laing DE5. The E. family. Curiously in MS Laing DE5, 'The ghost of the weed garden', Laing estimates that he spent 500 hours with Edith.

[50] Ibid., The E., 1954.

[51] Mullan, *Mad to be Normal*, p. 133.

[52] MS Laing DE5, Hospital case record. M[other]'s story to Dr MacNiven.

[53] Ibid., Hospital case record, Dr MacNiven's notes, p. 7.

She complained about the meals and how badly she was fed. She was unable to sleep at night and her mother slept with her. She had become a recluse. MacNiven prescribed a course of insulin therapy.

Laing met Edith in 1954 when she had been in Gartnavel Hospital for some years. He also interviewed her mother. He enquired about Edith's development as a baby. The mother reported that her daughter was a 'very poor eater' and was 'whinie' and 'girnie'.[54] She was, however, toilet-trained easily by the age of 15 months. As an infant, Edith was described as always 'excitable, sensitive, "hysterical" on the slightest provocation', and she was prone to temper tantrums and nail-biting.[55] However, her mother also commented that Edith 'always did what she was told' and that she 'never had any trouble with her'.[56] She said that Edith was always playing with dolls, which she kept doing until she was 17. Mr McGhie performed a battery of psychological tests on Mrs E. He was interested in the psychological profile of the mothers of children who suffered from schizophrenia. He concluded that Mrs E. was 'cold', had a 'suspicious nature', and had no 'warmth at all though superficially she is an affectionate mother'.[57]

Laing's notes give a detailed and verbatim record of his encounters with Edith. The notes give a good picture of his approach at this stage. He adopts a psychoanalytic perspective, and he is clearly influenced by the work of John Rosen. This passage is illustrative:

EDITH I've no tongue. I've a tongue but it's not my actual tongue.

LAING You have a tongue in your mouth anyway

EDITH Yes, I've a tongue in my mouth, but it's not my actual tongue. I've no actual tongue.

(I was a bit lost at this point.? tongue = nipple (= penis). Tongue = nipple seemed from yesterday to be more important. She had apparently lost her 'tongue' and hence 'couldn't speak'. Had she been weaned? Bitten off and swallowed nipple? How lost it? Castrated?) but what level of regression to work on?)

LAING Well I'm glad to hear that in a way. One tongue in your mouth is enough for anyone.

EDITH I've a tongue in my mouth (it peeks out from between her teeth rather coyly).

LAING You won't lose that tongue. The other tongue never really belonged to you anyway. You must have pinched it from somewhere . . . You've at least ten nipples anyway.

EDITH I was married.

LAING To your father?

EDITH To Dr Laing . . . Dr Laing cut out my tongue in Africa.

(I had previously suggested that her mother had cut out her tongue for marrying me in Africa—when she said 'Dr Laing cut out . . .' I was completely taken by surprise . . . silence for some time).[58]

54 Ibid. Data from M[other]'s Interview with Dr. Laing, p. 9.

55 Ibid., p. 9.

56 Ibid., p. 11.

57 Ibid., p. 18.

58 Ibid., p. 37.

Another bizarre exchange took place on 18 May 1954:

LAING I came here to see you but you were out with your mother and I had to go away. (reassurance)
EDITH Yes. They told me there was a hole in the ground. They are going to take my brains out.
I have beautiful teeth.
LAING And no one is going to take a razor to them.
EDITH I've no teeth.
LAING It's a terrible thing for a baby to dash her gums against granite breasts
EDITH Yes, it's a terrible thing. I was born in Poland this morning.
LAING If only you could have pinched your father's pole.
You're a baby piper.
EDITH My father *gave* me a kilt.
LAING And the bone under the kilt?[59]

In another interview Laing explained his approach:

During the whole interview the general line I took was as follows: 'Why should you be so scared? I'm fond of you. I won't hurt you. I won't smother you. You're smothered. I'm dragging that mother off you . . . You're a very special person. You're my sister. You're my daughter, you're my wife.'[60]

In another interview, Laing told her that her mother had cut her into little bits, but that she was dead to her now, Laing was going to be her new, good mother. In one interview, Edith was talking about tonsils and sucking. Laing interpreted this as meaning she wanted his penis in her mouth. She wanted his penis so she could be a boy. Her father's penis was damaging her.

Laing also used a doll as a means of encouraging Edith to talk. For example, he recorded:

I addressed myself to the doll mostly saying that her name is E. She's a beautiful little baby girl, she'll die if she's not loved: someone has to feed her milk, someone's got to take her to the bathroom. Someone has to change her nappies; and that she (the doll) has found a mummy who's going to do all these things.[61]

Laing frequently complimented Edith, telling her she was beautiful and that he liked her hair. At times Laing felt he was making little progress. He admitted that a 'great deal of what she says flows past me, as entirely incomprehensible'. Laing found that when he was spontaneous, rather than when he self-consciously reflected on what he was going to say, the interviews went better and there was more emotional contact between therapist and patient. There were times when he did feel she was improving. At one interview he told Edith a story about a little girl whose mother didn't want her. Because she was an unwanted child she went into a corner and died. Laing continued: 'And now she is the ghost of the weed garden. But I want that child and she's going to live for me.'[62]

---

[59] Ibid., p. 65.
[60] Ibid., p. 46.
[61] Ibid., p. 51.
[62] Ibid., p. 76.

Laing felt the effect was rather moving. Edith listened in silence and smiled at the phrase 'the ghost of the weed garden' which was her own. She remained silent for some time then looked at Laing and said simply, 'Thank you'.

As well as Laing's clinical notes we also have access to a draft paper he wrote about Edith E.[63] The paper is undated but was written sometime between 1954 and 1959, before the appearance of *The Divided Self*. It represents his further reflections on Edith and in particular on whether psychosis was understandable.

Laing started by admitting that it was difficult to present Edith's case without, on the one hand, imposing an order it did not possess, or, on the other, burdening the reader with 'an intolerable mass of incoherent data'.[64] He also admitted that the part he played in what she said to him must have been significant, although he added, 'I can say that I explicitly introduced no new ideas, however much her phantasies were provoked or activated by my presence and my feelings'.[65] At this stage, then, Laing acknowledged that the psychiatrist had the potential to influence how a patient behaved in an interview. The patient might pick up themes that the psychiatrist had suggested. However, Laing was convinced, or he convinced himself, that he had not brought new topics to the interview. However, when he came to write about Edith in *The Divided Self*, Laing did not refer to the potential of the clinician to contaminate what the patient said.

Laing's aim in his paper on Edith was to 'characterise her existence'. Initially Laing found her 'incomprehensible', but felt he slowly began to decode what she was saying. At times he considered that her language was 'more or less sane'. He also felt that, on occasions, she was able to 'translate' her language, which he termed 'schizophrenese', into his. As an example, Laing recounted that during one interview, he had told her in exasperation that he could not 'make head or tail' of what she was saying. He went on:

> She came over and sat down beside me taking my hand, addressed me as a teacher might spell out a lesson to a backward child 'well, for Christ's sake! Jesus Christ, all bloody mighty! I've been trying to tell you for bloody years—I died this morning in symbolly, in symbolly land of the symbolly race'.[66]

Here we see Laing employing a favourite conceit: the patient as mentor to the psychiatrist. He used this conceit in his autobiography when he described how an elderly female patient in the refractory ward had tutored him in the secret language of the ward inmates. Laing was guided by the belief that Edith's apparently obscure communications were actually meaningful if one had the right tools to break the code. In trying to understand her, Laing drew on a variety of different theories. He drew on existential thought to discuss her statement that she was dead. He used Freudian theory, especially as employed by John Rosen, to explain Edith's statements of a sexual nature. He referred to Federn's concept of the lack of ego boundaries when she talked

---

[63] Ibid., Paper entitled 'The ghost in the weed garden'.

[64] Ibid., p. 1.

[65] Ibid., p. 1.

[66] Ibid., no page numbers.

about merging into other people, and he brought in object relations theory when she talked about her mother.

In the paper, Laing quoted examples of Edith's statements and considered what the hidden meaning might be. He claimed that Edith spoke about her predicament in metaphor and puns. For example, when she said she was born in Warsaw, she meant she 'saw war', because her parents were always fighting. He also felt that there was a purpose to the way in which Edith chose to express herself: that her speech possessed intentionality. Her seemingly incoherent speech was a ploy, for example, to throw the listener off track or to keep her deepest fears hidden. In all this Laing was trying to make the case that Edith's communication should not be dismissed as nonsensical babble, but that it yielded meaning if psychiatrists were prepared to make an effort.

After he left Gartnavel, Laing wrote to Edith E.'s mother asking her permission to use her case anonymously in *The Divided Self*. She agreed and thanked him for 'the very real interest' which he had showed in Edith.[67] Sadly, however, she reported that Edith was little better.

'Julie' in *The Divided Self*

In *The Divided Self*, Laing began his account of Edith, whom he renamed 'Julie', by noting that she had been in hospital for nine years and had been given a diagnosis of schizophrenia.[68] She heard voices, struck bizarre postures, and was mainly mute. When she did speak, it was completely incomprehensible. She had been given a course of insulin with no improvement and 'no other specific attempts had been made to recall her to sanity'.[69] According to Laing, Julie complained that she was not a real person and that there was an invisible barrier between herself and others. She complained that her mother was smothering her, would not let her live, and had never wanted her. Laing stated that her 'basic psychotic statement' was that 'a child had been murdered'.[70] Julie was vague about the details. She thought the child could have been herself and she might have been murdered, either by her own hand or by her mother.

In explaining how Julie developed schizophrenia, Laing outlined three stages: the good; the bad; and, finally, the mad. First, the child is perceived by her parents as exhibiting exemplary behaviour. When the child tries to break out of this conformist strait-jacket, the parents see her as 'bad'. They then decide that their child is not deliberately misbehaving, and that she must be 'mad'. This absolves the child and also the parents of any responsibility for the predicament in which they find themselves. Laing sets out to see how Julie's parents defined these terms of 'good', 'bad', and 'mad'.

Laing first considers the 'good' phase. He finds that the mother describes Julie as 'good' because she was never a demanding baby: she was weaned without difficulty, was toilet-trained from an early age, and always did what she was told. Now for Laing,

---

[67] Ibid. Letter from Laing to Mrs. E. Letter from Mrs E. to Laing, 26 May 1959.

[68] Laing, *The Divided Self*, pp. 178–205.

[69] Ibid., p. 178.

[70] Ibid., p. 179.

this is evidence that the child has 'never come alive', because babies are usually much more unmanageable. While conceding that the mother's report might not be wholly accurate, Laing states that the crucial point is that those aspects that she takes to be evidence of 'goodness' in Julie as a baby—her passive obedience—are precisely those which he takes as evidence of 'an inner deadness'. Further, Laing claims that Julie's family are describing 'an existentially dead child' and that none of them 'know the difference between existential life and death'.

On the basis of what appears to be a fairly unremarkable account from Julie's mother that her child had been undemanding, Laing has built a great theoretical edifice, which makes many assumptions. While it is legitimate to analyse the mother's values, the same has to apply to Laing. He equates doing what one is told with existential death. This is rather an extravagant claim, and it is, by no means, immediately apparent why we should accept it, or even how we could assess if it was true or not. Laing's claim has its origins in his own theoretical background. Early on he had learnt from J.L. Halliday of the dangers of regimented child-rearing with its emphasis on enforced feeding and toilet-training. Laing associated breaking the rules with freedom of expression; the individual asserting themselves against the conforming masses. To this, he added existential notions of authenticity and 'bad faith'. His tone is one of condemnation.

Laing goes on to consider Julie's early development and draws on Freudian theories about instinctual needs. He interprets the mother's account that, as a baby Julie never finished a bottle and was always whining, as evidence of an 'almost total failure . . . to achieve self-instinctual gratification'. Worse, the mother completely fails to notice this, and Laing comments that this kind of interaction frequently occurs in 'the early beginnings of the relation of mother to schizophrenic child'. So, slowly Laing is building up a case against the mother as somehow being responsible for her daughter's subsequent psychosis. Next he interprets the fact that Julie was weaned without any trouble as evidence that she never developed 'autonomous self-being'. The fact that, until the age of three or four, Julie became very distressed when her mother was out of sight, seems to Laing, to confirm his conjectures.

Laing observes: 'It was now clear that from the time that this patient emerged beyond the early months of life she was without autonomy . . . Real satisfaction arising from real desire for the real breast had not occurred in the first instance'. One has to ask: How does Laing *know* all this? How does he know what Julie was thinking and feeling when she was a baby? The answer has to be that he could not possibly know. Instead he has built up a picture from what Julie's mother told him some twenty years later. He has approached her narrative armed with a preconceived theory: a theory that links early infant experience to the later development of schizophrenia. Thus Laing is able to see in apparently innocuous childhood events, the ominous warning signs of future psychosis. He is able to take the mother's account of her daughter's upbringing and decode what it *really* means, and thereby privilege his own version of events.

Laing next considers Julie's 'bad' phase. From the age of 15 onwards, she was encouraged by her mother to develop a social life but she refused to become involved with other people or in any activities. She did nothing or wandered the streets. She cherished a doll that the mother thought she should have grown out of. She swore repeatedly and made endless diatribes against her mother, whom she accused of never wanting her, of smothering her, and of not letting her be a person. On the face of it, Julie's behaviour sounds much like that of many adolescents. Her mother's attempts to encourage her to make friends seem understandable and even, dare we say, quite reasonable. For Laing, though, it signifies a more sinister agenda. The mother was trying to squash her daughter's attempts to assert herself.

In the final 'mad' phase, Julie's doll went missing and it was not clear whether she or her mother had thrown it out. Julie started to hear a voice that a child wearing her clothes had been beaten to a pulp by her mother. According to Laing the loss of the doll was 'catastrophic' because Julie was 'evidently closely identified with the doll'. Laing tells us that in her play with the doll, the doll was herself and she was its mother. Again we have to ask, how does Laing *know* this? He doesn't tell us, and we are left unsure as to whether Julie told him about her feelings for the doll, or whether he is just speculating as to what she *might* have felt. He goes on to suggest that 'it is possible that in her play she became more and more the bad mother who finally killed the doll'. It is certainly possible, but can we ever know if it is true?

Laing discusses Julie's case in the light of the concept of the 'schizophrenogenic' mother. This was a concept which postulated that a mother could induce schizophrenia in her child by the way she interacted with him or her. Laing's ex-colleague, Andrew McGhie was sceptical of such a concept and, in an article on the psychology of schizophrenia, concluded that research had not demonstrated its validity.[71] Laing, for his part, conceded that there had been a 'witch-hunt' quality to the idea, although it could be argued that his own chapter on Julie added to this atmosphere. Laing suggested that rather than just considering the mother, one should examine how the whole family functioned and how it might contribute to the development of psychosis in one of its members. He thought it was better to talk about 'schizophrenogenic' families and he went on to consider the behaviour of Julie's father, sister, and aunt. Nevertheless, Laing focused most of his attention on the mother: according to him, she denied Julie's right to be an autonomous person. The mother preferred her when she was 'compliant', which for Laing was an inauthentic way for Julie to be in the world. Juliet Mitchell has observed that Laing spent comparatively little time discussing Julie's father, thus giving the strong impression that the mother played a more a significant role in her daughter's subsequent psychosis.[72] She has noted that in his efforts to champion the schizophrenic patient, Laing tended to shift the problem to the family, and more particularly to the mother. There was a strong implication that the mother was to blame if her child went on to develop schizophrenia. Interestingly, when Laing does discuss the father, he reveals a disturbing episode which may have had a significant effect on Julie. When she was about 14, her father occasionally took her for a walk. Laing continues:

> On one occasion Julie came home from such a walk in tears. She never told her mother what had happened. Her mother . . . was sure that something awful had taken place

[71] McGhie, A. (1958). 'Psychological aspects of schizophrenia'. In Ferguson Roger, T., Mowbray, R.M. and Roy, J.R. (eds), *Topics in Psychiatry*. Cassell, London, pp. 35–46.

[72] Mitchell, J. (1974). *Psychoanalysis and Feminism*. Penguin Books, Harmondsworth. Reprinted with a new introduction, 2000.

between Julie and her husband but she had never discovered what. After this, Julie would have nothing to do with her father. She had, however, confided to her sister at the time that her father had taken her into a call-box and she had overheard a 'horrible' conversation between him and his mistress.[73]

While Laing concedes that this event must have been of 'very great importance' to Julie, he does not explore it further.

For Laing, Julie's delusion that she was being murdered expressed the existential truth that her own true possibilities were being smothered. Generally, in his account of her in *The Divided Self*, Laing tried to decode Julie's mad utterances as statements about her existential predicament. He saw her 'language as an expression of the way she experienced being-in-her-world'.[74] Julie was said to be describing in a cryptic way, what Laing called a 'death-in-life existence in a state approaching chaotic nonentity'.[75] In a celebrated passage Laing attempted to translate Julie's seemingly nonsensical speech. Julie says: 'She was born under a black sun. She's the occidental sun'.[76] One of Laing's notebooks suggests that the patient might not have used these exact words. Laing records:

'I was born under a black sun (E. S.) Sitwell.'
c.f. E[dith] . . . 'I was born under a hot sun—scorched prairie.'
Kierkegaard. 'Woe to the child whose mother blackens her breast'.[77]

Another set of notes does have Edith say 'black sun'.[78] Whether Laing changed 'hot' to 'black' for greater effect, or whether the patient made the original statement is difficult to determine. In the book, he goes on to offer this interpretation:

The ancient and very sinister image of the black sun arose quite independently of any reading . . . She always insisted that her mother had never wanted her, and had crushed her in some monstrous way rather than give birth to her normally. Her mother had 'wanted and not wanted' a son. She was 'an occidental sun', i.e. an accidental son whom her mother out of hate had turned into a girl. The rays of the black sun scorched and shrivelled her. Under the black sun she existed as a dead thing Thus,

'I'm the prairie.
She's a ruined city.'

The only living things in the prairie were wild beasts. Rats infested the ruined city. Her existence was depicted in images of utterly barren, arid desolation. This existential death, this death-in-life was her prevailing mode of being-in-the-world.

'She's the ghost in the weed garden.'[79]

Laing's approach here caught the imagination of writers, who were taken with his ingenious and apparently credible interpretation of Julie's language. How one responds

---

[73] Laing, *The Divided Self*, pp. 209–10.
[74] Ibid., p. 224.
[75] Ibid., p. 214.
[76] Ibid., p. 224.
[77] MS Laing K16. R.D. Laing: Notebook, July 1953 to August 1962, p. 10.
[78] MS Laing DE5. The ghost of the weed garden.
[79] Laing, *The Divided Self*, p. 224.

to Laing's quest to find meaning in madness depends on whether one is confident that he is, in the words of Gavin Miller, 'a reliable hermeneutic guide'.[80]

What are we to make of this case history of one of Laing's most famous patients? He spent a considerable amount of time with Julie and showed great dedication and diligence. His aim to try and make sense of what she was saying sprang from humanitarian motives. Laing tried to translate Julie's speech with the tools that were available to him at the time. These were psychoanalysis, existential therapy, and object relations theory. To these he added the writings of William Blake, who features several times throughout *The Divided Self*, and the example of Ophelia. Laing provides a plausible, poetic and, to some, compelling explanation of Julie's seemingly incomprehensible language and behaviour. But is it an accurate account of Julie's condition?

We have reasons for exercising some scepticism in our judgement of Laing's portrayal of Julie. We have seen from his clinical notes the nature of his exchanges with her. Guided by a notion of entering Julie's 'world', Laing spoke in a symbolic and metaphorical language, which was heavily influenced by Freudian notions of the sexual underpinning of mental pathology. Laing's approach was based on an established tradition as espoused by such therapists as Sechehaye and Rosen, but when one reads the transcripts, there is often a difficulty in deciding who is sane and who is insane. It is possible that some of the strange statements that Julie makes were shaped and influenced by what Laing was saying to her. In *The Divided Self*, Laing omits this important context: Julie's comments were not made in a vacuum but in response to his interjections, which were informed by his concept of schizophrenia. To what degree did Julie's observations about her predicament mirror Laing's existential and psychodynamic perspective? For example, Laing seems to spontaneously enter into a dialogue with Julie about the 'bad' mother. Was he merely following the lead of his patient or had he suggested the idea to her?

In Laing's account of her statements there seems to be a blurring between what she said and how he interpreted it. For example, Laing tells us that Julie mentions that she has 'ten nipples', but the transcripts suggest that it might have been Laing who originally made this claim. Laing also tells us that she usually regarded him as 'her brother', but Laing adopted various roles, such as mother or husband, so that it becomes confusing as to who initiated particular ideas. It does raise questions as to the value of the therapy. If the reader of the transcripts is confused, what about Julie? No doubt Laing's approach was sincerely meant and had some kind of theoretical basis, but did it make the patient better? Did it make her worse? These questions are difficult to answer, though we certainly have no evidence that Julie improved or left hospital.

When one examines the pages of interviews, one is impelled to ask: to what degree did Laing selectively edit the material? Did he highlight passages that fitted with his theory and ignore those that did not fit or were simply incomprehensible? Laing had eloquently criticized Binswanger's study of Ellen West, saying that he had buried the poor woman under 'a rubble of words'. The same charge could be levelled against

---

[80] Miller, G. (2008). 'Psychiatry as Hermeneutics: Laing's argument with Natural Science'. *Journal of Humanistic Psychology*, **48**, 42–60.

Laing with his complicated, albeit imaginative, attempts to bring meaning to the words of Julie.

Edith is one of the most famous of Laing's patients, and some commentators have judged the portrayal of Julie in *The Divided Self* as the highpoint of the book. Laing himself felt that the account of Julie, in which he attempted to capture 'the pathos' of her existence, was what gave the book its heart.[81] He remembered that she was 'very beautiful', but that 'she was wasting away with no chance of ever getting out of it'.[82] Somewhat unkindly he described her parents as 'just a total disaster'.

The chapter on Julie has been for many later commentators a good advertisement for Laing as an insightful and compassionate therapist. Howarth-Williams judged that it was 'a masterpiece of empathic understanding' and he was particularly impressed by 'the interpretation of the girl's speech, conventionally regarded as gibberish, but in Laing's hands, a mine of the most incredibly subtle yet illuminating puns, metaphors, double entendres etc'.[83] Writers, such as the playwright David Edgar were drawn to Laing's hermeneutic exegesis of Julie's speech. Juliet Mitchell also praised Laing's interpretation of his patient's psychotic language. Kotowicz was struck by Laing's sensitivity and his ability to penetrate 'Julie's' 'seemingly incomprehensible speech, her schizophrenese'.[84] He mockingly contrasted Laing's approach with what went before: 'She had very little "treatment", just a course of insulin, and thereafter she no more than just vegetated on the ward.' This is of course unfair as, according to Laing, Edith/Julie had been part the 'Rumpus Room' project and had been exposed to social interventions. As part of Laing's self-mythologizing strategy, it was important that others, staff and relatives, were portrayed as unimaginative if not downright inhumane. He could then appear as the hero-therapist who alone possessed an understanding of the patient. Many commentators, such as Kotowicz, have uncritically repeated this narrative.

But there is a problem here. A major concern of Laing's was to show that there was *not* an abyss of difference between the sane and the insane, that we are all 'simply human'. The implication is that psychiatrists should not write off patients with psychosis because communication is possible. However, we are being told that it was Laing's unique gifts that enabled him to make meaningful contact with individuals suffering from schizophrenia. So which is it? Does one need to possess the semi-magical qualities attributed to Laing, or is the task of communicating with a psychotic person relatively straightforward in view of the shared humanity of doctor and patient?

There is an interesting footnote to the case of Julie. In 1964 Laing wrote to MacNiven saying he was involved with people who wanted to make a short film about Edith E.[85] The actress Vanessa Redgrave was interested in playing the part of 'Julie'. It would be

---

[81] Mullan, *Mad to be Normal*, p. 266.

[82] Ibid., p. 266.

[83] Howarth-Williams, M. (1977). *R.D. Laing. His Work and its Relevance for Sociology*. Routledge and Kegan Paul, London, p. 13.

[84] Kotowicz, Z. (1997). *R.D. Laing and the Paths of Anti-Psychiatry*. Routledge, London, p. 26.

[85] Letter to Dr MacNiven from Laing, 12 May 1964.

a film that conveyed 'the inner or poetic reality' of her case. Laing asked if Peter Laurie, the writer involved with the project, could come and talk to Edith and record the conversation. In the event the request was turned down, though not by MacNiven, who was on holiday, but by his deputy, Dr McLatchey, who felt it would not be 'proper' for a lay person to interview a patient in the hospital.[86] This episode also highlights how far Laing had travelled in terms of fame during the intervening period. In 1954 he was an unknown junior doctor, administering to the mentally disturbed of Gartnavel. Ten years later, he was moving in celebrity circles in London and discussing making a film based on his first book.

Laing's clinical notes allow us to travel back over half a century and eavesdrop on his conversations with the mad people of Gartnavel Hospital, conversations which he conducted in the offices and in the noisy, over-crowded wards of this large and formidable Victorian institution. He comes across as astute, physically brave, and dedicated. He was influenced by the psychiatric ideas of the time, especially the belief that a modified psychoanalysis was the best approach to patients suffering from psychotic illnesses. What also comes across is the personality of the patient. More so than in his books, we hear the patient's voice directly. Many of these Gartnavel patients challenged Laing, opposed his interpretations of their symptoms, and suggested their own ideas as to the nature of their problems. Some clearly liked him and even flirted with him, while others were aggressive and abusive. In *The Divided Self*, some of the patients are described in a way that renders them as insubstantial as the mythical figures in the prophetic poems of William Blake. Here, though, in Laing's notes, they seem more real, more colourful, and more assertive. We see the clinical encounter as a two-way process, and we have a better idea of the context in which the patients expressed themselves.

---

[86] Letter to Dr Laing from Dr McClatchey, 15 May 1964.

Chapter 10

Laing at the Southern General Hospital

From February 1955 to September 1956, Laing was a senior registrar with Professor Ferguson Rodger at the University Department of the Southern General Hospital, in the Govan area of Glasgow. Thomas Ferguson Rodger was the first Professor of Psychological Medicine at Glasgow University. He had been an assistant to David Henderson at Gartnavel and had also worked with Adolph Meyer in America. During the Second World War, he had served with the Royal Army Medical Corps and became an international authority on the techniques of officer selection. He was appointed to the Chair of Psychological Medicine in 1949 and, along with the surgeon J Sloan Robertson, established the Southern General Hospital's reputation for combining psychological medicine with neurological sciences. During his time there, Laing was in charge of three male wards and was responsible for psychiatric problems arising on the medical and surgical wards of the hospital. He pursued individual and group out-patient therapy, and also attended the clinical case conferences which were held on a regular basis at the hospital.[1]

Southern General case conferences

It is useful to begin with an examination of the case conferences, as they provide a good idea of the psychiatric culture obtaining at the Southern General Hospital during Laing's time there. Case conferences were attended by Professor Ferguson Rodger, the other psychiatrists in the department, clinical psychologists, the nurses, and social workers.[2] These conferences were documented by the attending psychiatrists, who took turns to write up the discussions. They provide a fascinating view of not only the young Laing at work, but also of his colleagues and their approach to psychiatry during this period. Psychodynamic theory dominated the discussions, but there was also consideration of physical treatments, such as ECT, chlorpromazine, and leucotomy. In the reports, the purpose of the conference was outlined. This might be to reach a diagnosis, decide about treatment, or to plan 'disposal'. A case history would be presented and then the patient was interviewed before the audience. A discussion would

---

[1] Research Fellowship application for Foundations' Fund for Research in Psychiatry, 15 March 1960. Information contained in Laing's c.v.

[2] Case Conference Note-Book from 9-2-54 to 13-1-58. Unarchived document recently donated to Glasgow University Archive by Professor Sir Michael Bond.

follow, after which Professor Rodger would sum up and give the conference's decision on the patient.

A typical case conference was that of Mary M.[3] She had been admitted from the Vale of Leven Hospital following an overdose of sleeping tablets, and had an eight-year history of depression and 'occasional outbursts of excitement'. She had witnessed the death of her father in a street accident and her illness dated from that time. Mary expressed marked hostility towards her husband. As she had been treated before by Laing in Gartnavel, he led off the discussion:

> Patient is a hysteric and her underlying problem is a fear of sexual violation. She had a strong attachment to her father. She always conveyed the impression that she had a 'secret' and exhibited fears that Dr. Laing would penetrate her mind. Her reactions varied greatly. If the questioner remained silent she would attempt to provoke him . . . She frequently states that no one can help her. Her husband is a churlish individual and she also provokes him.

It is worth quoting the ensuing discussion in some detail as it gives an idea of the nature of these case conferences and of the psychiatric culture that Laing inhabited. After Laing spoke, it was recorded:

> *Doctor Clapham.* Manic episodes have been referred to but these sound more like hysterical excitement than true mania.
> *Miss Swann.* Suggests that the notes from the Psychiatric Social Worker at Gartnavel be obtained.
> *Dr Templeton.* Wonders if patient is guilty about this secret which she refers to.
> *Prof. Rodger.* Referred to an interference situation and this is in the nature of hysterical sexual behaviour, showing first enticement, followed by withdrawal and denial.
> *Sister McRury.* When the patient left the conference room she grasped me by both hands saying 'I could tell you some things but they would not be interesting to you'.
> *Prof. Rodger.* Because you are of the wrong sex probably. This again illustrates the typical enticement-withdrawal behaviour.
> *Doctor Roy.* Some of these past episodes may be due to drug addiction. On admission the patient herself suggested that she might get paraldehyde as a sedative. The symptoms which she had are those which would tend to lead to drug addiction. She has never had E.C.T.
> *Dr Small.* The trouble seems to date from the time of her marriage and is very chronic. She does not appear to be able to cope with her life situation. I do not think E.C.T. would help.
> *Dr Sclare.* Gets the impression that patient has immense genito-sexual problems. She has fears of intrusion (stated on admission that she wanted no talks). She is a hysterical character and exhibits the masochistic hysterics of Freud. She puts the therapist in the wrong by saying 'You can't help me'. A case of this nature is almost impossible to treat.

The doctors at the case conference agreed that Mary, M. showed hysterical behaviour. The professor summed up:

> *Prof. Rodger.* Equinil should be increased and paraldehyde stopped before the patient is dismissed. It is probably not an advantage to keep her too long. There is no indication for

---

[3] Ibid., pp. 77–8.

E.C.T. Her Doctor should be informed of the possibility of drug addiction and she should, therefore, be kept on Equinil rather than given barbiturates.

The discussion of the case of Annie C., a 31-year-old woman, reveals that Laing's contemporaries did not make the diagnosis of schizophrenia in an unthinking or dogmatic manner.[4] Dr Roy began the discussion by stating that he thought the patient had shown signs of schizophrenia from the beginning of her illness, but he also felt that depression occurring in someone of below average intelligence was a possibility. He suggested that Largactil should be considered. The conference continued:

> Dr. Laing said that he would hesitate to call the illness schizophrenic. He remarked on the distinct disturbance of ego feeling and of ego boundaries e.g. she had no feelings, everything felt hazy. She was not sure if her memories were real or imaginary. He noted that she spoke of thoughts characteristically, as if of concrete objects. e.g. her mind was a box in which a pendulum swings. She confused her identity with that of the doctor. He felt that there was no satisfactory clinical psychiatric label, but this was a predominently [sic] schizophrenic like illness. He felt that she should remain in the ward for a time, provided there was no nursing problem. He did not feel that deep insulin therapy was urgently required.

Dr Scott agreed, but Dr Clapham thought that 'it was stretching things too far' to call the patient schizophrenic. He did not feel she should be sent to a mental hospital, which would have a destructive effect on her illness, but rather she should be supported at home. Miss Maas, a social worker, said that there was much less support at home following the death of the patient's mother. Dr Sclare preferred to call this a 'schizoid state', rather than 'active psychotic state', whereas Dr Shenkin thought it was a case of 'agitated depression'. The conference concluded that the patient should remain in hospital meantime with no active treatment, but that consideration should be given to Largactil or ECT in the future.

At another case conference Laing presented a Sarah McD., a 36-year-old woman who suffered from a severe obsessional compulsive neurosis.[5] Her husband had a colostomy and both their lives had been dominated by the need to take precautions against contamination—bedding, clothing, carpets, and 'practically all household accessories'. She felt that something from her could do harm to things outside her. Laing added: 'She now feels that she is dead—that she is a robot which responds mechanically to commands issued by an inner voice.' In *The Divided Self*, Laing was to describe patients who felt that they were machines. In the discussion that ensued, supportive psychotherapy was recommended and it was considered that ECT was contra-indicated. Laing wrote:

> Some psychiatrists e.g. Minski might recommend leucotomy but such a course of action was not recommended. It was decided to try the effects of Largactil in large doses while maintaining her as an out-patient and that it would be valuable to report on what effect this drug had.

---

[4] Ibid., p. 50.
[5] Ibid., p. 32.

Interestingly, given his later hostility to psychotropic medication, we see Laing using it, seemingly without qualms. In the discussion of Mrs Helen F., one of the psychiatrists, Dr Clapham felt anxiety was a major factor in her high blood pressure and that a 'maternal Oedipal attachment' might be relevant to the case.[6] It was reported:

> Dr Laing felt it was a schizoid type of psychosis; he did not think she was depressed, but felt that she looked rather bewildered instead; that separation from her husband had precipitated an anxiety reaction and led to the rapid onset of this schizophrenic type of illness. He suggested deep insulin as a treatment.

This last suggestion by Laing is even more surprising than his recommendation of Largactil, as he had given a very negative account of insulin coma therapy in his autobiography. Professor Rodger concluded that the patient should have heavy sedation with sodium amytal and then a course of ECT.

Mrs Mary, H., a 36-year-old married woman, was interviewed at one conference and was found to speak rapidly and to be extremely agitated. A variety of treatments were discussed including ECT and psychotherapy. It was reported that Dr Laing wondered why she had married her husband.[7] The notes continued:

> He referred to her relationship with both parents and felt that the unconscious hatred of her husband expressed a hatred of males in general and must derive ultimately from her relationship with her father . . . He referred to the paranoid tinge of her symptoms and quasi psychotic features e.g. feelings of abdominal swelling, hatred turned against herself etc. and suggested a basis for these in sexual and sadistic phantasies, with regard to her father.

In summing up, Professor Rodger stated that he thought the patient was 'in purgatory' because she felt very guilty about rebelling against her church and being estranged from it. He suggested that she be treated with pentothal to help 'ventilate some of her underlying conflict', and thereafter be seen by a 'sympathetic priest'. Clearly Laing was not the only psychiatrist at this time who thought that spiritual aspects were important.

Rosina, K. was a 32-year-old woman who had the sensation that her dead father was in the house.[8] Initially she welcomed his presence but then became frightened by it. Dr Clapham felt that 'the libidinal investment in parents was greater than in marriage, that the patient was an immature, hysterical person, probably frigid'. Dr Laing agreed with this, commenting that she was 'partially depersonalised'. He thought that there might be an analogy between this symptomatology and that of her 'phantomania'. She could not relate to the phantom without victimizing herself. All the conference doctors agreed that she had an 'hysterical personality'.

Mr James, W. was a 46-year-old man who felt there was a bad smell coming from his 'back passage'.[9] He was a heavy drinker who had assaulted his wife when drunk. Dr Laing felt that, if he continued assaulting his wife, he should be admitted to hospital,

---

[6] Ibid., p. 44.

[7] Ibid., p. 48.

[8] Ibid., p. 65.

[9] Ibid., pp. 67–8.

and if he was not willing to come in, 'it would be reasonable enough to certify him'. Not all the psychiatrists agreed with Laing on this point, but it is interesting to see Laing, at this stage in his career, adopting a position of coercion.

Jean, R. was a 44-year-old woman who was in an excited state with delusions that she was being poisoned.[10] Dr Laing did not feel that any specific treatment would be helpful and that 'probably benign institutional care would be the best thing, if she were not able to return home'. Another doctor suggested Largactil. Professor Rodger observed that, just because the lady was suffering from a paranoid delusional state, it did not necessarily mean she should be in a mental hospital. Again Laing was adopting an interventionist and restrictive option, while it was Rodger who offered the more libertarian one.

Another conference featured the case of Brenda M., a 20-year-old woman who had not consummated her marriage and who initially presented with acute depression.[11] She was given ECT and after the fifth treatment she became 'hypomanic'. On the morning of the conference she had discarded her nightdress and wedding ring and repeated continuously 'I am dead'. It was reported:

> Dr Laing felt that her condition was predominantly manic-depressive and that a schizo-affective state would account for some of it. Her father was the parent who denied her most. All through her teens she had feelings that she could do nothing right. When married she is appalled to find she is like her father—when she would not buy food after her marriage her husband told her she was mean like her father. She had incorporated or introjected her father in an effort to get what was denied her by her real father. If she is like her father then she would like to be dead—the classical Freudian representation of depression. She plays at representing other people. Dr Laing felt that if one other person comes into her magical world and stays with her then she may play out her role on that one person and that would be a therapeutic measure . . . she was trying to wish herself dead in a magical way but not going the length of suicide.

In this passage we see Laing expressing a common belief of his, that people could 'play' at being mentally disturbed. He expanded on this theme in *The Divided Self*, especially in the chapter, entitled 'The self and the false self in a schizophrenic'. Most of the psychiatrists at this case conference favoured a psychotherapeutic approach and tried to account for the patient's hypomanic upswing in psychodynamic terms. Dr Shenkin felt that 'this immature dependent girl had taken flight from sex and found a refuge in hospital'. The conference decided that Dr Laing should take the patient on.

In another case discussion, Laing drew on object relations theory. Mrs Ethel H. was trying to cope with a disabled husband and two babies.[12] The conference notes state:

> Dr. Laing said he thought that the psychopathology was similar to that of depression, that is that the patient identified herself with her husband and treated the introjective object with hatred. The fact that she assumed the same illness as her husband, seemed to him to be very radically a pure hysteria. The secondary gain from her illness did not affect the

---

[10] Ibid., p. 73.

[11] Ibid., p. 53.

[12] Ibid., p. 54.

diagnosis and he suggested referral to a mental hospital . . . Dr. Laing thought her silences protected her against repressing her angry feelings, and that this was the depressing problem.[13]

Christina, M. was a 26-year-old married lady who had experienced two episodes of mania, which had been treated successfully with ECT.[14] However it was noted that her family relationships were extremely disturbed and that she expressed considerable hostility towards her mother, both when she was mentally unwell and after she had recovered. Various relatives had been interviewed and it was clear that there were severe tensions within the family circle. It was felt that if Mrs M. was sent home and exposed to these tensions that it was likely that a third episode of mania would be precipitated. Instead it was advised that she stay in hospital and it was recorded that:

> Dr. Laing felt that further treatment along semi-analytic lines with interpretations based on a transference situation were indicated, and that members of the family should be seen together and allowed to discuss their problems in an attempt to reduce the tensions that exist between them.[15]

This is an early example of Laing conceiving of mental illness in terms of not just the patient but the whole family.

James, M. was a 19-year-old man whose father was a Catholic and whose mother was a Protestant.[16] His parents had split up and his mother had moved him from his Catholic school to a Protestant one 'to spite' his father. The patient presented with 'indefinite fears'. The conference doctors considered a diagnosis of depression but also the possibility of 'homosexual conflicts'. It was reported:

> Dr Laing felt that he had a schizoid character disorder from his split family situation. He cannot identify himself with one side or the other. He has an apparent apathy with no affective response, he does not show feelings or form attachments . . .[17]

This sounds like the Laing of *The Divided Self* and this time in the context of West-coast Scotland sectarianism. It was decided that the patient could be seen as an outpatient. A more extended example of Laing anticipating the views expressed in his first book is the case of Francis, C. who suffered from depression and recurrent bouts of derealization.[18] In the discussion Laing brought in an existential perspective, as well as discussing mysticism. He also refers to ethology and it is clear that, at this stage, he was drawing on many diverse fields of knowledge to understand his patients. It is also apparent from the discussion that Laing's views were received sympathetically and accorded respect. The conference notes record:

> Dr. Laing spoke . . . of the existential concept of a universal desire to be like everyone else. He felt that people like this patient might play at being depersonalised, perhaps as a means

---

[13] Ibid., p. 54.
[14] Ibid., p. 46.
[15] Ibid., p. 46.
[16] Ibid., p. 59.
[17] Ibid., p. 59.
[18] Ibid., p. 49.

of dealing with anxiety, and then that this mechanism takes over in adult life and gets out of hand. He lined [sic] this on one hand with the child playing at being invisible, and on the other hand with camouflage in animals which he felt was the biological analogue of depersonalisation. He referred to the existentialist way of regarding depersonalisation as a sense of a lack of distincness [sic], a feeling of complete hopelessness and condition of naked horror.[19]

Laing's comments provoked interest and one doctor observed that there might be a parallel between depersonalization and mysticism, and wondered why this should be desirable to the mystic, yet an illness in patients. Laing replied: 'the mystic felt he was fused with God, whereas the depersonalised person felt guilt at being a person, actually occupying space, and the ultimate of depersonalisation is nothingness'. Professor Rodger concluded by saying that he was most interested in the existentialist interpretation and also in the analogy drawn between depersonalization and camouflage in animals. In *The Facts of Life*, Laing recounts introducing existential ideas to the Southern General case conferences, and it is possible that it was this one he had in mind, though in the book the patient is a young man who suffered from a sense of futility. Laing writes:

> I ventured (this was in 1956) to remark that the question whether life was worth living had been taken up quite a bit in recent European literature, indeed one could find considerations of it all over the place. I did not think it was a foregone conclusion that the sense of futility betokened psychopathology.[20]

Laing contrasts his view with that of his colleagues who, he maintains, were keen to discuss the young man's problems in terms of 'schizoid personality' or as the beginnings of 'a schizophrenic process of deterioration'. Whether or not Laing is writing about the same case conference, it is clear that his colleagues were more open to non-medical ways of looking at their patients than he suggests in his book. Indeed, in the same passage, he goes on to write that, after the conference, the 'head of department'—obviously Professor Rodger—asked Laing to his office and confided that 'he thought there was something in what I said'.[21] According to Laing, the head of department admits: 'even he, a professor of psychiatry, could remember two occasions in his life when he had "attacks" of futility'. In fact the second attack was that very morning. In a typical back-handed compliment, Laing writes of his former professor: 'He is a very well-intentioned person, and I respect and am fond of him, but he would rate in my book as in some respects more out of touch with reality than the patient was'.[22] Laing adds, in a passage in which he could be describing himself:

> And so it is with so many people who are subjected to such an inundation of desperate people seeking their help, and feel helpless in the face of all this misery they are supposed to do something about. Such people are always dreaming of a 'breakthrough' in treatment.[23]

---

[19] Ibid., p. 49.

[20] Laing, R.D. (1976). *The Facts of Life*. Penguin, London, pp. 110–11.

[21] Ibid., p. 111.

[22] Ibid., p. 111.

[23] Ibid., p. 111.

Phillip

In one case conference, Laing described a 15-year-old boy, Phillip, who we know more about because he went on to write about him in *Wisdom, Madness and Folly*. According to the notes the boy's case was brought to the conference because of the difficulties in arranging his placement after being discharged from hospital.

Phillip was an adopted son whose mother had died of a cerebral haemorrhage on 5 September 1955. His father committed suicide on 15 January 1955.[24] The boy had been the first to find his mother dying and was also the first person to discover his father's body. None of Phillip's relatives were prepared to have him stay with them since he suffered from faecal incontinence and there was a 'most unpleasant smell' constantly with him. He was enuretic from an early age and had been subject to 'nightstarts and nightmares'. He occasionally heard a voice, and he had fears, especially before he went to bed, of being attacked by a man from behind and had 'to take magical precautions against this danger'. In the conference notes, Laing also mentioned that:

> He has frightening experiences when he feels himself becoming remote while the distance between himself and other people seems to increase and other people and outer objects seem to become smaller.

It was felt that the best arrangement was for him to go and live with 'an understanding family'. It was also suggested that he look for employment in a laboratory.

In *Wisdom, Madness and Folly*, Laing goes into more detail than that contained in the case conference notes.[25] He states that the boy's mother died from a haemoptysis and had drowned in the blood she had vomited. This is slightly different from the account in the contemporary notes, and either Laing's memory is at fault or he thought that having the mother vomiting up blood was more dramatic. Laing states that, two months after the death of his mother, the boy came home to find his father hanging from the living room door. The conference notes however give the date of the father's suicide as occurring *before* the mother's death. It is possible that the notes are inaccurate and the chronology outlined in *Wisdom, Madness and Folly* is the correct one. If it is not, it does rather undermine Laing's depiction of Phillip's father blaming him for his wife's death. In the book Laing has the father saying that his son has caused the mother's death by 'being conceived, by exhausting her through pregnancy and his birth and his whole life'.[26] However the conference notes state that Phillip was adopted! What seems to be happening here is Laing's tendency to embellish a story for dramatic effect.

In his book Laing writes that, after he was admitted, Phillip gradually came to alienate everyone on the ward as a result of his smell and by the fact he didn't seem to care about its effect on others. Laing further states that:

> There was no question of the diagnosis. He was an acute (probably becoming chronic) catatonic schizophrenic . . . it was clear that he was hallucinated, very paranoid and very deluded.[27]

The conference notes however suggest that no formal diagnosis was given to the boy. Laing adds that the Phillip's presentation was so disturbing to others, in fact so

---

[24] *Case Conference*, p. 27.
[25] Laing, *Wisdom, Madness and Folly*, pp. 148–53.
[26] Ibid., p.148.
[27] Ibid., p. 149.

'obscene', he attracted a diagnosis of schizophrenia, when really it should have been an 'extreme schizophreniform reaction to catastrophic loss'. Laing writes that the patient was being considered for long-term care in a mental hospital, though the conference notes state he was being considered for discharge. Laing had been seeing the boy every day for psychotherapy and found that he was not incontinent in his office, but that he reverted to his usual pattern when he returned to the ward. Laing writes that he did not want to see the boy ending up in institutional care and volunteered to take him in to his own home, with his wife Anne and three children, who at this time were all under four years old. This proved to be a success and the boy's incontinence stopped almost immediately. Laing attributed the success to his wife who avoided any hypocrisy in her approach to Phillip. Three months later he was placed with foster-parents. Dr Hunter-Brown remembers Laing discussing the case of Phillip at a teaching session for junior psychiatrists.[28] She remembers that the boy felt that he no longer merited inclusion in the human race and did his best to make himself repellent. Even such a fierce critic of Laing as Hunter-Brown conceded that taking the boy into the family home had been 'life-saving'.

Once again we have a rather mixed picture. Laing spent a lot of time with Phillip and does seem to have been genuinely concerned about his plight. It was undoubtedly a generous and compassionate impulse to take Phillip home, though some may feel it was beyond the call of duty. However Laing, in his retrospective account, does rather present himself as the lone hero coming to the boy's rescue, in the face of the rejection by the rest of the staff, who just wanted rid of him. Laing appears to have exaggerated the severity of the boy's symptoms, so that he could be seen as saving him from a psychiatric career as a 'chronic schizophrenic'. Indeed Laing claimed that an orthodox psychiatric approach would have been damaging, in that it would seek to classify the boy rather than understand him. Laing writes in his autobiography that what Phillip said to him in their sessions 'would be taken by many, probably almost all, psychiatrists today as the very epitome of psychotic ideation'.[29] In contrast, Laing sought to make sense of Phillip's utterances and relate them to the predicament he was in. There is also the underlying implication in Laing's version, that the boy's 'mad' behaviour was to some extent under his control and that with sensitive handling by the therapist, psychosis could be avoided. In opposition to Laing's presentation of himself as the only psychiatrist who wanted to liberate Phillip from long-term care, is the documented record of the case conference which shows that the opinion of the staff was that the boy should be discharged from hospital and found a place with an understanding family. There is an interesting footnote to this story. Some years later Phillip wrote to Laing, who was now living in London, to describe his adventures since leaving Glasgow. In an undated letter, he records:[30]

> Dear Dr Laing,
> I hope this finds you and your wife and children in good health. I must ask you to forgive me not writing sooner but I lost your address and besides I have been travelling a

---

[28] Hunter-Brown, I. (2007). *R.D. Laing and Psychodynamic Psychiatry in 1950s Glasgow: A Reappraisal*. Free Association Books, London, pp. 190–1.

[29] Laing, *Wisdom, Madness and Folly*, p. 152.

[30] MS Laing DM102. Notes taken by R.D. Laing.

great deal in the past year. I have been down to London on numerous occasions but I was unable to find your address.

At present I am in Torquay <u>after being put on Probation</u> *for 3 years in connection* [underlined by Laing] with a 'Student Rag' in April of this year. I will perhaps tell you all about it should I ever be in London again . . .

For the past two years I have been living 'a la Boheme' and, though it may seem funny to you, I am '<u>writing</u>' [underlined by Phillip] when I have inspiration, though most of it is poetry 'vers libre' or free verse. I was told about one and a half months ago to see a Psychiatrist by the Probation Officer, but the only one available was the Prison Psychiatrist for Exeter, so I declined with profuse thanks . . .

[In London] I usually stay with a crowd of Bohemian Beatniks etc. Have you read any Colin Wilson or John Osborne, Jack Kerouac, Anatole Brayard etc.? How do [you] look upon the Angry Young Men? I myself am in the transitory stage, this fact possibly being due to the fact that I am young (19) and am still labelled as a Teenager, a title which I detest. I have since changed my name as I found it gave me a façade, a pseudo-personality which to my astonishment has worked like a charm . . . now I am known as ARMANDO P. CASOVA . . .

The last I heard your wife had just given birth to a baby boy you always said you had wanted a boy so I hope that you are all enjoying life. Give my regards to your wife and children.

I Remain

As Always

Yours affectionately.

The letter reveals that Phillip was still having difficulties, but it is also clear that he was trying to impress Laing with his discussion about art and his pose as a Bohemian. He also retained warm feelings for Laing and his family.

The case conference records demonstrate that, at this stage in his career, Laing was applying ideas from existential literature to his clinical practice, as well as from animal behaviour studies. However the records also demonstrate that Laing continued to be greatly influenced by psychodynamic theory, and that this was very much in keeping with the outlook of his Glasgow colleagues during this period. What emerges from these conference notes from the Southern General Hospital is just how conventional Laing was in his approach to psychiatric illness: at times, he adopted an even more coercive line than some of his colleagues. We find him advocating Largactil, ECT, insulin coma therapy, institutional care, and the use of compulsory detention. We have to remember that Laing was still a junior doctor at this point and would have had to ensure the good opinion of his superiors. It is quite possible that he entertained more radical views—his Army diaries would seem to indicate that he did—but he may have felt it prudent to conceal such thinking. Years later, Laing offered a more critical and rather cryptic perspective on these case conferences in *The Facts of Life*. He writes:

Clinical conference
She is in the hospital because every time her husband, a travelling salesman, comes home she starts to vomit and continues to do so until he leaves.
She denies being sick of him
Is she *really* sick of him,

can't admit it to herself
denies the thought,
but converted to a physical metaphor
it expresses itself as
an hysterical conversion symptom?
(genital sexual difficulties and early oral problems, no doubt)
. . . .
perhaps a birth trauma?
perhaps psychotherapy?
perhaps tranquillizers?
perhaps behaviour therapy?
perhaps an interview with the husband?
perhaps marital therapy?
. . .
right well how about a few bangs with the box before he comes home or before she starts
vomiting, it might break the coupling and the periodicity . . .
maybe we'll think about it[31]

In this prose poem, Laing captures the multiple suggestions and different perspectives that were brought to the Southern General case conferences, and he suggests that the final decision as to treatment was somewhat arbitrary. His tone is rather mocking, implying the absurdity of the process. Dr Hunter-Brown contends that this poem was based on an actual conference and that she attended it along with Laing.[32] She remembers that Laing did not contribute to the discussion but she thought, at the time, that he was silently contemptuous of the way the professor had abruptly decided that the patient should have ECT. Unfortunately no case discussion resembling Laing's account is to be found in the Southern General conference file, which is not to say that it did not happen but rather that we have no other sources for it except those by Laing and Hunter-Brown.

Outpatients

Elizabeth

In 1955, Laing was asked to see Elizabeth, who was to become 'Marie' in *The Divided Self*.[33] She was a 1st year medical student, who, despite being intelligent, was said to be vague and hopeless in her actual work.[34] She was prone to accesses of depression which rendered her unable to interest herself in her studies. She was aware she was becoming increasingly isolated. Laing saw her four or five times but she missed most appointments. She would phone the next day to say she had quite forgotten or that she could not get up in time. She said she did not want to be a patient. Laing discussed with Elizabeth her unpunctuality and failure to keep appointments. He said to her that it formed a pattern: it 'arrested her freedom' and 'underlined her own impermanence'.

[31] Laing, *The Facts of Life*, pp. 86–7.
[32] Hunter-Brown, *R.D. Laing*, pp. 188–9.
[33] Laing, *The Divided Self*, pp. 167–71.
[34] MS Laing DB86. Notes on Elizabeth, 16 February 1956.

At a further session Laing told her firmly that he thought she was becoming increasingly self-absorbed and was losing her way. She needed more help and he suggested referring her to Dr Abenheimer. However she had no money and Laing agreed to see her every two weeks.

After several appointments Elizabeth arrived one day 'largely transformed'. From being pale and wilting, she was now blossoming. She had 'lustrous' hair, make-up, lipstick, and red nails. She felt joyful. About three weeks earlier she had been to the film, *La Strada*. Although this was mentioned only in passing in the original clinical notes, Laing was to make much of this event when he discussed Elizabeth's case under the name of 'Marie' in *The Divided Self*. He felt his patient had identified with the girl in the film, but at the same time had contrasted herself with the actress. From the clinical point of view, Laing contended, her case could be seen as one of schizophrenia, but from the existential perspective 'she had stopped trying to murder herself'.[35] In the book Laing changed Elizabeth's location from Glasgow to London. Was this simply to protect her anonymity or did he think it enhanced the story? There are no direct references to Glasgow in *The Divided Self*, though later in his career Laing was to make repeated and specific references to his home town and his experiences there.

Elizabeth is one of the few patients, featured in Laing's published work, who has left an opinion of the way she was represented.[36] She contacted Laing after he had moved to London and asked to consult him again because he had been 'very helpful' before. She saw him for a period in 1960 and again in 1963. Laing recorded that Elizabeth had read *The Divided Self* for the first time in 1963 and recognized the account of herself in it. She felt it was 'not misleading' but criticized Laing for saying she was an only child when, in fact, she had three siblings and they played an important part in her life.[37]

Mrs D.

Laing saw Mrs D. for outpatient psychotherapy.[38] She was in an unhappy marriage and had financial problems. The encounter had sexual overtones from the outset. Laing first saw her in September 1955. Mrs D. was a Roman Catholic and she informed him that her brother-in-law had objections to her coming to see a psychiatrist. In the first session, she discussed being in a room with a religious picture on the wall and having to turn it around so it was facing the wall, in order that she could masturbate. She described some of her previous sexual experiences and told Laing about a dream where she was being held down by six men. In further sessions she discussed her sexual fantasies, including those about Laing. He felt that she had developed a positive transference towards him which was related to her bitterness and frustration with her husband. She was now feeling guilty about her feelings for Laing.

[35] Laing, *The Divided Self*, p. 156.
[36] MS Laing DN3. Letter from Elizabeth to Laing, 28 March 1960.
[37] Ibid. Note by Laing, circa 1963.
[38] MS Laing DD31. Clinical Notes, 1955. Mrs D.

In a subsequent session, Mrs D. told Laing that she thought that he had been annoyed with her the week before and that this had made her cry in her room. The following exchange took place:[39]

> LAING You feel I criticise you, I frighten you. You are critical of me.
> MRS D. Well I admit I'm afraid of you, always been afraid of sarcasm. I think if you really gave me my character I would not know where to go. I couldn't come back.
> LAING You must have feelings for me that you are guilty about.
> MRS D. You said that last week. I don't really think that I have that sort of feeling . . .

It is clear that Mrs D. had some kind of feelings for Laing as judged by the many letters she sent to him between appointments. She wrote page after page to him, sometimes staying up half the night to complete them. She asked Laing about his children and made personal comments. On one occasion she sent a letter to his home, rather than the hospital, having looked up the phone directory to find Laing's address. A social work report had stated that she was sexually attracted to Laing. Mrs D. was stung by this and, in a rambling letter in which she rather gave herself away, she responded:

> . . . but I defyded [sic] anyone apart from Mrs Laing to take Dr. L. to bed with those eyes looking into one's soul . . . you make a smashing 'Mephistos'. . . I'm afraid I attribute you with some of the Almighty's powers . . . it's funny, I feel more protective & worry about you. I said I didn't know what my dream meant about your anguished expression. I don't, but my conscious thought was, God help him, on his off days it must be hellish, knowing of so much misery & heart break in the world.[40]

We only have a partial record of Laing's encounter with Mrs D., so we have to be cautious about how we appraise it. In many ways it is familiar clinical narrative, in which strong feelings, at least on the part of the patient, are engendered. Psychoanalysts would, of course, see this as a manifestation of 'transference', and, as such, a useful phenomenon that can be of therapeutic benefit. The patient is re-enacting her problems from previous relationships, and this can be examined and possibly modified in therapy. However, this patient seems to have been somewhat disinhibited from the beginning and this, combined with a therapy which concentrates on the sexual, may have served only to further eroticize the situation. There is, it must be said, absolutely no evidence of impropriety on Laing's part.

John

Laing saw a young man, called John, who was to become 'Peter' in *The Divided Self*.[41] Laing presented his case at a psychotherapy seminar, entitled 'The Body for the Self, and the Body for the Other'. Dr Hunter-Brown attended the seminar and, at the end Laing gave her signed copy of his paper.[42] She remembers that the presentation was 'fascinating', and, although long, it was well received. Hunter-Brown writes: 'It has been thought that he put a lot of his personal experience into the description of Peter,

---

[39] Ibid.
[40] Ibid. Undated letter from Mrs D. to Laing.
[41] Laing, *The Divided Self*, pp. 130–48.
[42] Hunter-Brown, *R.D. Laing*, p. 186.

with his feeling unwanted and allegation that his mother had played with nor cuddled him as a baby.'[43] The surviving paper is very similar to the chapter which appeared in *The Divided Self*,[44] though it does not contain a discussion section. In the book, Laing drew on existentialism and also on object relations theory, particularly the notion of the 'false-self system'.

In the paper, Laing writes that John came to see him, complaining that there was a smell coming from himself, but he was not sure if anyone else could detect it. The smell came from the lower part of his body and genitals. In fresh air it was like the smell of burning, but usually it was the smell of 'something sour, rancid, old and decayed'. He compared it to the 'sooty, gritty, musty smell of a railway waiting room'; and it was also like the smell of the broken-down closes of the slum-tenements of the district in which he grew up.

Laing writes that he was given the following information from John's father's sister, although in the book, it is his father's brother. There are several minor changes from the original in the book, and these were most probably introduced to preserve anonymity. The parents were described by the aunt as not happy but they 'stuck close to each other'. They had been married for five years before John was born, though the book states it was ten years. Significantly, ten years was the period Laing's parents had been married before *he* was born, so perhaps there is some foundation to Hunter-Brown's speculation that Laing drew on his own experiences when writing about the case. The parents' greatest interest was cycling and they spent their holidays travelling around the country on a tandem. They had a small hut in the country not far from Glasgow, where they spent weekends, winter, and summer. They took the child in a crib on the tandem. These last details were not mentioned in the book, and, as we have seen, at this stage in his career, Laing seems to have been keen to excise any reference to Glasgow.

The boy slept in the same room as his parents until he left school, although given that the parents' flat consisted of only a bedroom and kitchen, like so many working-class homes during this period, this was not necessarily significant. This social detail was not mentioned in the version in the book, and as we have seen, Laing frequently moved his patients up the social scale when he came to write about them. The boy's parents were not so much unkind to him as treated him 'as though he wasn't there'. In a passage which certainly has parallels with his own upbringing, or at least his account of it, Laing writes:

> His mother, his aunt went on, never could give him affection, since she never got any herself. He was bottle fed, and was always crying as a baby. But he was never cuddled, or played with.
>
> His mother, however, did not openly reject him, or neglect him. He was adequately fed, and clothed and so on. He put on weight normally, and passed thro' his subsequent childhood and adolescence without any noticeable peculiarities. His mother, indeed, his aunt said, hardly noticed him at all. She was a pretty woman, and always fond of dressing up, and admiring herself.[45]

---

[43] Ibid., p. 186.

[44] MS Laing DR13.

[45] Ibid., p. 1.

The father was reported to be very fond of the boy in his own way, but was unable to show his affection. He tended to be gruff, fault-finding and occasionally 'trashed' him. John was a lonely child. When he was about eight, another older girl was blinded in an air raid. He spent a lot of time with her, helping her and taking her out. She was later to tell the aunt that she owed her life to him as he had been so supportive when no one else was interested.

In his last year at school, a female teacher took a special interest in him and helped him find a job in a shipping office. At the same time his father had 'contacted a rather ambiguous relation' with this teacher. In the book, this is not mentioned. John left the shipping office, worked in a bank, served in the RAF, but was unemployed at the time of his referral to the psychiatric clinic.

John felt that his parents had not wanted him and had never forgiven him for being born. He felt guilty 'simply for being in the world in the first place'.[46] At school he felt he was being put by everyone in a 'false position'. He was expected to be a success, but he felt he was worthless. He had his first attack of anxiety while he was working at the bank. He was in the habit of masturbating in the toilet and the object of his sexual fantasy was a female colleague, who happened to meet him just after one such performance. She looked directly at him and 'she seemed to look right through him into his secret self'. He was filled with panic because he could no longer be sure that he could conceal his thoughts and actions from other people.

Over the subsequent years he was able to maintain an outward appearance of normality and freedom from anxiety by 'intensifying the schizoid split between himself and himself in quite a deliberate way'. In the book, Laing changes the wording to refer to a split between his inner 'true' self and his outer 'false' self.[47] This split, however, had the consequence of increasing his sense of futility and his belief that he was a 'nobody'. Because he was a nobody, he decided he would do nothing and was 'bent on destroying his self'. He experienced a 'deadness' and the smell became worse. He had lost the feeling of his self. He explained how this had come about:

> I've been sort of dead in a way. I've cut myself off from other people and become shut up in myself. And I can see that you become dead in a way when you do this. You have to live in the world *with* other people. If you don't something dies inside.[48]

Laing was to use this quotation at the end of his chapter on 'Peter' in *The Divided Self*, and it is certainly an eloquent description of the schizoid experience. In the book, Laing writes: 'He had all along felt that he was, in his own words (which incidentally are also Heidegger's), "on the fringe of being".' Laing also writes of John/Peter's 'shut-upness', which is an expression from Kierkegaard's *The Concept of Dread*. He goes on to compare him to Kierkegaard in his inability to form a lasting relationship with the one girl he felt was 'pure'. When Laing was seeking permission from John to use his

[46] Ibid., p. 3.
[47] Laing, *The Divided Self*, p. 135.
[48] MS Laing DR13, p. 5.

case in *The Divided Self*, his former patient wrote back, saying 'I would like to thank you for all your patience when I was at S.G.'.[49]

Other patients

Although Laing was mainly involved in pursuing a psychotherapeutic approach with his patients, there were occasions when he considered physical treatments. For example, in May 1956, we find him assessing a Mr C., whom he considered was very depressed.[50] He advised ECT but the patient rejected this and reproached Laing for not giving him hypnotherapy or asking him 'penetrating' questions. Laing felt that ECT would not solve the patient's problems, but that it would alleviate his depression and 'that would be something'. Laing had other patients for whom he prescribed ECT during his time as a senior registrar at the Southern General Hospital in 1955.[51]

Laing also ran psychotherapy groups and stated that he was influenced by Wilfred Bion. One such group was an outpatient one, which began in June 1955 and ran for 38 sessions.[52] Laing selected the patients by individual interviews and gathered seven young men and women for the meetings. One young man was James, a 19 year old, who described various odd subjective experiences. He had 'attacks of extreme detachment . . . At times he wonders if he exists at all'.[53] He also said that he was homosexual and asked if there was any treatment. Laing was 'pessimistic' about the possibility of being able to change sexual orientation.

Laing ran this group on his own. His notes reveal that he saw his role as interpreting the 'transference' which the group developed towards him. At times the group was hostile to him, and perceived him to be unhelpful and not providing the 'answers'. On other occasions, the patients spoke about their sexual attraction to him. The group discussed dreams, and the subject of sex occurred quite frequently. Following a passionate discussion about football, Laing linked this to masturbation.

He noted that one man did most of the talking and Laing felt this was a defence against his anxiety. In contrast, another member of the group said practically nothing. Laing's original notes suggest that this group was the one described in his paper with Aaron Esterson on 'The Collusive function of Pairing in Analytic Groups' and subsequently in *The Self and Others*.[54] In these two versions, which we have already considered, Laing upgraded the social standing of the group members, describing them, with one exception, as 'quite successful middle class people'.[55] This social upgrading seems to have been the pattern in Laing's early published case studies, and it raises questions. Does it betray an element of snobbishness on his part? Did he think his middle-class audience would be more receptive to accounts of patients from

[49] MS Laing B49-50. Letter from John to Laing.
[50] MS Laing DD31. Misfiled notes on Mr C., in papers on Mrs D.
[51] MS Laing DS92 Southern General Hospital, Clinical Notes, 1955.
[52] MS Laing DS91, Southern General Hospital, 1955–1956.
[53] Ibid., James.
[54] Laing, *The Self and Others*, pp. 109–15.
[55] Laing, R.D. (1961). *The Self and Others*. Tavistock, London, p. 109.

similar backgrounds to their own? Or was he simply trying to protect the anonymity of his patients?

In 1955, whilst a senior registrar as the Southern General Hospital, Laing was approached by a couple he knew socially who were worried about their son.[56] The father was a professor of theology, the mother's occupation was not mentioned. Their son, David, was 27 years old and was the middle child of a family of five, who were all 'extremely brilliant'. Initially David, too, showed academic brilliance but he began having difficulties when he went to Oxford University. According to his father, he began to suffer from the 'weltschmerz', a German word meaning 'world-pain' and defined as 'a feeling of the overwhelming oppressiveness of existence'.[57] He developed his own theory of history and came to the conclusion that the whole of the Oxford school of historians were on the wrong lines. He was considered arrogant but with flashes of brilliance. He only achieved a Fourth.

He then began studying at New College in St Andrews. He had by this time read widely in psychology and existentialism. His father commented that New College was not the place for his son to find anyone who could understand 'that sort of thing'. At a lecture, he got down on his knees to pray for the lecturer before all the students. He joined the Iona Community, with which Laing was also associated. He proclaimed that George McLeod, the leader of the Community and a friend of Laing's, was a 'repressed homosexual' and he cursed him to his face. He also cursed his own father. He had been seen by doctors in Glasgow and York who had diagnosed schizophrenia. Laing referred him to Dr Karl Abenheimer. Laing's letter reveals something about his social network at the time and the patient's story reflects some typically Laingian themes—the rebellion against authority, the preoccupation with religious matters and existentialism.

Ministers' group

Laing was involved with a series of joint meetings with ministers when he worked at the Southern General Hospital.[58] The Department of Psychiatry had been approached by a group of ministers who wanted to be given a course on counselling and human relations. It was attended by Professor Ferguson Rodgers, Laing, a changing cast of psychiatrists, a number of local Protestant ministers, and a rabbi. The meetings were part of a 'Course on Pastoral Psychology'. Each week the group met and discussed chapters from *Pastoral Psychology*. Before each meeting a minister would meet with a patient, whose case would then be discussed by the group. The first meeting took place on 12 January 1956. The aim was to bring psychiatric and religious perspectives to bear on individual cases and provoke discussion. The discussion was frequently erudite and the group referred to Martin Buber, Tolstoy, and to the effects of industrial developments on society, especially its most vulnerable members.

---

[56] MS Laing DF70, Letter from Laing to Dr. Abenheimer, 12 October 1955.
[57] Bullock, A. and Woodings, R.B. (eds) (1983). *The New Fontana Dictionary of Modern Thought*. Fontana Press, London, p. 920.
[58] MS Laing DS90, Ministers' Group, 1956.

In the third meeting we find Laing attempting to explain the behaviour of a female patient with mania.[59] He stated that her outward, 'manifest' behaviour was a reflection of 'latent' problems within. Characteristically he concluded that if we understood her 'pathological' condition, it might deepen our knowledge of 'normal' people. The fourth meeting was of note because it discussed a subject that preoccupied Laing, namely that of love.[60] One minister had claimed that what was required of a counsellor was 'unconditional love'. Laing felt that it would be wise to clarify the way in which the word 'love' was being used, because in a certain sense unconditional love was impossible and even undesirable. He said that he liked Simone Weil's statement that 'to love was to recognise the existence of the other person', which as we have seen he quoted in his paper on Paul Tillich.

The fifth meeting[61] dealt with the subject of guilt. Professor Rodger stated that there was once a popular idea that psychiatrists, by removing the 'repressions' of their patients, were advocating a 'moral laissez faire', but that this notion was shared by only a 'few cranks' now. Laing was asked his opinion of the relationship between guilt in neurotic patients and sin. He replied that he thought that 'authentic' guilt could not be analysed away, but neurotic guilt was 'inauthentic' and led to personal impoverishment.

These meetings illustrate that Laing was not alone in his interest in the spiritual dimension, especially as it related to mental disturbance. Professor Rodger played a leading part in the meetings and the clinicians adopted a respectful attitude towards the clergy. Martin Buber's concept of 'I–thou' relationship was discussed, and Laing was able to introduce existential themes, seemingly without provoking hostility or incomprehension in other members of the group. In *Wisdom, Madness and Folly*, Laing looked back at this experience.[62] He wrote that it had driven home to him how little he knew about life. He felt that the ministers knew far more about human relations than he did. In response to his facile Freudian 'explanations' of people's behaviour, the ministers offered a more complex account of human foibles, borne of their long experience with human suffering. They were out in the 'real' world, while he spent all his days in hospitals or outpatient clinics. He concluded that: 'The answers to why a lot of people are in hospital are to be found only outside hospital'.

Child psychiatry

Parents' group

Laing was later to claim that he would have liked to have been able to practise *both* child *and* adult psychiatry.[63] While he was a senior registrar, he was given the opportunity to do so. Laing did sessions at The Notre Dame Child Guidance Clinic.

---

[59] MS Laing DS90, 26 January 1956.

[60] Ibid., 2 February 1956.

[61] Ibid., 9 February 1956.

[62] Laing, *Wisdom, Madness and Folly*, pp. 135–6.

[63] Ibid., p.140.

It had been set up in 1931[64] and was established on an American model which favoured a three-member team of psychiatrist, psychologist, and social worker. Laing took a parents' group along with a female family therapist. The group consisted of four sets of parents and ran weekly from October 1955 to May 1956. In hand-written notes, Laing outlined the philosophy behind the group.[65] The parents were told that the purpose of the group was to discuss their difficulties with their children or anything else they wanted. No advice was given, and no approval or disapproval was directly expressed. Questions and demands for help were interpreted. The therapists tried to examine what they thought were the emotions behind the parents' questions. The Group was run on broadly analytic lines. The group was principally concerned with the parents' relationship with their children. It was hoped that if the parents understood themselves better, their children would be happier in themselves and less of a problem. The therapists examined the parents' descriptions of their children's behaviour and suggested that they revealed aspects of their children's lives of which they were unaware. Laing wrote:

> Such comments were in themselves useless unless the parents were themselves able to see this. Their inability, or refusal, to see the obvious implications in their children's actions, was of course, a function of their own emotional problems with respect to their children (i.e. obvious to an outsider who did not require to deny them).

Laing believed that the parents' own infantile difficulties were re-activated and unconsciously they behaved like children in the group. The records of the meetings suggest that the parents were keen to obtain specific advice, while the therapists sometimes found it difficult to avoid doing so. Here is the opening of the group that met on 15 November 1955. Laing is described as 'M.T.', medical therapist:[66]

> Mrs. D. I'll start off. I'd like to ask Doctor for some advice. Bruce is now starting the game of not eating. How am I to deal with it?
> M.T. When did this start? (Appeared uncomfortable . . . cornered.)
> Mrs. D. It started last week. Perhaps it was because he was not getting out so much and had no appetite.
> M.T. What are you doing about it at the moment?
> Mrs. D. I just give small portions and then take the plate away when he comes to a full-stop.
> M.T. What do other people feel about it?

Individual children

Laing made extensive notes about a young male child called Rob. He wrote:

> . . . the sessions I had with him showed me 'interpretations' in the psychoanalytic sense were not always as important as a lot of analytically-orientated child therapists take them

---

[64] See: Stewart, J. (2006). An 'enigma to their parents': the founding and aims of the Notre Dame Child Guidance Clinic, Glasgow. *The Innes Review*, **57**, 54–76; Bryce, T.G.K. and Humes, W.M. (2003) *Scottish Education: Post-Devolution*. Edinburgh University Press, Edinburgh, p. 843.

[65] MS Laing DF66. Parents' Group, 1955–1956.

[66] Ibid., Nov 15th Parents' Group.

to be. I do not remember making a full-blown psychoanalytic interpretation in the course of our time together.[67]

Laing observed that Rob wanted to play by himself but that he wanted Laing to watch him. Laing saw the child's play as a dramatization of his emotional problems. He wondered if any aspects of psychosis 'have potentially this salutary function of play'.

From the outset of his career, Laing had been interested in the interface between neurology and psychiatry. One patient he made notes about was a young girl, called Nan whom he had encountered at the neurological unit at Killearn when he was a senior registrar at the Southern General Hospital.[68] He was later to write about her in *Wisdom, Madness and Folly*.[69] Joe Schorstein,[70] who liaised with Laing in the treatment of the patient, also wrote her up in a paper, entitled 'The Case of Nan'. When she was 15, Nan had run out in front of traffic and suffered a severe head injury. She lay in a coma for two months. Laing was intrigued as to the relationship between brain damage and the integrity of personality. Initially, Nan was in a 'vegetative state' and appeared to not be a 'person'. As she slowly improved there was a stage when staff and relatives judged 'she' had returned as a 'person', albeit in a very restricted sense. Laing was interested in how we make these judgements and concluded that it was based on the emergence of some kind of interpersonal interaction between the patient and others.

Laing contended that we can usually understand something of another person by the various means, verbal and non-verbal, by which they express themselves. In the case of a patient who is in a vegetative state we are denied this means of access. Laing felt there was a crucial turning point in Nan's recovery from when she was perceived as little more than a heart and lung-preparation lying there, to the stage when staff felt themselves being looked at by her. As Laing wrote:

> We were experienced by her as she was by us.
>
> Once this happened it was impossible for me not to be aware that purely objective observation of her, was an intentional act on my part whereby I denied or granted this aspect of my own experience of myself as qualified by her, in order to regard her as a thing.[71]

As Burston[72] has observed, this is an early example of Laing examining clinical situations in the light of existential and phenomenological concepts, such as intentionality, the construction of meaning, and the properties of the 'I' in the interpersonal context.

---

[67] MS Laing A718. Drafts.

[68] MS Laing A713. Nan 1955, rewritten 1981.

[69] Laing, *Wisdom, Madness and Folly*, pp. 129–34.

[70] Schorstein, J. (1961). The story of Nan: a case of severe head injury. *Physiotherapy*, **47**, 335–6.

[71] MS Laing A713, p. 5.

[72] Burston, D. (1996). *The Wing of Madness*. Harvard University Press, Cambridge, Massachusetts, p. 40.

Laing's time at the Southern General Hospital allowed him to extend his clinical repertoire. As well as seeing patients individually, he conducted groups, saw children and families, and continued his exploration of the interface between neurology and psychiatry. In the case conferences, we see him prepared to utilize all the standard psychiatric treatment available at the time, including medication, ECT, and even insulin coma therapy. Though he subsequently gave him scant mention, Professor Rodger seems to have been an important figure to Laing during this period, and, after he moved to London, he sent him a draft copy of *The Divided Self*. In fact the early drafts of this work were written while Laing was at the Southern General, and as we have seen, some of the patients from this hospital were to feature in the book.

Laing as a conservative revolutionary in clinical practice

In his clinical practice, Laing described himself as a 'conservative revolutionary'.[73] By this he meant that in the 1940s and 1950s when physical methods of treatment were being introduced, the older generation of psychiatrists were 'disgusted' by these techniques such as lobotomies, electrical shocks, and new types of medication. They saw themselves as humanitarian clinicians whose duty was to care for and protect their patients. Laing said he felt in sympathy with these men who were by now in their 60s and 70s. Laing felt he was involved in a revolution to bring back the old values. An idea of contemporary psychiatric culture can be gleaned from a book edited by Professor T. Ferguson Rodger, R.M. Mowbray, and J.R. Roy, entitled *Topics in Psychiatry*, which reported the proceedings of a conference on psychiatry, held in Glasgow on October 1957. It contained contributions from many leading Glasgow figures, such as Thomas Freeman, Andrew McGhie, A.B. Sclare, J.L. Halliday, and Hunter Gillies, as well as clinicians from further a field, such as Ivor Batchelor, Mayer-Gross, and L.S. Penrose. Dr Cramond, the Physician Superintendent of the Woodilee Mental Hospital in Lenzie, outlined the standard treatment of patients suffering from schizophrenia:

> . . . chlorpromazine and reserpine are our two main drugs in the mental hospital. E.C.T. remains our first choice for the disturbed schizophrenic . . . Insulin is still our first choice for the recent schizophrenic . . .[74]

If this failed, Cramond recommended leucotomy. It would however be misleading to portray the 1950s generation of psychiatrists as simply advocating physical treatments and nothing else. Cramond ended his chapter by stating that physical treatment was no substitute for the 'broad mental hospital principles of full employment, as much freedom as possible, and a psychotherapeutic approach either individually or in the group'. The book also contained chapters by Freeman on the psychoanalytical treatment of schizophrenia, and by McGhie on the psychological aspects of the condition. Batchelor emphasized the importance of the therapist's personality.

---

[73] Mullan, *Mad to be Normal*, p. 107.

[74] Cramond, W.A. (1958). 'Clinical experience of tranquillising drugs in the psychoses'. In Ferguson Rodger, T., Mowbray, R.M. and Roy, J.R. (eds), *Topics in Psychiatry*. Cassell and Company, London, pp. 176–86.

Laing's portrayal of the older generation of psychiatrists as averse to physical treatments may not be entirely accurate; we know, for example, that Angus MacNiven sent patients for lobotomies. Laing appeared to perceive all physical treatment, including the antipsychotic medication, as, somehow, inhumane. This is a little curious as, from the staff discussion meetings, there was a definite impression that chlorpromazine was helping certain patients. This fitted with the impression that was being gained in Britain, Europe, and America that patients were showing significant signs of improvement on the new medication. As David Healy[75] has documented, some patients seemed to make a dramatic recovery and emerge, Rip van Winkle-like, from the isolation of their psychosis.

Laing did not see it like that and we may ask why? Alongside his scepticism about all types of physical treatment, he was also imbued with the psychoanalytic culture of the time. This held that psychoanalytic therapy addressed a patient's problems in a profound way, dealing as it did with an in-depth examination of a person's psyche and early family experiences. Physical treatments were regarded as 'superficial' and offering only symptomatic relief. This type of argument would have appealed to Laing's intellectual vanity. In addition to psychoanalytic influences, Laing was also reading literature on existential psychiatry, which argued that physical treatments were dehumanizing and that their use was based on the faulty Cartesian premise of a mind–body dichotomy. Laing left the world of psychiatric hospitals in 1956 to work in outpatient clinics at the Tavistock and later in private practice. Thus his exposure to the effects of medication on psychotic patients was short-lived. In later interviews Laing admitted that he had left hospital psychiatry just as anti-psychotic medication was coming in and that he had lost touch with this aspect of clinical practice.[76] Whether his views would have changed had he stayed in hospital psychiatry is, however, debatable. In an interview towards the end of his life, Laing maintained that he did not have any objection in principle to the use of medication.[77] Rather, he was concerned about it being used indiscriminately and thoughtlessly.

[75] Healy, D. (2002). *The Creation of Psychopharmacology*. Cambridge, Massachusetts, Harvard University Press.

[76] Mullan, *Mad to be Normal*, pp. 150–1.

[77] Ibid., 131.

Chapter 11

Laing in London

In October 1956 Laing began his training in London at the Tavistock Clinic and at the Institute of Human Relations. The Tavistock Clinic had been established in 1920 as one of the first outpatients clinics in Britain to provide systematic psychodynamic psychotherapy for patients who could not afford private fees.[1] Its founding medical director was Hugh Crichton-Miller who had worked with 'shell-shock' victims in the First World War. He wished to bring Freudian theory to the civilian population and, in particular, to those suffering from neuroses and personality disorder. Crichton-Miller brought to the Clinic an eclectic approach which embraced a variety of different therapies, but in the years following the Second World War, orthodox psychoanalysis came to dominate the institution.[2] During this period, there also emerged the Tavistock Institute of Human Relations, which became responsible for teaching and research. At the Institute of Human Relations Laing began his training in psychoanalysis, undergoing personal analysis, and attending lectures, albeit sporadically.

Laing has left us with an account of a typical working day in London.[3] On 16 March 1960, Laing gives the following timetable:

7.30–8.20 analytic patient

8.30–9.20 analytic patient

9.30–10.20 analytic patient; dictation etc.

11.00–12.00 personal analysis

1.00–3.00

3.00–5.00 Conference on Family Interactions and Psychosis. Attended by psychiatrists from different hospitals.

6.30–8.00 Group of borderline patients

8.30–10.30 Meeting of study group working on translations

11.30–1.00 Writing

This timetable was contained in a research application to America and it is possible that Laing was making himself sound busier than he was. Nevertheless, it does seem a very arduous working day, even allowing for what seems to be a two hour lunch break. As Laing himself reported, he was seeing a very different kind of patient in London

---

[1] Dicks, H.V. (1970). *Fifty Years of the Tavistock Clinic*. Routledge & Kegan Paul, London.

[2] Pines, M. (1991). 'The development of the psychodynamic movement'. In Berrios, G.E. and Freeman, H. (eds), *150 Years of Psychiatry 1841–1991*. Gaskell, London, pp. 206–301.

[3] Research Fellowship Application by Laing to Foundations' Fund for Research in Psychiatry, 21 March, 1960, pp. 5–6.

from those he had seen in Glasgow. Gone were the disturbed and deluded patients, and in their place were predominantly well-behaved and more settled patients. Laing's clinical notes reflect his clientele's middle-class world of private schools, tennis, and theatre going.

Mr B.

Laing took on patients for individual analysis. We gain an impression of how he worked from his notes on a young man, Mr B., whom he began seeing in 1958 and continued to see for the next two years.[4] After a preliminary interview, Laing met with Mr B. for their first session. He began by gesturing to the couch and sitting himself down. The patient lay down and Laing told him to tell him anything he wanted.

Mr B. began by saying that he was trying to discover who he was. He suddenly sat up with a jerk and said that the situation felt strange. He was panicking about his identity. He then asked if he could smoke, to which Laing agreed. Mr B. said that he had been able to speak to Laing the week before as he had felt he was understanding and not rigid in his outlook. He'd preferred sitting on a chair and was disconcerted that he was made to lie on the couch. By ordering him on the couch, Laing had sacrificed him on the altar of orthodoxy. He felt rejected and said he had to be accepted as a person first. Laing replied that they would have to understand why lying on a couch spelt rejection to him so strongly. They went on to talk about Mr B.'s dreams, and themes of homosexuality, guilt, and matricide emerged. At this stage Laing was more or less abiding by the rules of psychoanalytic orthodoxy, using the couch and asking the patient to free associate.

In his 'Final Notes' on the case, Laing discussed the patient's strong transference needs in the light of losing his parents when he was 15 months old. He also commented on Mr B.'s destructive fantasies about him and 'his desire for homosexual intimacy', which Laing refused to reciprocate. He concluded: 'He has felt angered and sad, as well as grateful, in a qualified way for the experiences he has had with me.' Laing recorded that he had conducted 600 interviews with Mr B. and outlined what he had been trying to achieve:

> . . . What I hope has happened is that he has had a sufficient relationship with me to establish within himself an autonomy which is not one of isolation & longing, but which he will allow to be open to others, and to deepen his understanding of himself.[5]

We have a brief record by the patient of his impressions of the therapist.[6] Mr B. commented that 'Ron', as he called him, possessed 'warmth, interest, skill', as well as 'uncertainty' and 'puzzlement'. He added:

> He is not a person I could identify with . . . except in so far as I admire and envy his brilliance, and his capacity for work and achievement . . . I mustn't forget his sense of humor [sic] which has been invaluable.

---

4 MS Laing DB22. Handwritten notes taken by R.D. Laing. 1958–1961.
5 Ibid.
6 Ibid.

Diana

A year later, in 1959, Laing saw a young woman called Diana for psychotherapy.[7]
His notes on her are illuminating and reveal that Laing's approach to theory and
therapy was evolving. Here he adopts an existential perspective rather than an orthodox psychoanalytical one. He was also interested in the dynamics of the girl's family,
and in particular the role of the mother. Diana had a constant preoccupation with
death. She felt that she had no future and that it was a matter of luck whether her next
heart-beat took place. In his note Laing wrote:

> Her life was divided between her fantasy life and her actual living. She was pretty well
> engrossed most of the time with the fantasy of continual games of tennis, in which
> Christine Truman and Ann Haydon in particular were playing. She took every opportu-
> nity to watch them play in the flesh or in [sic] TV. She read about them whenever she
> could. She had met both of them briefly.[8]

Laing felt that the girl retreated into this fantasy game of tennis during lessons at
school, when she had exams, or when she was at home. She preferred her inner life to
getting involved in the real world of real relations. Laing records:

> It was in terms of the fact that her life in existential terms had actually come to a dead stop
> that I interpreted to her her fear of death. Her fear of dying was indeed more true than she
> realized herself, because while she remained congealed in this static state she had indeed
> no future, she was unable to make any project for her own life.[9]

Laing felt the communication patterns in the girl's family were significant. Diana's
mother, who suffered from a mental illness, had a constant fear of becoming mad
again. She repeatedly accused her daughter of trying to drive her mad and put her way
in a madhouse. Laing felt the family were 'split', as the mother and father did not get
on. Laing described the mother as being 'locked in a life or death struggle' with her
own mother, and both fought to win the affection of Diana. Diana's father was
described as a quiet man who tried to keep out of conflict but was provoked into
arguments by his wife.

Diana presented a picture of herself as a helpless victim of these family forces, but
she also entertained the fantasy that she was responsible for the whole family and
the mess it was in. She felt that every member of the family looked to her to keep it
together and to 'keep the peace'. Her mother had recurrent admissions to hospital
and, during these periods, Diana became, in her father's words, his 'little wife'. She did
the housework and bought the food. Her father became more outgoing and they both
felt much happier when the mother was away. Following her return, the mother
would accuse her daughter of being disappointed that she had been discharged so
soon, a point that Diana could not honestly disclaim. Nor could she easily deny her
mother's further accusation that she wanted her back in hospital.

---

[7] MS Laing DH67. Handwritten notes taken by R.D. Laing.
[8] Ibid., p. 1.
[9] Ibid., p. 1.

Diana was described as being unable to reach out to other people because she was plagued with the thought that she was being laughed at. Laing described this as a delusion of reference and felt it was a good development when the girl reached the conclusion people *were* talking about her. He felt Diana's unhappy and socially awkward demeanour made it likely that she *did* attract the comments of others. Laing felt that another encouraging development occurred when, instead of being a passive spectator of her own fantasies, Diana was able to enter into them, if only to a small extent. Laing writes:

> I repeatedly interpreted my feeling that she must want to be playing tennis herself, and to beat Christina Truman and Ann Haydon in fantasy . . . She began, indeed to play some fantasy games of tennis, and even to win.[10]

When Laing started seeing Diana, she was failing exams. Her mother exhorted her to work hard, but repeatedly told her that she would never be able to pass, and, in Laing's opinion, was effectively 'forbidding her to do so'. In a passage which could have come straight out of *The Divided Self*, Laing observes:

> She finally became aware that she had really, secretly and intentionally, brought her own life to a stop, that she had really decided that she could not live; in other words that she had to be dead, because if she really went out, had friends, played tennis, passed her exam, her mother would go crazy. She observed that her mother worked herself up into a terrible state any time she seemed to have moved in that direction, and what she thought her mother was basically saying was that by being happy she was driving her mad.[11]

In his notes, Laing reported that in the course of seeing him, Diana had eventually passed her exams, gone to college, and made friends. She was now able to 'participate much more in life' and had lost the intensity of her fear that she might die at any moment. Despite this, Laing felt that she still had not dealt with her dysfunctional family. In a revealing passage he describes his approach to Diana:

> . . . in the last three months of my seeing her I faced her squarely with the basic choice which she had to make, it seemed to me, between living or dying, acting in the real world or watching a play of shadows of her own fantasies, and that she had to make the decision about doing this in terms of the real possibility that this might be her mother's problem—it might quite well be that her mother could go crazy if she really got well. Also it might quite well be that the family shared the same fantasy that she had, that she somehow had to keep them together. If she was to live her life she also had to accept the possibility that her family might go to pieces or might have to establish a new centre of gravity.[12]

In this we see Laing emphasizing the existential belief that individuals had to make choices in their lives and that this extended to whether or not they chose to be mentally ill. Like many of the patients described in *The Divided Self*, Diana preferred her inner world to the external one, and Laing alludes to Plato in his description of her 'watching a play of shadows'. Laing was interested in families and the 'phantasies'

---

[10] Ibid., p. 3.

[11] Ibid., p. 3.

[12] Ibid., p. 3.

they entertained about themselves. He was to go on to explore this in his 1964 book, *Sanity, Madness and the Family*. The case of Diana and her family is in some ways an archetype for the families described in that book. In that work, a common sequence of events is depicted: the nominal 'patient' is a young woman who has been scapegoated by her family. By a series of ambiguous and contrary communications, they place the burden of all their difficulties on her. The young woman's attempt to deal with her disturbed family is seen by them and, subsequently, by psychiatrists as evidence of mental illness and she is given a diagnosis of schizophrenia. In the case of Diana, in order to become an authentic individual, she has to risk the mental collapse of her mother and, indeed, her family, but it is a price worth paying to achieve full selfhood and avoid madness. In Diana's family, the finger of accusation, as is so often the case in Laing's writing, is pointed most directly at the mother.

By the end of the course of therapy, Laing felt that Diana had tentatively 'settled for living'. Our knowledge of the case of Diana is entirely dependent on Laing's account of it. It is difficult to tell from his notes how mentally disturbed she was. Was she verging on psychotic illness like her mother? She was, after all, said to have 'delusions of reference'. Or was she going through an adolescent crisis and suffering from no more than shyness and exam nerves? By Laing's account, his intervention seems to have been of value, though, as he never saw her again, we do not know if the benefits were sustained.

David

Towards the end of 1958, Laing began seeing a school boy called David.[13] The main interest of the encounter lies in what it reveals about Laing's clinical technique. Before he saw David, Laing met with his parents. He writes:

> His parents arrived punctually. I met them as they came off the lift on the third floor, and after introductions we went into 3/4 and sat in a triangle in three easy chairs, father on my right and mother on the left. F. had hardly sat down when he said, 'We would both be very grateful if you could tell us what you intend to do to David. I hope nothing drastic is going to be done to him—no drastic psychotherapy like psycho-analysis or anything like that.' His voice was trembling and his difficulty in controlling his breathing was evident. He was evidently very tense and upset.[14]

Laing thought the mother was more relaxed, and that she looked 25 years younger than her husband. Laing writes:

> Throughout the interview she crossed her legs in such a way as to show quite an amount of thigh, and I had very much the feeling of being caught up in quite an eroticised triangular situation.[15]

Before Laing could answer the father's question, the mother said she had been told her son might 'retrogress' once he began psychotherapy. The father asked Laing what he thought the matter was with his son. Laing replied that he couldn't say very much

---

[13] MS Laing DM101. Notes taken by R.D. Laing.
[14] Ibid., p. 1.
[15] Ibid., p. 1.

about anything at this stage, as he just met them a minute ago and he had yet to see the boy. He went on:

> I gathered that what had happened was that David, who had seemed to have a good mind, had run into difficulties about being able to summarise things, put ideas together and think abstractly, and this was particularly evident in his inability to write essays and his difficulty in maths, and I thought they could help me more than I could help them at this point, if they could tell me what they thought of this.[16]

The father agreed that this was all that was the matter with his son, and added that the boy had a good chance of getting through his exams and hoped that the psychotherapy wouldn't be too 'drastic' and make his son too disturbed to study. The mother emphatically disagreed with this and Laing felt that there was a 'radical disharmony' in the parents' relationship. The mother said:

> Let's face it—the boy is an oddity—he hasn't been normal for years. Things went wrong right from the very beginnings of his upbringing, he has never been able to face up to things or to tolerate unpleasantness, and has always managed to push such things aside and now it is all catching up on him.[17]

Laing thought that she was making a dig at her husband and was expressing her irritation at the way that *he* evaded reality. Laing felt from the way that the mother addressed her concerns to him, that she was trying to draw him into an alliance against her husband. Laing felt uncomfortable about this and started to 'waffle'.

Laing went on to suggest that the boy's apparent problems might be symptomatic of deeper, long-standing ones. The parents agreed and Laing said that unless David himself really wanted help, he would have to think carefully about getting involved. The parents said that they were quite sure that their son desperately wanted to be helped. Laing felt he was making progress. The parents were now asking *him* for his help rather than Laing asking *them* for consent to see their son.

They then retuned to the nature of psychotherapy and Laing said that it wasn't a question of him saying things to David, but rather of letting him say things to Laing. He continued:

> I ad libbed an imaginary first five minutes. I said that I thought when David first came along he would be very charming and anxious to please me, if he could, and I would rather make a point of not giving him any indication of what line to adopt with me. I should think that he would then probably feel a bit lost and not quite know what to do if he didn't know what I wanted him to do, and that if I was put in that position by someone else I would probably feel a bit irritated, and I expected he would too . . .
>
> I said the next step might be for me to point out to David what had been going on . . . and we might get to the point where he might realise that he could use me perhaps in a way that he wanted to rather than thinking all the time of simply acting in a way that I wanted him to, and that there was nothing else in psychotherapy really than going on like that.[18]

---

16 Ibid., p. 2.
17 Ibid., p.2.
18 Ibid., pp. 5–6.

The parents were happy with this and the father said: 'Well, we mustn't keep Dr Laing any longer. He has been extremely helpful to us and relived our minds a lot.' Laing said to them that he would not make contact with them when he was seeing David unless something 'exceptional' happened. However, he hoped that they would feel free to get in touch with them. They thanked him profusely and Laing joked that gratitude was rather premature as he hadn't seen their son yet. The parents went out with 'the momentum of what seemed very positive feelings towards' Laing. As she was leaving, the mother remarked that she had heard that Laing had an LRAM and enquired as to what instrument he played. He replied, the piano, and he had the impression that she was trying to prolong the conversation on a 'quasi-personal level', but her husband hurried her out. Laing's assessment of what he was trying to do in the interview is interesting:

> The course of this interview was manipulated as hard as I could possibly do it. I wanted to get a strong positive personal feeling to me from the parents in the space of 50 minutes, knowing that they came along with very considerable misgivings. I didn't care very much how I did it or how much negative had to be denied or somehow shoved away in this process. It was designed in the hope that this positive feeling would persist and stand me and the boy in good stead subsequently, and judged by this criteria, as far as I can assess, it seemed to come off.[19]

Laing started seeing David on 14 November 1958.[20] When he ushered him into his office, the boy took the seat that was obviously Laing's as it had his pipe, tobacco, and ashtray beside it on the desk. This was against psychoanalytic orthodoxy, but instead of objecting, Laing gathered his belongings up and sat in another chair. He offered David a cigarette but he declined, saying he didn't smoke. They sat in silence and Laing realized he would have to 'make all the running'. There then followed a Pinteresque sequence of silences and somewhat terse responses from the boy.

Laing commented that he was the third therapist that the boy had seen and he was probably 'a bit fed up'. David replied: 'Yes, you are'.

Laing reassured David that anything he said would be treated in 'complete confidence'. He replied: 'Confidence, yes, I know what that word means.'

There was again silence. Laing said:

> Well, one thing I could do would be to ask you questions, then if you answered them you would be telling me what I might want to know, but you wouldn't necessarily be telling me what you want to tell me, so I think I won't ask you any questions, and so we can see if there is anything you want to say.[21]

This was followed by a lengthy period of complete silence. Laing finally broke the silence and David asked him if he would like him to tell him about himself. David told Laing about his family and his interest in religion. He then asked Laing about himself. Laing writes:

> To the questions he asked me I answered truthfully and factually . . . that I was a Scotsman, who was born in Glasgow and who was brought up as a Presbyterian, but was not now a

---

[19] Ibid., p.7.
[20] MS Laing DM101. Notes on David.
[21] Ibid., p. 2.

member of the church. I had gone to a grammar school which was private, with vacancies for bursars. I had done Latin and Greek at school. I liked music, including jazz, but not particularly bagpipes, 'for not all Scotsmen are the same'.[22]

At the end of the session David was very enthusiastic about coming back and thanked Laing excitedly and profusely for their talk.

At the next session David told Laing: 'You know, some people have a very old-fashioned view of psychology. They think psychology is all nonsense and a waste of time, but I don't think that at all.'[23] At a subsequent session, David reported that his parents had told him not to tell his brother he was seeing a psychiatrist, but that was asking him to tell a lie. What did Laing think he should do? Laing writes:

> . . . when one was 17 all one could be given was advice, and one could take it or leave it. He had the choice of going against his parents' advice or going against what he thought was right. That was up to him. It depended whether he felt that honouring his father and mother consisted in doing what they told or advised though it wasn't what he thought was the right thing to do. He said, 'Well, I think I'll tell him where I've been', on which I made no comment, but he gathered that he had my tacit 'support'.[24]

The question of telling the truth came up again when, on 13 February 1959, David's mother came to see Laing without telling her son. Laing was uneasy about this and they discussed whether she should tell David about her visit. The mother thought not, but Laing argued that she should. Laing writes:

> . . . we agreed that she should tell him that she had asked to see me and I had seen her . . . I said that I had promised David that I wouldn't tell anyone else any of the things that he had told me, and that I hadn't quite kept that promise with her. She undertook not to tell him any of the confidences I had broken with him.[25]

At the sixth session David began talking with some embarrassment about his compulsion to look at himself in the mirror. Laing records:

> I said when I was his age I found myself looking at myself in a mirror quite a bit. He was very interested in this, and talked for some while about what he was trying to do in this. He said that he thought he was trying to see himself from outside himself: 'Maybe I am being much too ambitious.'[26]

Laing was not just pretending that he too looked in the mirror extensively as a youth: it was true. In *The Facts of Life*, he writes:

> There was one full-length mirror in my home as a child, and I spent a lot of time looking into it. That's supposed (in some quarters) to be an early symptom of schizophrenia or at least ominous.[27]

---

[22] Ibid., first session, p. 3.

[23] Ibid., second session, p. 3.

[24] Ibid., 5 December 1958 session, pp. 2–3.

[25] Ibid., note by Laing.

[26] Ibid., sixth session, 9 January 1959, p. 3.

[27] Laing, *The Facts of Life*, p. 108.

Laing adds a passage that echoes the thoughts of David:

> Mirrors are very important . . . many people feel that they are somewhere or other behind
> a face which they can't see because they are on the side of it, but if they could see, if they
> could look in a mirror, or if they could get around in their imagination from behind and
> look at themselves from outside, then they would see their 'face'.[28]

In fact Laing was evidently preoccupied with the concept of the mirror, and the
same book has a long prose poem on the subject, which begins:

> **My Face**
> I see it in the mirror
> I take the mirror image, turning it round, and
> Place it in the space where it is now suspended,
> Between 'me', and the paper I am writing upon.
> I take off this visual mask, an inverted reversed
> image of reflection.
> What is my face now?[29]

At the seventh session, David began by asking Laing if he believed the story of Christ
driving out the moneylenders was true. David didn't think it was as He was not capable of violence. Laing asked David if he could imagine Jesus as a sexual being and the
rest of the session consisted of talking about aggression and sexuality. At the next
session, David asked Laing about his family:

> He asked me if I had any daughters and became very concerned lest I was too tolerant about
> letting them swear and wanted to know if I was bringing them up as Christians. I said that
> if they used words that I objected to them using, I would say so and say these were rude.[30]

At one session, David asked Laing if he could call him by his first name. After getting
permission, he did so repeatedly and in a 'rather strained way' at a subsequent session.[31]

In his contact with David, we see Laing pursuing a non-directive approach. When
asked to reveal personal details about himself, he chose, as his notes make clear, to give
them in a straightforward manner, rather than 'interpreting' the boy's behaviour.
There is a postscript to this case in the form of a letter that David wrote Laing on
22 June 1961. In it he reveals he has been in a psychiatric hospital:

> Dear Ronald,
> I am back at Winston House after six months in Fulbourn Hospital, where I have been get-
> ting over a nervous breakdown, which I had last Christmas. Dr Clarke prescribed Insulin
> Treatment, which has proved most effective. Many have said that I look very relaxed . . . at last
> I feel an ability to 'stick' to things . . . My stay in hospital has proved a useful experience . . .
> I trust that you are all well and that the children are growing out of the mischief stage!!!
> . . . I should look forward very much to seeing you again. I frequently come home at the
> weekends and perhaps I could come up and see you at Hampstead.

---

[28] Ibid.
[29] Ibid., p.20.
[30] MS Laing DM101. Notes on David. eighth session, p. 1.
[31] Ibid., session, 20 March 1959.

David uses Laing's first name and knows a little about his family. He is obviously grateful to Laing, though it appears that he had developed a major mental illness, possibly schizophrenia.

Billy

Billy was a 15-year-old boy who was preoccupied with the size of his nose. He had also been exposing himself.[32] Laing saw him at home on the evening of Friday 11 December 1959. He interviewed Billy while his colleague, Dr Lee, interviewed the boy's mother. Laing's account of the interview reveals his clinical technique, which comes across as a sensitive attempt to put the boy at his ease and encourage him to speak about his problems.

The beginning of the interview was difficult, as Billy sat in a chair, looking dejected, frightened, and unfriendly. Laing began by explaining why he was seeing him and he commented that they were complete strangers and this made the situation difficult for both of them. Billy agreed and said that he felt 'very anxious and sick in his stomach'.[33] Laing decided that he should begin with unthreatening subjects and he observed that Billy had been off school for the last week. This led to the boy saying he wanted to be a policeman. His mother supported this choice, but his father objected because 'it wasn't good enough'. Laing asked him about his father and Billy replied that he was a very successful salesman and very knowledgeable. Laing asked him about his friends and Billy told him about listening to music on the radio. It emerged that Billy's favourite radio programme was produced by a friend of Laing. Laing writes: 'I thought that he brightened up towards me considerably after I had linked myself with this interest'. They then talked about 'the relative popularity of "rock" and jazz'. Laing comments: 'By this time, I felt I had established sufficiently good rapport with him to lead him on to talking about more personal matters.' Laing continued:

> I began by asking him about his nose and he said his nose was, he felt, too big and that people had begun to think him too big-headed and too big for his boots generally. I remarked that he certainly was a big chap generally, certainly bigger than me, and he said that he was bigger than his father too. I wonder [sic] how his father felt about that, but he made no obvious response about it.[34]

The subject of sex came up and Billy said he knew all about 'the facts of life', but that it was 'all terribly dirty'. He was a virgin and Laing contrasted Billy's knowledge of sex with that of adults, like his father who knew about it in practice as well as in theory. Billy went on to say that he was terribly ashamed of himself because of his sexual thoughts and he began to talk about exposing himself. Laing writes:

> I asked him what was the kick he got out of this and he said it was showing his penis to an older woman. I made some remarks about his wanting an older woman to see that he really had got a penis and that it really was a big one. There was a moment when his

---

[32] MS Laing DM41. Interview with Billy.

[33] Ibid., p. 1.

[34] Ibid., p. 1.

depression and overall listlessness evaporated. He gave something like a smirk to this statement of mine.[35]

Billy then went on to talk about masturbation and admitted that he masturbated while sitting on the top deck of buses and he was frightened of being found out. Laing asked him about the 'sleeping arrangements' at home and this led to Billy quickly telling him that he had imagined that his parents were having sexual intercourse in the next room but he now realized that it was only the budgie or the wind. He also said that he had dreams in which the whole family except his mother were dead. He had thoughts that he was going to die. Laing offered him a cigarette which Billy accepted but said that he was worried that he might develop cancer. Laing said to him: 'in most families there are ups and downs and I expected there would be rows and disagreements in his house too'. Billy said there were rows but they were all about him and that it was all his fault. He had caused his parents to argue over him and he was terribly ashamed of himself. He burst into tears, went into the scullery, had a sip of water and came back in again, apologizing for all the trouble he had caused. Laing writes:

> About now I made an interpretation about what he had told me in which I said that it seemed to me that he had quite recently grown big, that it was not only his nose that was big, but it was his whole body, his whole self, and for that matter his penis, and that I thought he wanted this to be registered. He wanted his mother in particular to recognise this, to see that he was a big person now, having a big penis was a token of growing up. I also said that I thought it must be a bit confusing for him to know when sex was dirty or clean. He felt that it was dirty for him to have sexual fantasies, to imagine sexual things, and yet he compared his mom and dad who he knew did have sexual relations with each other to a couple of love birds and that was rather sweet. Still, all of this must be rather difficult and confusing.[36]

Billy denied there was a problem. He said that he knew right from wrong. His mother had explained to him that it was alright to have sexual relations once one was married. Also, he didn't feel there was any relationship between his nose and his penis. Laing observed that, although Billy had not agreed with much he had said, he seemed more relaxed and also relieved that he wasn't going nuts. He had been worried that Dr Laing and Dr Lee had come 'to take him away'. Laing told him that he thought he was 'very emotionally upset', but that he wasn't 'going nuts in the sense that he was using the term'. Billy said that because of his talk with Laing he felt he would be able to get back to school and make up with his parents for all the trouble he had caused. He did not think he needed to see Dr Laing again. Laing commented that he thought it might be useful if they did meet again, but he did not press the point. Instead he told Billy he could phone him if he became upset again. Billy was keen to take up this offer.

From Laing's account, it seems that he skillfully developed rapport with his 15-year-old patient. Within a short space of time he managed to get Billy to talk about intimate personal matters. He treated him as a grown-up, offering him cigarettes and discussing music. Laing adopted a Freudian perspective. He judged that he should make an

---

[35] Ibid., p. 2.
[36] Ibid., p. 2.

'interpretation' after Billy had been stirred up emotionally and, in theory, more susceptible to psychoanalytic probing. In questioning Billy about the domestic 'sleeping arrangements', Laing was pursuing the Freudian notion of the 'primal scene', whereby the child witnesses his parents having sex, either in reality or in fantasy. The image is misunderstood by the child as a scene of violence, but it also provokes sexual excitement. The experience is held to be traumatic to the child and disturbs his sexual development, possibly leading to neurosis in later life. Several times in the interview Laing tried to encourage Billy to express his feelings about his father in the hope of drawing out Oedipal conflicts. Laing made an orthodox Freudian interpretation when he suggested that the boy's preoccupation with his nose was really about his penis. Laing was honest enough to record that Billy did not accept his linking of his concerns about his nose to sex. Nevertheless, he felt the comments had had some effect. We only have Laing's description of his encounter with Billy; nevertheless, he emerges as an empathic and interested therapist.

Immediately after the interview, Laing and Billy met with Dr Lee and the mother, joined later by the father, who had arrived late. The two therapists explored the boy's difficulties in the context of relationships within the family. The chief interest in the subsequent clinical notes is that Laing and his colleague focused on the communication style of the family and that they made reference to the 'double bind' theory. This theory had been advanced by Gregory Bateson, whose paper Laing was to quote in his first two books, although he only began discussing the concept of the 'double bind' in his second work, *The Self and Others*. Bateson and his colleagues had defined the double bind as 'a situation in which no matter what a person does, he "can't win" '.[37] For example, a child is told to do something, but the parent's emotional tone suggests the opposite is intended. The child is left in a quandary as to what to do, and Bateson suggests that if this experience is repeated frequently, the child may go on to develop schizophrenia. In their clinical notes, Laing and Lee concluded that Billy's parents displayed many examples of the double bind in their interaction with him. They write:

> The mother stated to the son, 'Go ahead and talk; say it', in a way which really prevented the son from talking truthfully . . .
>
> There was a strong statement to the effect, 'I want you to get well but also I'm glad you got ill if it draws us closer', made primarily by his mother.[38]

In *The Self and Others*, Laing was to use an example that he was later to admit was taken from his own childhood.[39] In the book a mother offers to embrace her son, but freezes when he approaches her.

Group psychotherapy

In London, Laing conducted outpatient psychotherapy groups. Typed notes were completed after each week's session. One group met on Tuesday evenings at 6.30 p.m.

---

[37] Bateson, G., Jackson, D.D., Haley, J. and Weakland, J. (1956). 'Towards a theory of schizophrenia'. *Behavioural Science*, **1**, 251–64.

[38] MS Laing DM41, p. 12.

[39] Laing, *The Self and Others*, p. 139.

and catered for young adults. It is worth examining the records of this group in a little detail as they provide a picture of the young Laing in clinical action, as well as describing the types of problems the patients experienced and the general cultural atmosphere of London in the late 1950s.

Members of the group referred to contemporary cultural phenomena, such as the 'Angry Young Men', the production of Harold Pinter's *The Entertainer*, Gurdieff whose mystical writings was then in vogue, and to political events, such as the Suez Crisis and the Hungarian Revolution. At the session held on 22 October 1957, the typed account reported:

> Dr Laing said that the discussion in the political sphere might be a way of expressing their feelings about their parents and the efforts, energy and expense to which their parents had gone in order to develop their children's resources. Did they, as children, have a right to overthrow or ignore the efforts of their parents, and go their own way?[40]

Laing was using a standard psychodynamic technique of relating external events to the internal world of the patient. Laing was not necessarily advocating that group members adopt a conservative, respectful attitude towards their patients—he was after all only suggesting that they, themselves, might have these feelings—but his remark does echo the type of Christian inculcation he received as a school boy at Hutchesons', where he was reminded that *his* parents had worked hard to pay for his fees. A subsequent meeting returned to the theme. The group had begun by discussing Colin Wilson's book, *The Outsider*, as well as other writers such as Kingsley Amis and John Osborne. They were critical of these writers. We know from Adrian Laing's biography that his father was very put out, not only by the publication of Wilson's book but also by its instant success.[41] Perhaps this influenced the remarks he made to the group. His fraught relationship with his *own* parents may have also coloured his views. The account read:

> Dr Laing said that their reference to and criticism of these angry young men was in marked contrast to their talk of expression of anger during the session. He thought this related to their feelings about their parents, since they had often expressed dissatisfaction at their relationships with their parents. He thought that the theme expressed by these angry young writers was that there was no parental figure about 25 years older who had shown them what to do, how to behave or to whom they could turn for advice and sympathy. This same lack of an adequate parent was a problem with which the group members were coping by not expressing their anger at their parents. Perhaps they even envied the ability of these angry young writers to express their anger with parental figures . . . they probably felt they were not getting the things from Dr Laing for which they came.[42]

Elsewhere, we find Laing making fairly orthodox interpretations about individual members of the group:

> Dr Laing said that if Miss H.'s mother continued to live on inside her, then her mother had never really died, and Miss H. had never accepted nor felt any grief for her mother's death.

---

[40] MS Laing DF67. Dr Laing's Tuesday 6.30 group, 22 October 1957.

[41] Interestingly, Wilson was to review Adrian Laing's biography of his father and was generally sympathetic to R.D. Laing.

[42] MS Laing DF67. Dr Laing's Tuesday 6.30 group, 5 November 1957.

> One way to prevent thoughts and feelings of matricide was to adopt some of the mother's
> habits, thus preserving her internally.[43]

The records of this group reveal Laing diligently taking the group each week, and, as he was in the midst of his analytical training, it is no great surprise that he seems to have adopted a fairly traditional psychodynamic line in his interactions with group members.

During this period in London, Laing received instruction in the formal techniques of psychoanalysis and had the opportunity to put these techniques into practice. He gradually experimented with conducting less formal therapy and finding a style that reflected his own outlook and which seemed to him a more effective way of being and behaving with patients. Thus, contrary to the notion of the analyst as a blank screen on to which the analysand projected their fantasies, Laing gave personal details about himself when asked and he did not rigidly insist that the patient behave in the manner dictated by analytic orthodoxy.

From the clinical notes to the published report

The second half of this book has looked at Laing in clinical practice. It has utilized primary source material, made up of Laing's medical notes and institutional records, to build up a picture of the young psychiatrist at work. It has gone some way to answering the question: what did Laing actually *do* in therapy. We see Laing interacting with his patients and trying different therapeutic strategies, such as interpreting symptoms, giving advice, or adopting a confrontational stance. He records his attempts to make sense of these encounters, and the feelings of fear, frustration, bemusement, sympathy, and human solidarity that they engendered. We also see Laing with his immediate peers, discussing medication and psychotherapy in staff meetings at Gartnavel, and making wide-ranging suggestions about treatment in case conferences at the Southern General Hospital in Glasgow.

Crucially, we are able to examine the ways Laing used his original clinical records when he came to write his books. As we have noted, there is often a discrepancy between how Laing describes his patients in print and how they appear in the original clinical notes. As we have suggested, the potential reasons for these discrepancies are various. Most simply, the demands of anonymity may have led to details being changed. The original records may be incomplete and Laing may have possessed more information about the patient than appeared in his notes. When he came to write his books, his memory may have been at fault. The need to construct a satisfying and coherent narrative may have out-weighed the need to adhere strictly to the 'facts'. What constitutes the 'facts' of the case may be open to interpretation. As Laing well knew, a particular perspective, clinical or philosophical, may determine how the 'facts' are seen. Less generously, was Laing guilty of deliberately changing the details of his reported case histories? After all, we have seen that when it came to describing his *own* life story, he created a particular narrative of himself as the Hero. Was Laing tempted to change the narratives of his patients in order to better illustrate his theories, to make

---

[43] Ibid., 29 October 1957.

them more convincing? Were changes made as part of the self-mythologizing project of presenting R. D. Laing to the outside world; for example, in the case of Phillip, the young boy in *Wisdom, Madness and Folly* whom he apparently rescued from a career as a long-term patient? These are difficult questions to answer, and Laing is not alone in having the accuracy of his published case reports challenged. For example, Freud's published cases have been examined and found to be suspect, either in misleadingly claiming therapeutic success when none transpired,[44] or in manipulating the testimony of the patient so that it appears to confirm to the tenets of psychoanalysis.[45] In the case of Laing, one has to avoid, at one extreme, entirely discounting many of his clinical studies as fabricated, or, at the other, claiming he was articulating some kind of poetic truth about the nature of his patient's madness which was superior to the prosaic details of their actual histories. In fact, the picture is a mixed one, and some of Laing's published cases, such as 'John' in *The Divided Self*, are little different from those found in the original clinical notes. In the accounts where there are discrepancies, it is likely that several of the factors discussed above were involved: the need for anonymity, faulty memory, artistic embellishment, and seeing the patient through the lens of a particular theory. The extent of the impact of these factors on the published case varied from patient to patient. It has to be said in Laing's favour that, whatever one concludes about the veracity of his published case histories, a great many readers, patients, psychiatrists, and lay public, responded positively to *The Divided Self*, and felt that his depiction of extreme mental states bore the mark of authenticity. It is to *The Divided Self* that we now turn.

---

[44] Sulloway, F.J. (1979). *Freud, Biologist of Mind. Beyond the Psychoanalytic Legend.* Basic Books, New York; Clare, A. (1985). 'Freud's cases: the clinical basis of psychoanalysis'. In Bynum, W.F., Porter, R. and Shepherd, M. (eds), *The Anatomy of Madness. Essays in the History of Madness.* Volume 1, pp. 271–88. London: Tavistock Publications.

[45] Berkenkotter, C. (2008). *Patient Tales. Case Histories and the Uses of Narrative in Psychiatry.* The University of South Carolina Press, South Carolina.

Chapter 12

The Divided Self

The intense labours that R.D. Laing had undertaken during his early years as a young psychiatrist finally bore fruition with the publication of *The Divided Self* in 1960. In this book Laing brought together his extensive reading in psychiatry, psychoanalysis, philosophy, literature, and religion to describe the patients he had encountered in the mental hospitals of Glasgow and in the psychiatric units of the British Army. From his adolescence, Laing had set himself the goal of having his first book published by the time he was 30. Although he was a few years behind schedule—a fact that Laing tended to obscure in his subsequent accounts—the publication of *The Divided Self* was still an important personal milestone, and one that was to have not only a major impact on his career, but also a profound influence on the world of psychiatry and the public perception of the mentally ill. For the rest of his life, Laing was to return to his first work, commenting on it in interviews and in subsequent publications, writing a revised preface for the 1965 paperback edition, and, as late as the 1980s, making annotations on his copy of the book. In this chapter we look at early drafts of *The Divided Self*, the comments of his colleagues to whom he sent his work in progress, the published book itself, and the response of others to its appearance. We will also look at Laing's subsequent opinions of the book and how it has been judged since its publication. We will ask if Laing's work can be seen as belonging to a Scottish cultural tradition, and briefly consider the effects on him of attaining fame and then losing it.

Early drafts

We can follow the emergence of *The Divided Self* from the various drafts and outlines that Laing composed in the years leading up to its publication. Laing began writing *The Divided Self* in Glasgow when he was a senior registrar. As he later observed, *The Divided Self* was almost entirely based on his experiences of psychiatry in Glasgow, and, in particular, his time at Gartnavel,[1] though, as we have seen, patients from his Army days were also included. The manuscript was initially typed at the Southern General Hospital and subsequent drafts were typed by one of the secretaries at the Tavistock after he had moved to London.[2] At one stage Laing considered that *The Divided Self* would be the first in a series of books, with *The Self and Others* forming the second volume. In a letter to Donald Winnicott on 30 May 1958, Laing outlined

---

[1] Mullan, B. (1995). *Mad to be Normal. Conversations with R.D. Laing.* Free Association Books, London, p. 151.
[2] Ibid., p. 264.

yet another plan which would involve three volumes.[3] Volume one was to be *The Divided Self*, volume two was to be an historical, critical examination of the concept of schizophrenia from 1911 to the present day, while volume three was to describe treatment. The last volume would have been especially interesting, because Laing never left an extended account of his method of therapy.

In a draft outline of *The Divided Self*,[4] Laing envisaged that there would be another chapter after 'The ghost of the weed garden'. This was to be entitled 'Infancy and ontological security'. Certainly the book as published seems to end abruptly and might have benefited from a concluding chapter. An early draft which seeks to explain how schizophrenia develops, contains many of the key ideas that Laing was to articulate in *The Divided Self*.[5] Here he adopted an existentialist perspective, but he also drew on Winnicott's account of the development of the personality. This attempt to bring together existential philosophy and object relations theory forms the backbone of *The Divided Self*. In the draft Laing began by observing that some people felt a split between their mind and body, and, as a consequence, experienced themselves divided into two different and distinct substances. Rather than regarding mind and body as separate, Laing, alluding to the writings of the German theologian, Rudolf Bultmann, suggested that spirit and flesh were different modes of being, as opposed to the view that they were independent entities. An individual was free to choose either a spiritual mode of being or a life of the flesh. Laing referred to Winnicott's claim that the crucial factor in the development of a fully integrated personality was the infant's early experience with their mother. A mother who provided a continuity of care enabled her child to develop a 'continuity' of being or to 'become a real whole person'.

Laing felt that knowledge of both mind–body relations and the infant's interaction with the mother was necessary if 'the schizophrenic way of existing' was to be understood. In his discussion of the subject he used 'being', 'mind', 'self', 'soul', and 'spirit' interchangeably. This presented problems in his exposition, because, at this stage, he never really defined the terms and this led to a sense of vagueness and wooliness in what he was trying to say. Laing contended that psychiatry did not have an appropriate framework to make sense of the schizophrenic experience. He maintained that people with schizophrenia had problems with experiencing themselves as fully integrated in mind and body. For example, they might experience their self as a substance which was detachable from the body. It was a short step to conclude that they had been robbed of their self, or that it had been extinguished. Laing drew on the example of Daniel Schreber, the German judge who believed that his soul had been 'murdered'. Laing suggested that people with schizophrenia could lose their soul or self without undergoing biological death. In this draft, Laing attempted to account for what he saw as the core problem in individuals who suffered from schizophrenia: they had never achieved, or they had lost the possibility of being a 'real integrated person'.

---

[3] MS Laing B43. Letter from Laing to Dr Winnicott, 30 May 1958.
[4] MS Laing A590/1Draft Outline of *The Divided Self*.
[5] MS Laing DE5. The ghost of the weed garden.

The language of madness

Laing was fascinated with language, and in a preparatory paper written in relation to the chapter entitled 'The ghost of the weed garden', he examined psychotic communication.[6] Laing commented on the contemporary psychiatric approach to the speech of patients with schizophrenia. Most clinicians, he wrote, assumed that language was a relatively non-distorting medium which served to reflect fairly accurately what an individual thought and felt. These assumptions applied not only to the definition of what constituted a metaphor or a simile, but also to the syntactical structure of language. Laing observed: 'It is quite obvious that if we judge schizophrenese from the standpoint of our sanity we will find that it is a mass of absurdities, incongruities and so on.'[7] This is a typical Laingian view. He repeatedly contended that we have to see psychosis through the eyes of the sufferer if we are to understand it. Laing felt that using psychoanalytic concepts, such as the 'primary process', did not address the problem. Analytic theory held that there were two types of mental functioning, 'primary' and 'secondary' processes, representing, respectively, the unconscious and the conscious.[8] Primary process thinking was characterized by fusing words and images together, and by the use of symbolization, whereby items replaced or represented other ones. It ignored the categories of space and time, and was governed by the 'pleasure principle'. In contrast, secondary process thinking obeyed the laws of grammar and logic, and was governed by the 'reality principle'. Although Laing was convinced that 'schizophrenese' undoubtedly exhibited the characteristics of primary process thinking, he thought that it did not explain why a person with schizophrenia spoke in that way. What was the speaker's intention?

Laing maintained that psychiatrists thought it was not sensible to speak in terms of the 'intention' of the schizophrenic speaker, and that the speech of many patients was simply incomprehensible. According to this view, 'one would really be exercising misplaced ingenuity in attempting to discover a meaningful unity behind what is being said, where no such unity in fact exists'.[9] Laing felt that this view was profoundly mistaken. This debate, as to whether madness was understandable or not, goes to the heart of Laing's work. He repeatedly argued that the utterances of the mentally ill made much more sense than psychiatrists allowed. However, he was aware, as the previous quotation makes clear, that others felt that such a view was misguided, that it was a Quixotic search for meaning where none could be found.

Laing speculated as to why the communication of patients with schizophrenia seemed obscure. He felt that obscurity was to some extent intended. The psychotic person felt vulnerable and wanted to protect themselves by disguising what was going on inside them. In an interesting passage, Laing wrote:

> There exists a terrible sense of loneliness and a desire to reach out for some companionship, coexistent with the feeling of themselves as superior and above other people, which leads them to look down contemptuously at the pedestrian, ordinary, mediocre,

---

[6] Ibid., The ghost of the weed garden. Section headed 'Language'. No page numbers.

[7] Ibid.

[8] Rycroft, C. (1995). *A Critical Dictionary of Psychoanalysis* (2nd edn.). Penguin Books, London.

[9] MS Laing DE5. The ghost of the weed garden. Section headed 'Language'. No page numbers.

commonplace—and derive a certain sardonic satisfaction out of speaking in hidden meanings, concealed puns, equivocations, and so on.[10]

This is interesting for two reasons. First, Laing conceives of a model of madness wherein the symptoms are under the control of the patient, at least to some degree. From his existential perspective, he felt that mentally ill individuals had some choice as to how they conducted themselves in the world. For example, they could choose to manufacture disturbed speech if it fulfilled an existential need. Secondly, when Laing referred to the mad person feeling superior and contemptuous of ordinary people, the similarity to his own outlook seems evident. In his notebooks he commented on his feelings of loneliness, of not being able to find like-minded people. In this context he discussed the dilemma of the modern artist, who combined a feeling of being alienated from society with a desire to have their work seen and heard by others. Laing had used the word 'equivocation' to describe the way *he* sometimes dealt with questions about himself, particularly in regard to his spiritual beliefs. In explaining how apparently disturbed speech emerged, Laing argued that, where once the individual had deliberately adopted a strategy of misleading the listener, they eventually became so estranged from the world and themselves that their speech was now a way of signalling to others the desperation of their predicament.

Manuscript

Laing sent the manuscript of *The Divided Self* to friends and colleagues in Glasgow and London. Professor Ferguson Rodger replied that Laing had produced 'a very important work',[11] but thought the chapter on the origins of insecurity was weak. He wanted Laing to emphasize the connection between infantile experience and adulthood. He went on to suggest that he might ask Henricus Cornelis Rumke, a Dutch professor of psychiatry, who had worked with Eugen Bleuler, to write the foreword to the book. Rumke, who has been described as a 'metaphysical romantic', maintained that schizophrenia was diagnosed, not by examining the patient but by examining one's own inner world.[12] Laing cited one of Rumke's papers in the book but made no reference to him in the text. Ferguson Rodger added: 'I feel that one of the virtues of your book is that it bridges the gap between Continental and British and American psychiatry in a most attractive fashion.' Henry Chalk, a former colleague at the Southern General Hospital, wrote back to say the manuscript was being passed around the department, and that he felt it was 'a fine piece of work'.[13]

Joe Schorstein felt it was a bit pompous of Laing to be publishing a book so early in his career.[14] He thought of it as a private PhD thesis, which was good practice for later, mature work. Schorstein gave Karl Abenheimer the manuscript and he wrote to Laing

---

[10] Ibid.

[11] MS Laing B45. Letter from Ferguson Rodger to Laing, 30 June 1958.

[12] Neeleman, J. (1990). (trans. and introduction). Classic Texts No 3. 'The nuclear symptoms of schizophrenia and the praecox feeling. By H C Rumke'. *History of Psychiatry*, 1, 331–41.

[13] MS Laing B46. Letter from Henry Chalk to Laing, 9 September 1958.

[14] Mullan, *Mad to be Normal*, p. 266.

to give his opinion.[15] Abenheimer felt it was 'a fine start' with its emphasis on the self being the central problem in schizophrenia. However, he felt the manuscript needed much rewriting. He took Laing to task about his understanding of certain concepts, such as the self and false-self systems. He was particularly critical of the last chapter on the case of Julie. He ended: 'I would be glad to be assistance to you because your book has the potential of a good book in it and I would hate that it adds to the existing muddle instead of clearing it up.' We do not have a record of Laing's response to this, but a second letter by Abenheimer, five days later, apologizes for his previous 'sharpness of tone' and is more conciliatory. He repeated his offer to help Laing 'improve' the book.[16] Years later Laing recalled that Abenheimer had thought the book was immature and that it was not sophisticated enough.[17]

Laing sent the manuscript to Winnicott, who wrote back to say that he was so excited on reading it that he had tried to ring Laing immediately. However, he added: 'It is possible that at the beginning you are talking to yourself quite a bit . . . I did not really get interested until I was about a third of the way through. I hope that the book gets published soon and that from there you may get on to making a more concise theoretical statement'.[18] John Bowlby liked *The Divided Self*, but thought that first two chapters contained 'too many long words'.[19] He thought it would be greatly improved by the deletion of the words 'existential' and 'phenomenology'. He was not sure of 'ontology' either.[20] Charles Rycroft thought it was very good but needlessly repetitive. Marion Milner felt it contained 'vivid descriptions' of patients.[21]

Laing sent the manuscript to several publishers before it was finally accepted. These included Penguin, Allen and Unwin, Pantheon, and Kegan Paul.[22] One of the first publishers that Laing tried was Gollancz. In a revealing letter to Victor Gollancz on 3 September 1959, Laing wrote:

> . . . It has been read by . . . Dr D.W. Winnicott (President, British Psycho-Analytic Association) Dr Marion Milner, Dr J.D. Sutherland (Director of the Tavistock Clinic), and T. Ferguson Rodger (Professor of Psychiatry at Glasgow University). Everyone who has read it has regarded it as highly controversial . . . In Professor Rodger's view, as expressed to me, it is the greatest contribution to psychiatry since Freud.[23]

We have access to the publisher's readers' reports. One reader objected to the constant use of the words 'existential' and 'ontological'.[24] Another reader found it very stimulating, but thought that an American audience would be more receptive than a

---

[15] MS Laing B47. Letter from Karl Abenheimer to Laing, 10 September 1958.

[16] MS Laing B48. Letter from Karl Abenheimer to Laing, 15 September 1958.

[17] Mullan, *Mad to be Normal*, pp. 264–5.

[18] MS Laing B44. Letter from Dr Winnicott to Laing, 28 July 1958.

[19] Laing, A. (1994). *R.D. Laing. A Biography*. Peter Owen, London, p. 69.

[20] MS Laing A685, p. 2.

[21] A Laing, *Biography*, p. 69.

[22] Mullan, *Mad to be Normal*, p. 266.

[23] MS Laing B33. Letter from Laing to Victor Gollancz, 3 September, 1959.

[24] MS Laing B54. Reader's report on *The Divided Self*.

British one, which was not very interested in existential therapy.[25] This reader, however, thought there should be more clarification of terms, in particular the use of the word 'self'. Interestingly, one reader commented that the last chapter was theoretical and would have been better placed at the beginning. As we know, *The Divided Self* ends somewhat abruptly with the case history of Julie, so perhaps Laing changed the order of the chapters in response to the publishers. The book was eventually published by Tavistock in 1960.

The book

We have already considered many of the elements that contributed to *The Divided Self*. We have examined existential-phenomenology, object relations theory, psychiatric approaches to the treatment of psychosis, and the artistic and religious traditions that Laing drew on in writing the book. We have traced the original clinical accounts of the majority of the patients who were described in *The Divided Self*, and looked at how Laing modified them for the book.

Laing took his title for *The Divided Self* from the eighth lecture of William James' *The Variety of Religious Experience*. In this chapter James considered descriptions of mystical experiences by saints and mystics, and concluded that they were divided selves, who were responding not to God, but to their own guilt. Adrian Laing writes that Lionel Trilling's *The Opposing Self*[26] influenced his father's book and certainly there is a lengthy quotation from it in *The Divided Self*. Trilling, a distinguished American literary critic, was concerned with 'the idea of the self',[27] and contended that the modern self was distinguished by its 'intense and adverse imagination of the culture in which it has its being'.[28] The modern self, he maintained, was born in a prison and denounced its oppressor. Trilling felt that Hegel in his *Philosophy of History* gave the best account of the conflict between the self and modern culture. It was a conflict which led to the alienation of the self. Such ideas chimed with those of Laing.

Laing claimed that, stylistically he had been influenced by T.S. Eliot.[29] Part of the appeal of *The Divided Self* to many people was the quality of the writing. Commentators, such as Elaine Showalter, Roy Porter, Lisa Appignanesi, and Tom Leonard, have praised Laing's prose style. The text is replete with literary references and allusions, and eloquent turns of phrase. For example, Laing describes a young patient as 'an adolescent Kierkegaard played by Danny Kaye'.[30] Elsewhere he evokes the 'sooty, gritty, musty smell of a railway waiting room'.[31] Early in the book, Laing examined the clinical technique of Emil Kraepelin in a passage we have already considered from an existential-phenomenological perspective. Here we note that it serves a highly

---

25 MS Laing B53. Reader's report on *The Divided Self*.
26 Trilling, L. (1955). *The Opposing Self*. Harcourt Brace Jovanich, New York and London.
27 Ibid., Preface, p. 1.
28 Ibid., Preface, p. 1.
29 Clay, J. (1996). *R.D. Laing. A Divided Self*. Hodder & Stoughton, London, p. 59.
30 Laing, R.D. (1960). *The Divided Self. A Study of Sanity and Madness*. Tavistock Publications, London, p. 73.
31 Ibid., p. 130.

effective polemical strategy. The reader feels emotionally bound to side with the patient and to view Kraepelin as an insensitive brute. Jones[32] has called this kind of strategy an 'anti-psychiatric parable'. Scales fall from the reader's eyes and the meaning of the encounter is reversed so that the patient becomes a truth-telling victim and the clinician an unfeeling bully. Sedgwick felt that Laing showed great originality in making use of a text that had been in the public domain for fifty years without comment.[33] Theodore Lidz, however, claimed that Laing had set up a 'straw man', because contemporary psychiatrists did not behave like Kraepelin and had not done so for many years.[34] Whether one agrees with Lidz or not, Laing's technique is undeniably memorable.

Early in the book, Laing makes a disarming confession:

> I must confess here to a certain personal difficulty I have in being a psychiatrist, which lies behind a great deal of this book. This is that except in the case of chronic schizophrenics I have difficulty in actually discovering the 'signs and symptoms' of psychosis in persons I am myself interviewing. I used to think that this was some deficiency on my part, that I was not clever enough to get at hallucinations and delusions and so on. If I compared my experience with psychotics with the accounts given of psychosis in the standard textbooks, I found that the authors were not giving a description of the way these people behaved with me.[35]

Laing goes on to suggest that the behaviour of the patient is to some extent a product of the behaviour of the psychiatrist. If the psychiatrist behaves in a 'standard' way, so then will the patient. Such an approach, as exemplified by Kraepelin, ignores the emotional and existential aspects of the encounter between doctor and patient. Although this argument has an element of self-promotion, in that Laing is suggesting that he does not behave in a 'standard' manner, and consequently his patients do not either, he is nevertheless making a serious point about the limitations of the conventional psychiatric examination. Anthony Clare expressed some sympathy with Laing's difficulty and conceded that it might have been widely shared by other clinicians.[36] Clare quoted with approval the clinical axiom, 'The better a clinician knows a patient, the harder it is to make a diagnosis.' But he contended that the reason that Laing was not seeing patients whose presentation fitted the 'standard textbook' descriptions was because the advances in modern treatment had prevented such florid conditions developing. However, as we have seen, Laing began to work in psychiatric hospitals at a time when there were still many patients who had not been treated with the new medication.

In the preface to *The Divided Self*, Laing wrote that it was a study of schizoid and schizophrenic persons. Its basic purpose was to make madness and the process of going mad comprehensible. He was keen to stress what the book was *not* about. It did

---

[32] Jones, C. (1998). 'Raising the anti: Jan Foudraine, Ronald Laing and anti-psychiatry'. In Gijswijt, M. and Porter, R. (eds), *Cultures of Psychiatry and Mental Health Care in Postwar Britain and the Netherlands*. Rodopi, Amsterdam, pp. 283–94.

[33] Sedgwick, P. (1982). *Psychopolitics*. Pluto Press, London.

[34] Lidz, T. (1972). 'Schizophrenia, R.D. Laing and the contemporary treatment of psychosis'. In Boyers, R. and Orrill, R. (eds), *Laing and Anti-Psychiatry*, Penguin, London, pp. 123–56.

[35] Laing, *The Divided Self*, p. 28.

[36] Clare, A. (1980). *Psychiatry in Dissent. Controversial Issues in Thought and Practice* (second edn). Tavistock, London, p. 148.

not aim to give an all-encompassing theory of schizophrenia; nor did it attempt to explore organic or constitutional factors. Such a statement implied that, at this stage, Laing felt that such factors were not entirely irrelevant. Laing claimed that a further purpose of the book was to give in plain English an account in *existential* terms of some forms of madness. Once again Laing was at pains to stress what he was *not* trying to do. It was not a direct application of any established form of existential philosophy, but he acknowledged that his 'main intellectual' debt was to the 'existential tradition'. Laing claimed that his book was the first existential study in English of the ways that schizoid patients experienced themselves in the world.[37] Laing also stated that the book did not describe his method of therapy nor his relationship with his patients.

Laing aimed to explain how schizophrenia developed. His central thesis was that schizophrenia, or at least certain types of it, emerged from individuals with a schizoid personality. In an eloquent statement that opens *The Divided Self*, Laing writes:

> The term schizoid refers to an individual the totality of whose experience is split in two main ways: in the first place, there is a rent in his relation with his world and, in the second, there is a disruption of his relation with himself.[38]

Laing began by exploring the nature of the disturbances in schizoid individuals, and went on to speculate that schizophrenia developed when these disturbances grew more intense. He stated: 'The mad things said and done by the schizophrenic will remain essentially a closed book if one does not understand their existential context'.[39]

Laing maintained that the basic premise of *The Divided Self* rested on the concept of 'ontological security', the feeling of being at home in the world and with oneself and one's body. According to Laing, most people experienced themselves as real, alive, and more or less worthwhile. They possessed ontological security which they took for granted. They were comfortable with their being-in-the-world. However, there were those whose basic ontological position was one of insecurity. Such individuals could not take their realness and aliveness for granted. They were preoccupied with finding ways of 'trying to be real' in order to preserve their identity and to prevent the loss of their self. As we have seen, Laing referred to Franz Kafka as an example of a person who suffered from 'ontological insecurity'.

Laing outlined three forms of anxiety, which he maintained were experienced by the ontologically insecure person: 'engulfment', 'implosion', and 'petrification'. Engulfment was defined as a dread of human interaction, which it was feared would lead to loss of identity and of autonomy. The individual dealt with this fear by isolating themselves from others. Implosion referred to the fear that, at any moment, the world could crash in and obliterate one's identity. Petrification was the fear of being turned to stone, of being deprived of one's subjectivity, and becoming an object. The schizoid individual used the mechanism of petrification to turn other people into objects in order to make them less threatening. And here Laing referred to Sartre's discussion of this concept in *Being and Nothingness*.

---

[37] MS Laing A590/1. Draft outline of *The Divided Self*.
[38] Laing, *The Divided Self*, p. 15.
[39] Ibid., p. 15.

Laing went on to consider the nature of the relation that ontologically insecure people had with themselves. He contended that they primarily saw themselves as split into mind and body. Further, they most closely identified with the 'mind'. If this split became extreme, the individual was at risk of developing psychosis. In this context, Laing referred to Rudolf Bultmann and his description of Gnosticism, which conceived of the body as a prison from which the soul needed to escape.[40] Miller has argued that the work of Bultmann strongly influenced Laing in *The Divided Self*, especially his depiction of the schizoid condition.[41]

Laing stated that ontologically insecure individuals tended to have a sense of self which was disembodied, rather than embodied. This self was felt to be their 'true' self, and it was often cherished as upholding the ideals of inner freedom, honesty, omnipotence, and creativity. However, because this true self was disembodied, it had no direct contact with real people or real things. In order to communicate with the outside world, the person constructed a 'false self', which was identified with the body. However, this way of operating in the world was doomed, because it was impossible to maintain. The true self, which was shut away and isolated, was not enriched by outer experience, and, as a consequence, the person's inner world became impoverished. It became unreal, empty, dead, and split. It lost its anchor in reality. It had the ability to be any figure it wanted to be in its imagination, but was unable to be anyone in reality. We have discussed Dostoyevsky's description of this experience in his short story, *White Nights*. The divorce of the true self from the body occurred as a means of defence against the anxieties of participating in the outside world. The true self longed to be reconciled with the body, but at the same time feared being placed in a situation of danger from which it could not escape. It began to hate but also envy the outside world.

The false self was moulded by the expectations of others. There was a tendency for the false self to assume more and more of the characteristics of other people. The false self gradually became more autonomous, but this was accompanied by it becoming more unreal and more mechanical. The estrangement of the true self from the body had the potential to lead to psychosis, because the body was viewed as there to comply with others and to be under their control. Perceptions were regarded as false, because the world was being seen through the eyes of others.

With the stage set for impending psychosis, Laing held that it could arrive by two routes. First, the true self might decide it had had enough of the deceit and subterfuge of its representative on earth, the false self. If the true self decided to reveal itself, it was by now an entirely imagined self, which had no relation with the outside world. Its sudden appearance would appear psychotic to others. Psychosis represented the sudden lifting of the veil of the false self, which had long since failed to reflect the state of the true self. Secondly, the person might decide to 'murder' his self. Laing admitted that this was the 'ultimate and most paradoxically absurd defence possible'. It involved the person killing his or her 'self' in order to avoid being killed. It was, wrote Laing: '*the denial of being, as a means of preserving being*' (Laing's italics).[42] Laing stated that

---

[40] Ibid., p. 69.

[41] Miller, G. (2009). 'R.D. Laing and theology: the influence of Christian existentialism on *The Divided Self*. *History of the Human Sciences*, **22**, 1–21.

[42] Laing, *The Divided Self*, p. 163.

psychosis might be an attempt to preserve being by magical refuge in non-being. When a patient said that he had murdered his self, psychiatrists usually regarded this as evidence of a delusion. But for Laing, the patient spoke an 'existential truth', which was 'literally true within the terms of reference of the individual who makes them'.[43] Laing speculated that the fragmentation of the self led to warring 'inner phantoms'. The self's hiding place became a prison, where it was tortured by fragmented bits of itself. Laing suggested that the disintegration of the self led to the experiences of fragmented selves being treated as hallucinations by the true self.

Once schizophrenia developed, Laing maintained, patients frequently played at being psychotic or pretended to be so. This was done to keep the true self hidden and free of danger. Laing claimed that what was perceived as a disturbance of language and communication was, in fact, a deliberate strategy on the part of the schizophrenic patient. He wrote:

> A good deal of schizophrenia is simply nonsense, red-herring speech, prolonged filibustering to throw dangerous people off the scent, to create boredom and futility in others . . . He is playing at being mad to avoid at all costs the possibility of being held *responsible* for a single coherent idea, or intention.[44]

As an aside Laing commented: 'I am quite sure that a good number of "cures" of psychotics consist in the fact that the patient has decided, for one reason or other, once more to *play at being sane*' (Laing's italics).[45] As we have repeatedly seen, Laing contended that being mad was a role that an individual was free to take on or relinquish.

In the chapter, entitled 'The self and the false self in a schizophrenic', Laing used the case of a young woman which had been described by two American authors in the journal *Psychiatric Quarterly*.[46] Hayward and Taylor described in great detail the case of Joan, a 26-year-old white woman. Laing wrote that he chose the case because it seemed to strikingly confirm his own theories. He pointed out that he had come across the paper *after* he had written most of his book. He was interested in the fact that paper had devoted so much space to the patient's own account of her illness. He felt that Joan's account avoided a possible criticism of *his* case descriptions that his patients were merely repeating his theories parrot-wise. Laing felt that Joan's words were very much her own way of looking at herself and had not been imposed upon her or suggested to her by the authors. However, Joan's account does seem to be very much imbued by the psychiatric theorizing of her time. For example, she writes:

> It's hellish misery to see the breast being offered gladly with love, but to know that getting close to it will make you hate it as you hated your mother's. It makes you feel hellish guilt because, before you can love, you have to be able to feel the hate too . . . It's hell to want the milk so much but to be torn by guilt for hating the breast at the same time. Consequently, the schizophrenic has to try to do three things at once. He's trying to get the breast but he's also trying to die. A third part of him is trying not die.

[43] Ibid., p. 162.
[44] Ibid., p. 179.
[45] Ibid., p. 162.
[46] Hayward, M.L. and Taylor, J.E. (1956). 'A schizophrenic patient describes the action of intensive psychotherapy'. *Psychiatric Quarterly*, **30**, 211–48.

Although Laing stated he would not be discussing treatment, he makes occasional mention of the subject. For example he writes:

> Psychotherapy is an activity in which that aspect of the patient's being, his relatedness to others, is used for therapeutic ends. The therapist acts on the principle that, since relatedness is potentially present in everyone, then he may not be wasting his time in sitting for hours with a silent catatonic who gives every evidence that he does not recognise his existence.[47]

Elsewhere he states that the task of psychotherapy is to make 'an appeal to the freedom of the patient'.[48] He also claims: 'The task in therapy' is 'to make contact with the original "self" of the individual'.[49] And in a passage that bears the influence of the ideas of Ferenczi and Suttie, Laing says: 'The main agent . . . is the physician's love, a love that recognizes the patient's total being, and accepts it, with no strings attached'.[50]

Laing on *The Divided Self*

Laing continued to discuss *The Divided Self* for the rest of his career. In a letter written on 7 September 1960 to a former colleague in Glasgow, Laing was at pains to explain the relation between schizophrenia and the schizoid state:

> I think it would be advisable to say [of schizophrenia] 'its possible precursor, the schizoid state'. My method was to give an account only of those life histories where the person was either very schizoid and sane, or when the psychosis had undoubtedly issued out of a prior schizoid state . . . if schizophrenia is diagnosed in one way, the pre-psychotic schizoid personalities are probably in a minority. This was, incidentally, another reason why I made a point of disclaiming any attempt to present a comprehensive theory of schizophrenia.[51]

These caveats are important and emphasize that, initially at least, Laing was clear about the limitations of his work. He was not trying to explain all types of schizophrenia, nor was he saying that the condition always emerged from the schizoid state. In time, these caveats would be ignored by others, including Laing, and *The Divided Self* would be seen as offering a more wide-ranging explanation of madness in general.

In 1965 in the Preface to the Pelican edition of his first book, Laing gave his opinion:

> I wanted to convey above all that it was far more possible than is generally supposed to understand people diagnosed as psychotic. Although this entailed understanding the social context, especially the power situation within the family, today I feel that, even in focusing upon and attempting to delineate a certain type of schizoid existence, I was already partially falling into the trap I was seeking to avoid. I am still writing in this book too much about Them, and too little about Us.[52]

---

[47] Laing, *The Divided Self*, pp. 25–6.

[48] Ibid., p. 64.

[49] Ibid., p. 173.

[50] Ibid., p. 180.

[51] MS Laing GD42/50. Letter from Laing to S.A. Barnett, Zoology Department, University of Glasgow, 7 September 1960.

[52] Laing, R.D. (1965). *The Divided Self*. Pelican, London, preface.

In this comment, written when he was enjoying popular success as a counter-culture guru, Laing feels he was originally too influenced by the standard psychiatric approach which saw the patient as an object to be studied. He expanded on this in *Wisdom, Madness and Folly*:

> In my first book, *The Divided Self*, I tried to show the situation here. The attribution (the patient is autistic) is made by a person in the role of diagnosing psychiatrist, about a person, in the role of patient-to-be diagnosed. It is made across a gulf *between* them. The sense of a human bond with that patient may well be absent in the psychiatrist who diagnoses the patient as incapable of any such bond with anyone . . . Some enhanced understanding of what is going on between psychiatrist and patient does not preclude a scientific explanation of what is going on in the patient alone, and such a scientific explanation does not need to be a way to cut off a cut-off person from the possibility of human reunion, communion and renewal.[53]

In the margins of a 1983 edition of *The Divided Self*, Laing had written: '"We want a term" to match the original experience'.[54] In his contribution to the 1987 edition of *The Oxford Companion to Mind*, Laing (writing about himself in the third person) stated that in *The Divided Self*:

> . . . he offered a personal understanding of the scientist's scientific explanation and construed it as, unwittingly, a way of cutting off the cut-off person from the possibility of reunion and renewal.[55]

Further, he contended:

> The psychiatric diagnostic look is itself a depersonalised and depersonalising cut-of look . . . It is a way of seeing *things*, and the relation between things, by subtracting all personal experience.

Laing was later to describe *The Divided Self* as occupying the 'soft edge between psychoanalysis and existentialism', and he felt the nearest similarity to any author was Ludwig Binswanger, although Medard Boss, too, was writing in the same tradition.[56]

Responses to *The Divided Self*

What did Laing's colleagues make of *The Divided Self*? His old professor, Ferguson Rodger wrote to say the book deserved to become a psychiatric classic and that he was glad that Toynbee had given it such a favourable review in *The Observer*.[57] His former colleague from Gartnavel, Thomas Freeman gave the book a rather negative review, commenting that the existential-phenomenological approach militated against speculating about unconscious mechanisms, but that Laing had been unable to conform to

[53] Laing, *Wisdom, Madness and Folly*, p. 9.

[54] Glasgow University Library Special Collections. Laing's personal library. 14. *The Divided Self*, annotation on p. 19.

[55] Gregory, R. (ed.) (1987). 'Laing's understanding of interpersonal experience'. In *The Oxford Companion to Mind*. Oxford University Press, Oxford, pp. 417–8.

[56] Mullan, *Mad to be Normal*, p. 159.

[57] MS Laing GD42/20. Letter from Ferguson Rodger to Laing, 4 June 1960.

this discipline.[58] He had brought in psychoanalytic concepts to phenomenology, and, as a result, had provided an unsatisfactory mixture of interpretation and description. His London colleague, Peter Lomas thought it was a 'breath of fresh air'.[59] Winnicott felt he should have been given more credit for the notion of the false self. Laing pointed out to him that many of his concepts had long been a part of the Western intellectual tradition. He remembers Winnicott telling him, 'You may never write anything like that again'.[60] Writing about this remark some twenty years later, Laing observed: 'This is a good example of a Winnicotticism. A congenial compliment wrapped up in an uncongenial prediction.'[61] Laing was evidently stung by this remark as he still remembered it a long time afterwards and felt he had to prove Winnicott wrong.

What of the response of the wider world? *The Divided Self* was not an instant success. In its first four years it sold a mere 1600 copies.[62] It was only later in 1965 when it was published as a Penguin paperback that it became popular with the public. However, on its first appearance, it attracted several positive reviews. *The Times Literary Supplement* praised the quality of the writing and observed of Laing that 'his patients were singularly fortunate in their physician'.[63] The psychoanalyst, Marjorie Brierley found it 'a most interesting book' and wrote: 'the young author is an acute and empathetic observer, well endowed both intellectually and intuitively'.[64] Philip Toynbee in the *Observer* wrote: 'Dr Laing is saying something very important indeed. He is defining sanity and madness by means of a relationship between persons.'[65] The eminent London psychiatrist, Michael Shepherd stated: '. . . the book is written with sufficient clarity and sympathy to convey something of the way in which patients with schizophrenic or near schizophrenic disorders view the world. Anyone with a professional or humanitarian interest in these unhappy people will learn something from it.'[66]

According to Douglas Kirsner, *The Divided Self* was the first major book on existential therapy to make a mark on the English-speaking world.[67] *Existence*, edited by May, Angel, and Ellenberger, had appeared two years earlier but its influence did not extend beyond a limited circle of psychotherapists and academics.[68] Kirsner claimed: 'Laing did for the psychotic what Freud had done for the neurotic—he listened to psychotic

[58] Freeman, T. (1961). 'Review of *The Divided Self*. *British Journal of Medical Psychology*, **34**, 79–80.

[59] Lomas, P. (1973). *True and False Experience*. Allen Lane, London, p. 74.

[60] MS Laing A685, p. 4.

[61] Ibid., p. 4.

[62] Clay, *R.D. Laing*, p. 62.

[63] Ibid., p. 73.

[64] Brierley, M. (1961). 'Review of *The Divided Self*. *International Journal of Psychoanalysis*, **42**, 228–9.

[65] Toynbee, P. (1960). 'Review of *The Divided Self*. *Observer*, quoted on the back cover of *The Self and Others*.

[66] Shepherd, M. (1960). 'Review of *The Divided Self*. *Medical World*, quoted on back cover of *The Self and Others*.

[67] Kirsner, D. (2005). 'Laing and Philosophy'. In Raschid, S. (ed.) *R.D. Laing. Contemporary Perspectives*. Free Association Books, London, pp. 154–74.

[68] May, R., Angel, E., and Ellenberger, H.F. (eds) (1958). *Existence. A New Dimension in Psychiatry and Psychology*. Basic Books, New York.

patients and treated their speech and actions as potentially understandable and meaningful.'[69] However, he felt that Laing almost certainly overrated the magnitude of the patient's choices in schizophrenia. James Hood, a fellow medical graduate, observed that Laing wrote most of the book in Glasgow when he was working in a supportive and familiar environment, and he pointed to the presence of Schorstein and Abenheimer as being of particular importance.[70] Hood regarded *The Divided Self* as marking a turning point in British psychiatry and he felt its success was because Laing had been able to bring together ideas that were already current or latent in Europe and North America. By combining a clear exposition of such ideas with clinical examples, Laing made a compelling case for his approach to madness.

The response of Anthony Clare to *The Divided Self* was typical of his generation of psychiatrists. Clare writes:

> I first read the book as a medical student . . . in the early 1960s. It made an immense impact on me because of the lucid and convincing way in which it demystified madness, ruptured the divide between the mad and the sane and offered a meaningful explanation of much so-called 'pathological' symptoms and behaviour. In the words of one of his colleagues and supporters, Joe Berke, Laing 'put the person back into the patient'.[71]

Many other psychiatrists have ventured similar opinions. In a series, entitled 'Ten books' in the *British Journal of Psychiatry*, senior clinicians are asked to discuss books that have influenced them. One of the most commonly cited book is *The Divided Self*, which many say inspired them to become psychiatrists. Though they do not necessarily continue to agree with Laing's perspective, there was something about his first book that a generation of psychiatrists found appealing.

Critique

The Divided Self was a bold and innovative attempt to bring together existential philosophy, psychiatry, psychoanalysis, and literature in order to understand schizophrenia. Even one of Laing's most trenchant critics, Peter Sedgwick, judged: 'One of the most difficult of philosophies was brought to bear on one of the most baffling of mental conditions, in a manner, which, somewhat surprisingly, helped to clarify both.'[72] However, the very boldness in attempting to bring together disparate disciplines inevitably led to certain difficulties.

The self

The first concerns the notion of the self, which some modern thinkers dispute even exists. In an historical survey of ideas about the self, Roy Porter presents what he calls

---

[69] Kirsner, *Laing and Philosophy*.

[70] Hood, J. (2001). 'The Young R.D. Laing: a personal memoir and some hypotheses'. In Steiner, R. and Johns, J. (eds), *Within Time & Beyond Time. A Festschrift for Pearl King*. Karnac, London, p. 48, pp. 39–53.

[71] Clare, A. (1993). *In the Psychiatrist's Chair*. Mandarin, London, p. 201.

[72] Sedgwick, *Psychopolitics*, p. 74.

the 'standard' version of the story, before examining modern critiques of it.[73] The standard version embodies core Western values and stresses authenticity and individuality. It presupposes that there is some real 'inner self' which needs to be nourished if the person is to achieve fulfilment. The Renaissance is highlighted as the era in which man became centre stage for the first time. The Renaissance witnessed new cultural developments, such as the self-portrait, the diary, and the autobiography, which all reflected the growing preoccupation with individuality. Reformation Protestantism is seen as continuing this trend: believers were implored to search their souls and to keep spiritual diaries. In the standard version, Rene Descartes occupies an important place. In his *Discourse on Method* of 1637, Descartes made the famous statement, 'I am thinking, therefore I am'. He declared that his own consciousness was the only thing he could be sure of. As a result of the work of Descartes, the conscious self became the subject of a great deal of attention from philosophers, such as John Locke, who argued that the mind did not possess innate ideas but developed in response to experience and education. The self evolved, rather than being in a fixed state from birth. Later the Romantics hailed self-development as the primary goal of life, while Freud saw self-discovery as a voyage into inner space. Porter traces the standard history of the self up to the twentieth century and existentialism, which 'stressed the paramount need to combat the "bad faith" of the unexamined life, and all its duplicitous deceptions'.[74] He then considers thinkers such as Derrida and Foucault who have challenged this standard narrative and have suggested that the self is 'just a construct, a trick of language, a rhetorical ruse'.[75] Such writers challenged the liberal belief in human agency and individuality. Feminist thinkers have criticized the standard story of the emergence of the self, because it is entirely about the masculine self and reinforces stereotypes of male and female.

From a philosophical perspective, Bennett and Hacker have also argued that the notion of the self is illusory, that it is a 'pseudo-entity'.[76] They contend that it has been created in part by language: We have taken the reflexive pronouns such as 'myself' and 'yourself', and inserted a space in the words to yield 'my self' and 'your self'. It now appears that we have discovered a mysterious entity, the self, whose nature we proceed to investigate. Bennett and Hacker object to the philosophical tradition, derived from Descartes and Locke, of conceiving of the self as an 'inner' subject and the 'owner of experience'. In like manner, the Oxford philosopher, P.F. Strawson has emphasized that the individual is a person, not an 'animated body' or an 'embodied anima'. In his classic book, *Individuals*, which Laing had read, Strawson maintained that a person was a fundamental and irreducible category of being, and was distinctive in having both physical and psychological attributes.

In their conceptual history of the self in psychiatry, Berrios and Markova also contend that the self is a construct, that it is not a natural entity situated somewhere in the

---

[73] Porter, R. (ed.) (1997). *Rewriting the Self. Histories from the Renaissance to the Present*. Routledge, London.

[74] Ibid., p. 7.

[75] Ibid., p. 12.

[76] Bennett, M.R., Hacker and PMS (2003). *Philosophical Foundations of Neuroscience*. Blackwell, Oxford.

human mind or brain.[77] Ideas about the self are shaped by culture. The Western concept of self stresses individualism and autonomy, whereas other cultures have a more collective concept of self, which revolves around the family or clan. They observe that it was originally meant by Saint Augustine to be a metaphorical or virtual space for the interplay of responsibility, guilt, and sin. In the nineteenth century, the self was transformed into a psychological entity and was, effectively, reified. It was considered to really exist inside the mind and brain. It was also believed that the self could be affected by pathological lesions and diseases. Schizophrenia came to be viewed by psychiatrists as primarily a disorder of the self.

John Heaton was critical of Laing's concept of the self, arguing that he treated it as a reified entity.[78] By talking about selves rather than persons, Laing was compelled, at times, to write in a tortuous manner, which illustrates the difficulty, if not absurdity, of the enterprise. For example, he writes:

> . . . the *other self* is the basis of a hallucination. An hallucination is an as-if perception of a fragment of the disintegrated 'other' self by a remnant (self-focus) retaining residual I-sense . . .[79]

Laing constructed a complicated theory of the disintegration of the self, in which fragmented selves did battle with each other. Although he criticized Freud's mechanical model of the mind as 'ghostly hydraulics', his own model was also susceptible to the charge of reification: that he had taken abstract concepts and treated them as real entities. Like Freud, Laing's model has a Cartesian division between mind and body.

Kotowicz maintains that Laing's notion of the 'true self' has analogies with Freud's account of the unconscious, because it is a conception of selfhood, formed round some essential but never experienced inner core.[80] He argues that it has no more validity than the Freudian unconscious and that it might feed the illusion that there is a real self waiting to thrive once the false self has been discarded, whereas there is probably no such thing. Kotowicz suggests that the true self and false-self system led to a cul-de-sac because it posited two distinct realms.[81]

Phenomenology and existential philosophy

A second concern is that of phenomenology, as Thomas Freeman had noted. Laing claimed that he was using the phenomenological method, but this involves putting one's preconceptions and theories aside in order to describe the patient's experience. Admittedly this is extremely difficult, if not impossible, to achieve, as Laing readily conceded in his paper on 'Existential analysis'. However, Laing had a great many preconceptions, which had been shaped by the psychiatric and philosophical culture

---

[77] Berrios, G.E. and Markova, I. (2003). 'The self and psychiatry: a conceptual history'. In Kircher, T. and David, A. (eds), *The Self in Neuroscience and Psychiatry*. Cambridge University Press, Cambridge, pp. 9–39.

[78] Heaton, J. (1991). 'The Divided Self: Kierkegaard or Winnicott?' *Journal of the Society for Existential Analysis*, **2**, 30–7.

[79] Laing, *The Divided Self*, pp. 172–3.

[80] Kotowicz, Z. (1997). *R.D. Laing and the Paths of Anti-Psychiatry*. Routledge, London, p. 25.

[81] Ibid., p. 68.

he inhabited, and he brought these to his encounters with patients. This in turn affected what patients said to him and how they behaved. We have seen that he considered that the account of 'Joan' by two American psychiatrists represented the 'pure' voice of the patient, but it seems apparent that she spoke in a language heavily influenced by contemporary analytical ideas about mental illness. In the extract about *The Divided Self* from *Wisdom, Madness and Folly*, previously quoted, Laing recognized that the presence of the psychiatrist played a part in how the patient responded, but here he was criticizing what he saw as the alienating effect of the clinician adopting the disease model. In *The Divided Self*, he did not consider how his own clinical approach, imbued by existential and psychoanalytic theory, influenced the patient's presentation. Friedenberg perceptively imagines what the encounter with Laing might have been like for the patient:

> Laing's humane acceptance of persons otherwise deemed psychotic must, therefore, have posed characteristic problems for them of a kind that, in a period of major status disloca-tions throughout society, has become familiar: the problem of how to respond to the sweet-talking liberal who sincerely wants to be on your side but who cannot really imagine the amount of misery he would have to go through if he really lived there. Retaining the support of such people requires special but time-honoured social skills: it is necessary to convey to them a sense of underlying competence and self-respect and a gratitude to them for understanding and caring about the hell you are in, and wanting to help you get out of it. But at the same time, it is absolutely imperative to remember that they don't really understand it; that their image of what it must be like is almost certainly romanticised precisely because they romanticise *you*.[82]

Another concern is the application of existential philosophy to mental illness. Laing stated that he was applying existential principles to the understanding of psychiatric conditions, but existentialism holds that there is no fixed human essence. Laing's con-cept of the self would seem to contradict this. Kirsner maintains that object relations theory is incompatible with existential philosophy, which asserts that there is no human nature and no essential self. As we have seen, John Heaton also considered that Laing's ambition to reconcile a psychological theory with a philosophical tradition, was beset with problems.

Derzen-Smith[83] felt that ontological insecurity, which was such a central feature in *The Divided Self*, did not just apply to mentally disturbed people but was a universal experience. She felt that if Laing had made this point in his book, he might have avoided the difficulties he encountered later. He had attached an aspect of ordinary human experience to a pathological condition. In tandem, Collier also maintained that the experience of ontological insecurity was common amongst many people who were not mentally ill.[84] In fact, Alan Tyson judged that *The Divided Self* struck a chord

[82] Friedenberg, E.Z. (1973). *Laing*. Fontana/Collins, London, p. 17.

[83] Van Derzen-Smith, E. (1991). 'Ontological insecurity revisited'. *Journal of the Society for Existential Analysis*, **2**, 38–48.

[84] Collier, A. (1977). *R.D. Laing: The Philosophy and Politics of Psychotherapy*. The Harvester Press, Hassocks, Sussex, p. 8.

with thousands because schizoid feelings were so prevalent and intense in our society.[85]

Howarth-Williams argued that in *The Divided Self* Laing focused almost entirely on the individual and his or her relation to the world, rather than the mutual inter-relatedness of two or more individuals, a point that Sedgwick also made.[86] The world was seen through the eyes of the patient, and Laing tried to gain access to this experience. Collier was concerned that, although an admirable ambition, it had implications for therapy. If the psychiatrist felt that the patient's world view was distorted or, in some way pathological, should it be challenged, indeed, could it be challenged? If the patient was articulating his or her 'existential truth', surely that was valid and not in need of 'correction'. What was the role of the psychiatrist in this situation? In fact did the psychiatrist have a role? It could be argued that the logic of the existential position dictated that the psychiatrist did not, in fact, have a role. Laing had written that '. . . one has to be able to orientate oneself as a person in the other's scheme of things . . . One must be able to effect this reorientation without prejudging who is right and who is wrong'.[87] Whereas the disease model allowed the psychiatrist to intervene with physical treatments, and the psychoanalytic model permitted the analyst to try and modify the patient's psychic defences, it is not so clear what an existential therapist is supposed to do. This ambiguity may have contributed to Laing's difficulty in giving a detailed account of what existential therapy entailed. In the wake of *The Divided Self*, he was to experiment with many different approaches to mental disorder. Burston has argued that, although Laing was attempting to take a neutral stance with regard to the experiences of schizoid patients in *The Divided Self*, he was actually implying that, by rejecting the bodily and communal aspects of existence, they were 'in flight from their basic humanity'.[88] Burston considers that there are unacknowledged tensions in Laing's approach between attempting to change the patient and being accepting of them. Burston compares this to the contrast between therapy inspired by Martin Buber which seeks communion but also confrontation, and the therapy inspired by Martin Heidegger, which is more passive and 'lets Being be'.[89] Burston speculates that Laing adopted one or either position, depending on how disturbed the patient was.

Feminist critiques

Feminist thinkers have been attracted to Laing's early work as it appeared to suggest that female insanity was a violation of the expectations of the gender role. Juliet Mitchell considers that Laing's writing provided women with the vocabulary to protest

[85] Tyson, A. (1971). 'Homage to Catatonia'. *New York Review of Books*, **16**, 3–6.

[86] Howarth-Williams, M. (1977). *R.D. Laing. His Work and its Relevance for Sociology*. Routledge and Kegan Paul, London, p. 85.

[87] Laing, *The Divided Self*, p. 25.

[88] Burston, D. (1996). *The Wing of Madness. The Life and Work of R.D. Laing*. Harvard University Press, Cambridge, Massachusetts, p. 187.

[89] Burston, D. (2000). *The Crucible of Experience. R.D. Laing and the Crisis of Psychotherapy*. Harvard University Press, Cambridge, Massachusetts, pp. 52–4.

against the restrictions of their role.[90] Mitchell locates Laing's work in the context of what she sees as the British post-war restructuring of the family and the rise to prominence of the adolescent, whose central dilemma was 'the crisis of leaving home'. She judges that Laing's case histories are 'models of readability' and 'fascinating in their revelations of how we operate in our most intimate relationships'. Because females formed the majority of the cases, Mitchell maintains that they served to highlight the essential feminine predicament: the conflict of the daughter leaving home and the mother letting go. Mitchell observes that Laing left the father out of the picture, for example, in his account of Julie, and, as a consequence, the mother was given the blame for the plight of the daughter. Mitchell felt that Laing was not even aware of the 'prejudice' he held against the mother. Despite this, she sees Laing's work as making an important contribution to feminism.

While feminist critics have been much exercised by a work outside the focus of this book, namely *Sanity, Madness and the Family*, which appeared in 1964, they have also commented on *The Divided Self*. In her discussion of 'anti-psychiatry' in *The Female Malady*, Elaine Showalter complains that generally women play the role of patient, while the male gets the job of therapist.[91] However, in *The Divided Self*, there are several male patients, such as David, James, and Peter, and Laing makes reference to many female therapists, such as Fromm-Reichmann, Sechehaye, Klein, and Segal. Later feminist writers have found Showalter's contention that mental illness is a peculiarly 'female malady' unsupported by the evidence.[92] For Showalter, the case studies in *The Divided Self* vividly describe women struggling with the family's conflicting messages about femininity, but she criticizes Laing for not exploring this further and examining how gender expectations contributed to their mental distress. She maintains that Mrs R. is infantilized by her dependence on male approval and that Mrs D.'s anger towards her husband is not taken seriously by Laing, who dismisses it as 'unaccountable'. However, in the book it is the patient who says her anger is unaccountable, not Laing. The passage reads: 'She complained . . . of unaccountable accesses of anger towards her husband'.[93] Showalter also observes that both Julie and Joan have parents who wanted them to be boys, and she finds Laing guilty of ignoring the possible psychological consequences of such an upbringing. Showalter's final judgment on Laing is a mixed one. On one hand, she concedes:

> It is impossible to write as a feminist about R. D. Laing without acknowledging the importance of his analysis of madness as a female strategy within the family. For a whole generation of women, Laing's work was a significant validation of perceptions that found

[90] Mitchell, J. (1974). *Psychoanalysis and Feminism*. Penguin Books, Harmondsworth. Reprinted with a new introduction, 2000.

[91] Showalter, E. (1987). *The Female Malady. Women, Madness and English Culture, 1830–1980*. Virago Press, London, pp. 231–2.

[92] Tomes, N. (1994). 'Feminist histories of psychiatry'. In Micale, M.S. and Porter, R. (eds), *Discovering the History of Psychiatry*. Oxford University Press, Oxford, pp. 348–84.; Busfield, J. (1996). *Men, Women and Madness. Understanding Gender and Mental Disorder*. Macmillan Press, London.

[93] Laing, *The Divided Self*, p. 62.

little social support elsewhere. In the academy, too, Laing's work has been important to feminist critics, his theory of 'ontological insecurity' providing a valuable method of understanding the *representation* of women . . .[94]

On the other hand, she concludes that Laing did not provide a 'coherent analysis' of the particular problems of women, nor did his work lead to a restructuring of the social forces that kept females in their place. Lisa Appignanesi, while giving a more sympathetic and positive account of Laing, agrees with Showalter that his case studies dramatized the very specific plight of women, but that he did not attend to the implications of the role of gender in their mental breakdown.[95]

How Scottish was R.D. Laing?

Gavin Miller has recently asked, 'How Scottish was R.D. Laing?'[96] The question was first addressed by Craig Beveridge and Ronald Turnbull in their 1989 book, *The Eclipse of Scottish Culture*.[97] With some justification, they noted that accounts of Laing and his writing up until that time had entirely ignored his Scottish background, or, if it was mentioned at all, it was only to denigrate it, or express surprise that from scenes like these, from lowly and uninspiring beginnings, he was able to bring forth work of such intellectual breadth and sophistication. Beveridge and Turnbull see the neglect of Laing's Scottish heritage as part of a wider malaise, which they diagnose as an 'inferiorist' mentality, created by the relentlessly negative images of the country served up by historians and cultural commentators, both within and without Scotland. They observe that when Laing's Scottish origins are acknowledged, it is usually to declare that he is part of a native tradition preoccupied with divided personalities—a tradition that reflects the supposed profound schism in the Scottish psyche and society. They quote an article from the *Guardian* which demonstrates this type of thinking:

> Clearly Dr Laing is himself somewhat divided, as are so many Scotsmen. Highlands and Lowlands, cold rationalists and Calvinist fanatics, Glasgow and Edinburgh, teetotallers and dram-drinkers. Perhaps *Divided Self* should be seen in a tradition that includes such other works by Scots as Stevenson's *Dr Jekyll and Mr Hyde* and Hogg's *Confessions of a Justified Sinner*.[98]

The authors strenuously object to this picture of Scotland which they find 'freakish and pathological'. Instead they maintain that Laing can be seen as part of a thriving native intellectual tradition. We have already made reference to this tradition, which includes the philosophers, J.J. Russell and John Macmurray, as well as the theologians

---

[94] Showalter, *The Female Malady*, p. 246.

[95] Appignanesi, L. (2008). *Mad, Bad and Sad. A History of Women and the Mind Doctors from 1800 to the Present*. Virago, London, p. 368.

[96] Miller, G. (2009). 'How Scottish was R.D. Laing?' *History of Psychiatry*, 20(2), 226–32.

[97] Beveridge, C. and Turnbull, R. (1989). *The Eclipse of Scottish Culture. Inferiorism and the Intellectuals*. Polygon, Edinburgh; See also Turnbull, R. and Beveridge, C. (1988). 'Laing and Scottish philosophy'. *Edinburgh Review*, **78**(7), 119–28.

[98] Beveridge and Turnbull, *The Eclipse*, p. 106. Quotes J. Richard Boston, 'The Divided Self', *The Guardian*, 3 August, 1976.

John Baillie and John Macquarrie, and of course the Schorstein-Abenheimer group. Beveridge and Turnbull emphasize that the influence of this tradition is apparent in Laing's work. They summarize the common features:

> A foregrounding of the phenomenon of personhood; an insistence that knowledge is not exhausted in scientific cognition; hostility to the disestimation of important aspects of human experience which the triumphs of science have encouraged . . .[99]

Inspired by Beveridge and Turnbull's thesis, Miller has sought to uncover and examine in more detail the particularly Scottish factors in Laing's work.[100] He has looked at the influence of the philosopher, John Macmurray, but also at the impact of Scottish psychoanalysts, such as Fairbairn and Ian Suttie, on Laing. These were all writers whom Laing cited in his early writings, but Miller goes on to consider more seemingly tangential influences such as David Hume.[101] Laing certainly read Hume, and we have seen from his notebooks that he was keen to immerse himself in the work of the thinkers of the Scottish Enlightenment and beyond. His colleague John Heaton reveals that Laing was a great admirer of Hume and also the Scottish Common Sense School.[102] Heaton contends that if commentators were more aware of Laing's debt to the Scottish philosophical tradition, then his 'intellectual itinerary' would become clearer. In particular, he maintains that both Hume and Laing argued that the human world was understood through social participation, in contrast to the world of physical sciences which was determined by observation and theorizing. Both argued that social participation should involve interaction with females, and Laing felt strongly that those philosophers, such as Kierkegaard and Nietzsche, who had not experienced a sustained heterosexual relationship, were thereby limited in their perspective on the world.

Miller also examines the possible influence on Laing of J.B. Baillie, the early twentieth century Scottish philosopher, whose translation of Hegel's *The Phenomenology of Mind* is referred to in *The Divided Self*, and William Robertson Smith, the Victorian social anthropologist, who receives no mention. The argument for widening the net to include writers whom Laing might not have studied, is that particular cultures are permeated by the theories and assumptions of thinkers who are not necessarily read by the public, but whose ideas are nonetheless part of the common discourse. Sigmund Freud and Friedrich Nietzsche would be good examples of this phenomenon; their writings have had a profound impact on European culture and its citizens, despite being unread by the great majority of them.

However, Carthy has expressed some reservations about Miller's thesis, in particular the extent of the influence of Macmurray on Laing.[103] He points out that there was

---

[99] Ibid., p. 107.

[100] Miller, G. (2004). *R.D. Laing*. Edinburgh Review in Association with Edinburgh University Press, Edinburgh.

[101] Miller, G. (2001). 'Cognition and community: The Scottish philosophical context of the "divided self"'. *Janus Head* **4**, 104–29.

[102] Heaton, J.M. (2005). 'Laing and psychotherapy'. In Raschid, S. (ed.) *R.D. Laing. Contemporary Perspectives*. Free Association Book, London, pp. 313–25.

[103] Carthy, I. (2008). 'Book Review: Gavin Miller, R.D. Laing'. *History of Psychiatry*, **19**(2), 237–9.

a crucial ideological difference between Macmurray and Laing, and that this rested on their respective attitudes to the mentally ill. Whereas Macmurray felt that the utterances of mad people were essentially unintelligible, Laing spent much of his professional career emphasizing that they were potentially meaningful. Macmurray felt that it was impossible to form a personal relationship with a mentally ill person. He took as an example the situation where a psychologist finds that his pupil is in an 'abnormal state of mind'. Macmuray writes that for the psychologist: 'the relation has changed from a personal to an impersonal one; he adopts an *objective* attitude, and the pupil takes on the character of an object to be studied, with the purpose of determining the causation of his behaviour'.[104] This was precisely the attitude that Laing condemned when he discerned it in his psychiatric colleagues.

Not everybody has accepted Beveridge and Turnbull's thesis of the 'eclipse of Scottish culture', either, and, for example, the sociologist, David McCrone has criticized the notion that there is some essentialist Scottish culture waiting to be reclaimed and restored.[105] McCrone argues that there is not a single definition of Scottish identity, but rather many, which individuals adopt and discard as the occasion demands. In fact, they may inhabit several identities simultaneously. Beveridge and Turnbull have countered that McCrone's vision of a postmodern self that exists in a limbo out with history and tradition, is a vision of a self in a state of profound disorder.[106] It resembles, they suggest, Emile Durkheim's concept of the state of *anomie*, said to arise when an individual is estranged from any sort of social community. This debate echoes the previous discussion as to whether the self is real or whether it is a metaphor.

This debate is also relevant to the question: 'How Scottish was R.D. Laing?' We have to ask, what do we mean by 'Scottish'? If we subscribe to the postmodern view, the question is largely meaningless. The individual is free to choose what identity they adopt, and, anyway, 'Scottishness' is just a cultural construct which fluctuates over time, buffeted about by changing fashions and having no permanent anchor in human experience. If we reject this position, we then measure Laing against our definitions of what it is to be Scottish, whether this involves particular personality traits, or being part of a unique intellectual and cultural tradition. We look for aspects of his personality that fit with what we define as the national character, and we look for continuities in Laing's work with what went before. Do we, however, need to choose between these two opposing viewpoints? Can we concede that there is a large element of cultural construction in the notion of national identity? Can we further concede that that these constructs fluctuate and that individuals exercise some degree of choice in the personas they inhabit? After all, existentialists maintain that there is no human essence, and we are free to choose who we become. But, to divorce Laing entirely from his national background, from its language, religion, education system, art, literature, philosophy, ethical codes, and ways of life, seems perverse and self-defeating. Nations may well be

---

104 Macmurray, J. (1961). *Persons in Relation*. Faber & Faber, London, p. 29.

105 McCrone, D. (1992). *Understanding Scotland. The Sociology of a Stateless Nation*. Routledge, London.

106 Beveridge, C. and Turnbull, R. (1997). *Scotland After Enlightenment. Image and Tradition in Modern Scottish Culture*. Polygon, Edinburgh.

'imagined communities' as Benedict Anderson[107] has famously suggested, but they nevertheless exercise a profound influence on their members. In her recent history of modern Scotland, Catriona Macdonald concludes that the notion of 'Scottish' identity has remained meaningful to most of its citizens throughout the twentieth century.[108]

If we need to ask what we mean by 'Scottish', we also need to ask what we mean by 'R.D. Laing'. This is not a fatuous question. As we have seen, Laing was aware that he often played the role of 'R.D. Laing', as he made clear in his interview with Bob Mullan. In fact, Douglas Kirsner, who met with Laing observed: 'Laing was too star-struck by his own image, overawed by his own reputation and role . . . he seemed to have the delusion that he was "R.D. Laing".'[109] One of his biographers, John Clay has described Laing as a 'divided self', but Mullan feels this is too parsimonious, stating that Laing had many selves. Certainly the testimonies of those who knew him give contradictory and conflicting views of the man. Even during our period of study–Laing as a young man–we have seen a contrast between the public figure of the well-respected and companionable doctor, and the private one, who expressed contempt for his colleagues and who struggled with melancholy and despair. Of course, none of this is unique to Laing: we all have several sides to ourselves, and have public and private personas. But, in Laing's case, these contrasts seem more extreme than in many people, and it does make answering the question: 'How Scottish was R.D. Laing?' more complex.

If we return to the question of locating Laing in Scottish culture, we have seen that one response is to see his first book as part of a literary tradition of doubles and doppelgangers, and to see this tradition as a reflection of the divisions in the Scottish psyche and society. We have seen that Beveridge and Turnbull have objected to this approach, as denigrating Scottish culture. It is worth looking briefly at the literary history of the subject. In 1919, G. Gregory Smith, a Professor of English at Queen's College, Belfast, wrote one of the most famous books of Scottish literary criticism, *Scottish Literature: Character and Influence*.[110] In it he argued for the distinctive nature of Scottish literature, and put forward his highly influential thesis of the 'Caledonian Antisyzgy'. This was the term he coined to describe what he saw as the 'zigzag of contradictions', which he claimed were characteristic of Scottish literature. Gregory Smith maintained that there were two poles, those of realism and of fantasy. These two propensities could co-exist with a 'sudden jostling of contraries', and he traced such a tendency from the time of the medieval 'makars' or poets to the late nineteenth century. James Hogg's *Private Memoirs and Confessions of a Justified Sinner* and Robert Louis Stevenson's *Dr Jekyll and Mr Hyde* are seen as being part of this tradition. The poet, Hugh McDiarmid, whom Laing had invited to the Socratic Club when he was a student, was an enthusiast for the idea of the Caledonian Antisyzgy, which he perceived

---

[107] Anderson, B. (2006). *Imagined Communities. Reflections on the Origin and Spread of Nationalism*. (revised edn) Verso, London.

[108] Macdonald, C.M.M. (2009). *Whaur Extremes Meet. Scotland's Twentieth Century*. John Donald, Edinburgh.

[109] Mullan, *Mad to be Normal*, pp. 30–1.

[110] Gregory Smith, G. (1919). *Scottish Literature: Character and Influence*. Macmillan, London.

as giving him a licence for creative disruption.[111] In his great poem *A Drunk Man Looks at the Thistle*, he claimed he was 'aye to be whaur extremes meet', a sentiment that could apply equally well to Laing. Modern literary critics, however, have objected to what they see as Smith's over-arching generalizations, which leave little room for individual creativity. Gerard Carruthers has written that such an attempt to argue too strongly for the cultural distinctiveness of a nation risks separating it from the rest of world culture and its interactions with it.[112] Carla Sassi has pointed out that the theme of the double is common in European and American literature, but, nevertheless, in view of the frequency with which it occurs in Scottish writing, she feels it is especially relevant to Scotland.[113]

If we accept, like Sassi, that the concept of divisions and doubles does have some relevance to Scottish culture, then *pace* Beveridge and Turnbull, Laing and *The Divided Self* can be seen in this tradition. We have noted that Laing was described by contemporaries as 'mercurial'. To this we could add: his mood swings from exuberance to depressive despair; his radical reputation, but his description of himself as a conservative; and his championing of the marginalized, alongside his contempt for much of humanity. Clearly, *The Divided Self* deals in divisions: between the 'true' and the 'false' selves: between the mind and body; between the outside world and the inner one; and between official psychiatric language and that of the patient. In a later work we find this passage:

> Two men sit facing each other and both of them are me. Quietly, meticulously, systematically, they are blowing out each other's brains, with pistols. They look perfectly intact. Inside devastation.[114]

The Glasgow poet, Tom Leonard has spoken of Laing as part of the European existential tradition, but he also locates him in a Scottish tradition.[115] In this, Leonard includes James Thompson, the nineteenth century author of the long pessimistic poem, *The City of Dreadful Night*, Robert Owen's *New Lanark*, Alasdair Gray's *Lanark*, and Ian Hamilton Finlay's garden at Stonypath. What unites them with Laing, Leonard judges, is that they have all created: 'Places of authentic being, or allegories of inauthentic structure'.

We also have to consider the argument that notions of national identity change over time, as it is especially relevant to case of Laing. What did being 'Scottish' mean in the 1940s and 1950s? We have seen that in his first entry onto the world stage with the appearance of *The Divided Self*, Laing played down the book's Scottish origins. There is very little, on superficial acquaintance with the book, to suggest that the author was Scottish. There are only two references to Scottish writers, Fairbairn and Macmurray, and we have seen that the case histories were shorn of their Scottish context. Although issues of

---

[111] Carruthers, G. (2009). *Scottish Literature*. Edinburgh University Press, Edinburgh.

[112] Ibid.

[113] Sassi, C. (2005). *Why Scottish Literature Matters*. The Saltire Society, Edinburgh.

[114] Laing, R.D. (1967). *The Politics of Experience and the Bird of Paradise*. Penguin Books, London, p. 147.

[115] Mullan, B. (1997). *R.D. Laing. Creative Destroyer*. Cassell, London.

patient confidentiality undoubtedly contributed to this decision, it might not have been the only factor. Did being Scottish at this time evoke any negative response? Did Laing calculate that his career would be better served by downplaying his origins? Certainly by 1967, with the publication of *The Bird of Paradise*, Laing was openly celebrating his Scottish background, more particularly his native town of Glasgow. This piece contains affectionate observations, memories, and jokes, which paint a picture of a Glasgow of tenements, tramcars, pubs, medical students, psychiatric patients, and American sailors chatting up the local women. One passage gives a flavour of the earthy humour:

> Jimmy MacKenzie was a bloody pest at the mental hospital because he went around shouting back at his voices. We could only hear one end of the conservation, of course, but the other end could be inferred in general terms at least from:
>
> 'Away tae fuck, ye filthy-minded bastards . . .'
>
> It was decided at one and the same time to alleviate his distress and ours, by giving him the benefit of leucotomy.
>
> An improvement in his condition was noted.
>
> After the operation he went around no longer shouting abuse at his voices, but: 'What's that you say? Say that again! Speak up ye buggers, I cannae hear ye!'[116]

In *The Bird of Paradise*, Laing presents his home city as a place of poverty, squalor, and heavy drinking, but also as a place of human warmth and resilience, where humour is used as a means of survival. At this later period, in the mid 1960s when the Beatles had made their home town very fashionable, did coming from Glasgow, which had many similarities with Liverpool, carry some cachet? Later writers, such as Elaine Showalter and Clancy Sigal, both Americans, have bought into the Glasgow stereotype, and, despite their criticisms of him, have accorded Laing respect for his supposed gritty authenticity. Showalter describes Laing (misleadingly) as a 'working class Marxist' from the deepest, darkest Gorbals, while Sigal, in his novel *Zone of the Interior*, bases his character, Dr Willie Last, on Laing.[117] While Sigal changes Dr Last's home town to Dundee, he has all the characteristics associated with the Glasgow stereotype: working class, left-wing, hard drinking, and authentic. We learn that Last was inspired to study medicine by reading A.J. Cronin's novel *The Citadel* about a 'poor Scottish lad who becomes a rich society doctor'.[118] Sigal has Dr Last talk in a Scottish dialect, for example, he tells his patient, who is a fictional representation of the author:

> 'You've done this neat li'l trick on yirself'. Dr Last said. 'Internalised yir maw's fear an' hatred of you, treatin' yirself as yir maw treated ye. Ye're nae bein' so guid tae yir own li'l bairn, th'yew within yew. Take more pity on yirself, mon.'[119]

Now Laing did not speak like this, as films and audio recordings of him attest. Sigal has written a comic novel and was not striving for complete verisimilitude.

---

[116] Laing, *The Politics of Experience*, p. 146.

[117] Sigal, C. (2005). *Zone of the Interior*. Pomona Books, Hebden Bridge (first published in 1976).

[118] Ibid., p. 6.

[119] Ibid., p. 8.

However, he clearly intends for Dr Last's language to be perceived as amusing and for it to fulfil the task of rendering the character somewhat ridiculous, which is often the task that the appearance of dialect language in a novel, written in standard English, performs. In fairness, Laing was capable of playing the Glasgow stereotype, as the description of him as 'gallus' by one of his contemporaries indicates. Late in his life, he told Anthony Clare, when asked about his drinking: 'I'm not sure that I'm prepared to accept a type of heavy drinking, ageing Scotsman as a sort of character type.'[120] This remark reveals both that Laing was well aware of Scottish stereotypes, and that he felt he was able to choose whether or not to adopt them.

Against the argument about the essential Scottishness of R.D. Laing is the fact that a great deal of his reading and the work he cites in his books come from outside Scotland, and in particular from Europe. This supports the view that too much emphasis on the distinctiveness of Scottish culture neglects its links with the wider world and creates an excessively parochial vision. The term 'parochial' could never be applied to Laing, steeped as he was in Continental literature and Eastern religions. However, some might argue that an engagement with European thought is, itself, a feature of the Scottish cultural tradition, and one that distinguishes it from that of the supposedly insular and anti-intellectual English.[121] However, the effort to maintain what one critic has called 'Caledonian pure breeding' risks extending the definition of what counts as Scottish to be so all-encompassing as to be rendered meaningless.[122] Thus the answer to the question, 'How Scottish was R.D. Laing?' is not a simple one. He was well versed in Continental philosophy, which was the main inspiration for *The Divided Self*, but he can also be located in a Scottish literary and philosophical tradition. The emphasis he put on his Scottishness fluctuated throughout his career, and there was an interplay between how others felt Scottish people should behave, and Laing's adoption of the 'gallus' Glaswegian persona.

Laing's influence on Scottish culture

In his book, *From Trocchi to Trainspotting*, Michael Gardiner portrays Laing's work as dealing with the same issues as that of Muriel Spark, James Kelman, Alasdair Gray, Janice Galloway, and, of course, Alexander Trocchi.[123] Laing was to meet Trocchi, who shared his interest in Breton and Artaud. Trocchi was a Glaswegian writer whose 1950s novel, *Young Adam*, is often described as Camus's *Outsider,* relocated to Glasgow. What, though, of Laing's influence on Scottish culture? Judging by how often his name and his ideas appear in Scottish literature, his influence has been sizeable.

---

[120] Clare, *In the Psychiatrist's Chair*, p. 114.

[121] See Miller, G. (2009). 'Scotland's authentic plurality: The New Essentialism in Scottish studies'. *Scottish Literary Review*, **1/1**, 157–74. Miller provides a comprehensive account of the current debate about whether Scottish culture is 'essentialist' or 'pluralist'.

[122] Hayward, R. (2007). 'Recovering R.D. Laing'. *Metascience*, **16**, 525–7.

[123] Gardiner, M. (2006). *From Trocchi to Trainspotting. Scottish Critical Theory since 1960.* Edinburgh University Press, Edinburgh.

The Glasgow poet, Tom Leonard, who knew Laing, was an admirer of *The Divided Self*, which he reveals had a liberating effect on him and his writing.[124] He sees it as part of a tradition that includes Kierkegaard's *Either/Or*, Beckett's novels, Sartre's *Nauseau*, Robbe-Grillet, and Gabriel Marcel's *Being and Having*. Leonard, whose own work has wittily portrayed how non-standard English is perceived, is particularly interested in what Laing has to say about language. He contends that Laing had examined the nature of the complicity in relationships within institutional structures. He had shown how the mad person could be viewed as 'other', because their language was deemed invalid. Leonard sees parallels between Laing's account of the negation of the voice of the mad with the way non-standard English is portrayed in imaginative literature. Just as schizophrenic language is perceived by the doctor and the relatives of the patient as inferior, so the perception of dialect language in literature is regarded as a sign that the character employing it is second-rate. When the dialect speaker appears in a narrative, Leonard maintains, there is a conspiracy between the writer and the reader to view the speaker as 'other'. They are not considered to be on the same footing as the author or reader. Laing had shown that language could be used to invalidate others, whether it was the mentally ill or, indeed, anyone who did not 'speak the right language'. All were denied their full existence.

There are a host of other Scottish writers where the influence of Laing can be discerned. Alasdair Gray has spoken of the influence of Laing on his work, and Miller has performed a Laingian analysis of his writing, particularly focusing on the novel, *Lanark*.[125] William MacIlvanney's Laidlaw is an existentialist detective who keeps the works of continental philosophy in his desk at work. In his fictional account of his mental breakdown, *In the Middle of the Wood*, Iain Crichton Smith, who has spoken of himself as a 'double man', has the main character, Ralph refer to Laing.[126] Prior to his admission to a psychiatric hospital, Ralph, feels he knows about mental illness because he has read the work of the Scottish psychiatrist. John Burnside, who has had psychotic episodes requiring hospital admission, takes a distinctively Laingian view of madness, seeing it as a visionary experience, superior to the grey mundaniety of 'normal' society. His two volumes of autobiography, *A Lie about My Father* and *Waking Up in Toytown* explore this view. In *The Trick is to Keep Breathing*, Janice Galloway depicts the depressive breakdown of woman called Joy, in existential terms. After the death of her lover, she cannot find anyone to acknowledge her existence. In his novel, *Surviving*, about a group of alcoholics, Allan Massie, himself a recovered alcoholic, has a character read Laing and declare: 'Laing was only half a charlatan, the other half genius'.[127] In *The Book of Scotlands*, the musician and writer, Momus imagines: 'The Scotland in which every schoolchild can recite, by heart, the table talk of R.D. Laing.'[128] Divided selves are portrayed in: Alasdair Gray's short story *The Spread*

[124] Mullan, *Creative Destroyer*, pp. 89–91.

[125] Miller, G. (2005). *Alasdair Gray. The Fiction of Communion*. Rodopi, Amsterdam.

[126] Crichton Smith, I. (1987). *In the Middle of the Wood*. Victor Gollancz, London.

[127] Massie, A. (2009). *Surviving*. An Rubha, Vagabond Voices, p. 93.

[128] Momus (2010). *The Book of Scotlands*. Sternberg Press (place of publication not given), p. 47.

of Ian Nicol and his novel *Poor Things*; Brain McCabe's *The Real McCoy*; Irvine Welsh's *Filth*; James Robertson's *The Fanatic* and *The Ordeal of Gideon Mack*; and Angus MacAllister's *The Canongate Strangler*. 'Divided Selves' is also the title of a recent survey of the Scottish self-portrait, which takes its inspiration from Laing and devotes a chapter to him.[129]

Aftermath

After the publication of *The Divided Self*, Laing wrote *The Self and Others*, which appeared in 1961 and endeavoured to extend the discussion from the individual to their relationships with other people. It again featured patients Laing had seen in Glasgow and in the Army. Like *The Divided Self*, it drew on existential phenomenology, but Laing was clearly interested in other matters and *The Self and Others* also contains an attempt to describe human communication in terms of mathematics. His subsequent books are marked by this restless engagement with diverse systems of thought, ranging from the 'double bind' theory of family communication to notions of 're-birthing', via psychoanalysis, Sartrean dialectical reason, and Eastern religion. Some critics have pointed to the irreconcilability of the models that Laing later adopted.[130] It could be argued that the existential position Laing adopted in *The Divided Self* left him nowhere to go. After all, existentialism argues against systems. One should not impose an abstract theory on a patient's lived experience. By doing so one denies the person's full humanity and turns him into an object. John Macmurray had predicted Laing's dilemma. In *The Self as Agent*, he had observed:

> The existentialists, determined to grapple with the real problems—and their sensitiveness to the darkness of human despair leads them to discover the emergent problem of our time—find no formal analysis that is adequate to the task. They are constrained to quit the beaten track; to wallow in metaphor and suggestion; to look to drama and the novel to provide an expression, albeit an aesthetic expression, for their discoveries.[131]

As we know, Laing increasingly turned to literature, especially poetry, to express himself. In their book *Chronic Schizophrenia*, Laing's old colleagues, Freeman, Cameron, and McGhie had discussed the need to have a theory, but also the problems it presented:

> . . . an observer must have some theoretical framework by means of which he can order his clinical observations. With it he is subject to a certain bias; without it he is overwhelmed by a meaningless mass of clinical data . . . If we assume that the independent observer believes that there is a meaning in what confronts him, then we are faced with a new problem. This arises from the fact that several psychopathological systems vie with one another in explanation of clinical phenomena. One clinical observation can be interpreted in many different ways.[132]

[129] Hare, B. and Bielecka, P. (eds) (2006). *Divided Selves. The Scottish Self-Portrait from the 17th Century to the Present*. The Fleming-Wyfold Art Foundation, London.

[130] Siegler, M., Osmond, H. and Mann, H. (1972). 'Laing's models of madness'. In Boyers, R. and Orrill, R. (eds), *Laing and Anti-Psychiatry*. Penguin Books, London, pp. 99–122.

[131] Macmurray, J. (1957). *The Self as Agent*. Faber & Faber, London, pp. 27–8.

[132] Freeman, T., Cameron, J.L. and McGhie, A. (1958). *Chronic Schizophrenia*. Tavistock, London, p. 5.

This again describes something of the dilemma Laing faced: how to understand and make sense of the patient without a theoretical framework. If one decides that theory is important, there are several, competing systems of explanation on offer. Looking back at his work, Laing admitted that, although he had tried to be 'scientific', he could never find a method of investigating human passion and relationships that satisfied the rigours of 'hard scientific objectivity'.[133] However, he did not think that such aspects of the human experience should be ignored or that they were unimportant. When he tried to be 'scientific' in *The Self and Others* with the use mathematical models to describe interpersonal interaction, it was not particularly successful. Peter Lomas perceptively commented:

> There is a dilemma in that all descriptions of human behaviour that depart from ordinary language are in danger of leading us into the very kind of arid, atomistic, mechanistic world which the existentialists are so anxious to avoid.[134]

Kotowicz agrees.[135] He was sceptical about the mathematical notations of *The Self and Others*, and, like Lomas, thought that it was as estranging as the psychiatric language that Laing had criticized in his first book. He noted that in *The Divided Self*, Laing was aiming to create a 'science of persons', and that in subsequent works he constantly adopted a new method to attain this. In later years, Laing admitted that there was no Laingian School, though, after his death, one of his followers, Anthony Lunt attempted to describe the core principles.[136] Another colleague, M. Guy Thompson has argued that Laing really behaved as a psychoanalyst, both in his outlook and clinical approach. Although he upturned many of its conventions, he was still guided by the tenets of psychoanalysis.[137] Thompson has attempted to reconcile the twin strands of existential and analytic thought in Laing's work. He maintains that Laing's conception of psychoanalysis rested on two fundamental principles, which could be seen as common to both analytic and existential schools of thought: all human knowledge is rooted in human experience; and the weight of experience is so painful that people seek to avoid it by self-deception.

However, Scott Bortle has argued that the unsystematic nature of Laing's ideas is actually their strength.[138] Bortle sees Laing as a 'negative thinker', who was sceptical of all-encompassing explanatory theories or 'grand narratives', such as Marxism or Freudianism. Laing's existential-phenomenology was a *method* of enquiry, not a closed philosophical system that sought to account for every aspect of the world. In fact,

---

[133] MS Laing A662.

[134] Lomas, P. (1968). 'Psychoanalysis–Freudian or existential'. In Rycroft, C. (ed.) *Psychoanalysis Observed*. Pelican, London, p. 143.

[135] Kotowicz, *Laing and the Paths of Anti-Psychiatry*, pp. 40–1.

[136] Lunt, A. (1990). *Apollo Versus the Echomaker. A Laingian Approach to Psychotherapy, Dreams and Shamanism*. Element Books, Longmead. Mullan also discusses Laing's approach to therapy and the difficulty in giving a description of it, in Mullan, B. (1999). *R.D. Laing. A Personal View*. Duckworth, London, pp. 120–5.

[137] Thompson, M.G. (2000). 'The heart of the matter. R.D. Laing's enigmatic relationship with psychoanalysis'. *Psychoanalytic Review*, **87**, 483–509.

[138] Bortle, S. (2001). 'Laing as a negative thinker'. *Janus Head*, **4**, 130–58.

Bortle argues that Laing was being true to his phenomenological perspective by resisting the lure of reductionist theorizing. In a similar vein, Bracken has suggested that Laing's early exploration of phenomenology might have been responsible for leading him away from psychiatry and even challenging its very legitimacy.[139] Phenomenology opened up ways of understanding psychosis that were opposed to any 'technical ordering of experience'.

Laing's existential-phenomenological stance militated against constructing a formal system of psychotherapy, and he was left with the notion of clinical 'style'. This is by no means an unimportant quality, and, in fact, it goes to the heart of psychotherapy. His colleague, John Heaton has written about Laing's style:

> What struck me on first meeting Ronnie was his style; he stood out from most people because of his unique way of being. This was not a matter of the way he dressed, the music he liked, his conversation, his looks, and his rather dry and sometimes cruel humour; rather, his style conveyed something of great importance. It was crucial in his psychotherapy, and one of the things he can teach us is the vitality of style in the practice of psychotherapy and counselling.[140]

Laing was sceptical of formal techniques in psychotherapy, and, in this, Heaton feels he was ahead of his time, as research has subsequently shown that the crucial ingredient in therapy is not the particular school to which the therapist belongs, but rather their personality and ability to form a relationship with the patient. John Macquarrie had observed that existentialism did not provide a system of philosophy, but rather an *attitude*. This would seem to fit with Laing's approach, which was concerned with the human encounter, not with rigidly following the instructions of a textbook of psychotherapy. Laing was later to give a definition of psychotherapy: 'Essentially psychotherapy is an authentic meeting between human beings.'[141]

Fame

This book covers the period *before* Laing became famous, a development that arguably sent him off the rails. His colleague, James Hood noticed a great change in Laing following the publication of *The Divided Self*:

> The R.D.L. I perceived then was visibly and in his predominant mood very different from the Ronald whose company I had enjoyed . . . during my visits to London prior to 1959, when I moved south from Glasgow. Then he had been relaxed, cheerful, appropriately sensitive or celebratory, and in full command of his personal resources.[142]

His good friend John Duffy also noted that Laing changed as he grew older. He recalls: 'When we were younger he was always different—he was outstanding . . . He was a lovely gentle, and caring person. What saddened me most of all—was that he

---

[139] Bracken, P.J. (1999). 'Phenomenology and psychiatry'. *Current Opinion in Psychiatry*, **12**, 593–6.

[140] Heaton, J. (2000). 'On R.D. Laing: style, sorcery, alienation'. *The Psychoanalytic Review*, **87**, 511–26.

[141] Mullan, B. (1997). *R.D. Laing. Creative Destroyer.* Cassell, London, p. 279.

[142] Hood, *The Young R.D. Laing*, p. 50.

became a bit of a bastard'.[143] In a revealing interview with Peter Mezan in 1976, Laing discussed fame:

> Fame is 'that last infirmity of noble mind', he [Laing] quoted from Milton's *Lycidas*, and for few minutes he was silent. I suppose what that means is that fame is the last thing seducing the noble mind into pursuing worldly aims rather than recognizing its true ones, which are unworldly—the last symptom of the mind's disease . . . When it comes to fame, it become spiritualised somehow. There's a spiritual narcissism—one wants to be higher up the spiritual hierarchy, a bit nearer to the centre of the cosmic real estate. One wants at least to be among the cherubim or seraphim, or near the throne itself, sitting at the right hand of the Father, or the Father himself, omnipotent, omniscient, and so on. I remember Sartre used to say in the old days that man's aim, his impossible passion, was to be God. Perhaps fame is the subtlest form of that.[144]

As we have seen, from an early age Laing had set himself the goal of becoming famous. He admitted looking at the *Oxford Dictionary of National Biography* and comparing who fared best in terms of status accorded. Burston has suggested that Laing's drive for intellectual success was a means of making up for the unconditional love he felt he was never given as a child. He was torn between 'his craving for success and his humanistic values, between his public and private selves'.[145] Peter Lomas felt that Laing's 'narcissistic drive to become famous at all costs' was ultimately his undoing.[146] Laing not only had to cope with fame, but he had to cope with the loss of it. It must have been difficult for Laing that his first book, written in his late 20s and early 30s, was considered his best, and that his later work attracted increasingly negative reviews. In addition, the personal problems that Laing alluded to in his early notebooks, his tendency to melancholy and excessive drinking, became very much worse in middle age.

The outsider

Ingleby[147] sees Laing's relationship to the psychiatric profession as that of an outsider, who deliberately sought out other, marginalized people. Alasdair Gray feels that Laing extended a great tolerance to the mad, but was intolerant of the sane.[148] Kotowicz[149] has observed that Laing's work presented an unpalatable dilemma: choosing a grey constricting 'normality', or the wretchedness of madness. Laing never resolved this dilemma. Kirsner maintains that Laing was essentially a Romantic: he believed that

---

[143] Mullan, *Creative Destroyer*, p. 100.

[144] Mezan, P. (1976). 'Portrait of a twentieth-century sceptic by Peter Mezan'. In Evans, R.I. (ed.), *R.D. Laing. The Man and his Ideas*. E.P. Dutton & Co., New York, pp. xxii–lxxv.

[145] Burston, D. (1996). *The Wing of Madness*. Harvard University Press, Cambridge, Massachusetts, p. 19.

[146] Mullan, *Creative Destroyer,* p. 19.

[147] Ingleby, D. (1998). 'The view from the North Sea'. In Gijswijt-Hofstra, M. and Porter, R. (eds), *Cultures of Psychiatry and Mental Health Care in Postwar Britain and the Netherlands*. Rodopi, Amsterdam, pp. 295–314.

[148] Interview with Alasdair Gray, *In the Footsteps of R.D. Laing*. Radio Scotland, 2009.

[149] Kotowicz, *Laing and the Paths of Anti-Psychiatry*, p. 116.

people were basically good and that it was only an oppressive social system that made them bad or mad.[150] He compares Laing to Jean-Jacques Rousseau, who had hailed the natural goodness of the 'noble savage', uncorrupted by civilization. Mischler has called Laing a 'survivor poet', a term he borrowed from Stephen Spender to describe those who saw themselves as survivors of an already destroyed civilization, to whose demise they bore testimony.[151] Laing's old colleague Karl Abenheimer[152] had observed: 'Like so many champions of the misunderstood, the despised and the unprivileged, [Laing] is inclined to turn the tables completely'. Abenheimer felt that Laing had moved from a position of compassionate regard for the mentally ill to one where they were seen as existing in a superior realm to that of the merely sane. Jenni Diski, who herself suffered from psychiatric problems and encountered Laing in the 1960s, has written that he portrayed the mad person as a type of hero:

> The mad—the word became a banner of resistance—were outcast, prophets, speakers of unspeakable truths, and were pronounced heroes. Pushed by malign normality, the mad, on behalf of those of us who hadn't the courage, took a journey to the furthest depths of the human psyche to look at what was really there, and who we really were. They trod the lonely hero's journey . . . beyond the boundaries of society to places most of us dared not go, and they returned changed but with news of the truth they had found and brought back for us if we would just pay proper attention.[153]

A colleague, the psychiatrist Joseph Berke, thought Laing saw patients as 'a sort of emotional proletariat', fighting to survive an unjust family or society, but that he tended to 'idealise' the mad and to ignore the very real difficulties their behaviour could cause others.[154] Further, he ignored the emotional damage his patients wrought on *him*. This last point is important, and Laing, in a late interview with Anthony Clare, conceded that he had difficulty in protecting himself from the enormous demands and pressures of the clinical encounter. He observed: 'I haven't been able to do what a lot of doctors are able to do . . . which is to keep their sensitivity within a fairly formally ordered frame of conduct. I get tossed and turned.'[155]

Concluding remarks

In standard accounts of the development of modern psychiatry, Laing, if he is mentioned at all, is allotted a small role. He is seen as a part of the 'anti-psychiatry' movement of the 1960s, though he, himself, objected to the term. His ideas about schizophrenia are regarded as erroneous, and now disproved by the findings of the neurosciences

[150] Kirsner, *Laing and Philosophy*.
[151] Mischler, E.G. (1973). 'Man, morality, and madness: Critical perspectives on the work of R.D. Laing'. In Rubinstein, B.B. (ed.), *Psychoanalysis and Contemporary Science*, Vol 2. Macmillan, New York, pp. 369–94.
[152] Quoted in Calder, R. (1988). 'Abenheimer and Laing–some notes'. *Edinburgh Review*, **78–9**, 108–16.
[153] Diski, J. (2010). *The Sixties*. Profile Books, London, pp. 127–8.
[154] Berke, J. (1990). 'R.D. Laing'. *British Journal of Psychotherapy*, **7**, 175–7.
[155] Clare, *In the Psychiatrist's Chair*, p. 209.

and genetics. His exploration of the connection between disturbed family communication and schizophrenia is viewed, at best, as misguided, and, at worst, as serving to scapegoat parents, already severely stressed by having a mentally ill child. However, despite the great advances in the field, many commentators contend that the neurosciences do not fully explain psychiatric illness. As Broome and Borlotti have noted, the end of the 'decade of the brain' in the 1990s paradoxically led to a realization that social factors play an important part in the aetiology of mental illness.[156] On philosophical grounds, Ratcliffe argues that neurobiological approaches can only ever offer a limited account of psychiatric disorders; they cannot tell us what it is like to experience mental distress.[157] Psychiatric conditions that involve alternations in the sense of reality, he maintains, require a 'phenomenological stance' and he draws on Laing's *The Divided Self*, as well as other works, to examine existential changes that occur in mental illness.

The psychologist Richard Bentall has examined Laing's work in the light of contemporary research and finds support for some of his ideas, for example, his contention that psychotic patients make more sense than psychiatrists often allow.[158] Bentall quotes research which finds that, generally, schizophrenic patients are quite clear in their speech, but, if they are upset, then emotional-laden ideas intermingle with their normal communication, making comprehension difficult. Bentall also finds support for Laing's contention that sanity and insanity are on a spectrum, rather than there being a sharp division between the two. He approves of Laing's criticism of the Kraepelinian diagnostic model: that it reflects the social relations inherent in the psychiatric interview rather than representing the objective description of mental 'pathology' in the patient. Bentall reports that there is some evidence that dysfunctional parents may contribute to the development of psychosis in their offspring. Research, he reveals, has also found a link between psychosis and creativity, but Bentall feels that Laing overly romanticized the positive aspects of madness, which is more often a terrible blight than a blessing. He concludes that Laing's greatest contribution was to make people 'change their point of reference in order to see the world from the viewpoint of the patient defined as psychotic'.

Commentators from within the psychiatric establishment, such as Anthony Clare and Digby Tantam, while considering his views on schizophrenia entirely redundant, nevertheless grant Laing a prime place in highlighting the plight of the mentally ill and persuading the wider society to recognize the essential humanity of psychiatric patients. Clare wrote:

> Yet the fact remains that this complicated, contradictory, agonised and spiritually tortured man exacted a formidable effect on British and on world psychiatry. He dragged

---

[156] Broome, M.R. and Borlotti (eds) (2009). *Psychiatry as Cognitive Neuroscience. Philosophical Perspectives*. Oxford University Press, Oxford.

[157] Ratcliffe, M. (2009). 'Understanding existential changes in psychiatric illness: the indispensability of phenomenology'. In Broome, M.R. and Borlotti (eds), *Psychiatry as Cognitive Neuroscience. Philosophical Perspectives*. Oxford University Press, Oxford, pp. 223–45; see also Ratcliffe, M. (2008). *Feelings of Being. Phenomenology, Psychiatry and the Sense of Reality*. Oxford University Press, Oxford.

[158] Bentall, R.P. (2005). 'R.D. Laing: An appraisal in the light of recent research'. In Raschid, S. (ed.) *R.D. Laing. Contemporary Perspectives*. Free Association Books, London, pp. 222–45.

psychiatric illness and those who suffered from it right on to the front cover of newspapers and magazines where they have remained ever since and he gave the most powerful and eloquent of voices to those who until then had been mute in their isolation.[159]

Tantam agreed: 'For all Laing's faults, he had the fierce determination that psychosis mattered, and for a while, persuaded other people that it did. For that we should honour him.'[160]

To follow Laing's early career is to embark on an intellectual roller-coaster, taking in a bewildering number of cultural, literary, and philosophical works. One cannot fail to be impressed by the sheer breadth of his reading and his range of interests. The early Laing was an attractive figure, curious, driven, astute, and possessed of wit and charm. The records of his clinical encounters reveal a young doctor who was highly serious about his work, going to great lengths to try and understand his patients. Laing's notes also illuminate the mid-twentieth century world of psychiatry and reveal an exciting time of change, when the role of large mental institutions was being challenged, social theories of madness were being advanced, and new medication was being introduced. Laing's clinical notes also allow us to meet many of the psychiatric patients of the era and to hear their voice.

While Laing has not left a school of psychotherapy that bears his name, and while some of his ideas about the nature and origins of psychosis have been discounted, many of his preoccupations are now part of the mainstream, and it is to here that we should look for evidence of his legacy. Thus Laing's immersion in philosophy finds an echo in today's proliferation of books, papers, and conferences on philosophy and phenomenology. This has been fuelled by the belief that biological psychiatry does not provide all the answers, and that we have to critically examine its assumptions and claims about what it is to be human. Laing's interest in the arts finds its modern day equivalent in the rise of the medical humanities, which holds that the arts can inform and improve clinical practice. We have also seen the emergence of narrative-based medicine with its contention that, as well as relating their symptoms, patients are also telling a unique story about their predicament. Laing's anguished engagement with religious questions finds its present-day heirs amongst the many who feel that there is a spiritual dimension to madness that cannot be ignored. Most importantly, Laing's burning interest in the patient as a person, as a fellow human being whose utterances should be listened to attentively, rather than dismissed as nonsensical babble, has had a major impact on the attitudes of society to the mentally ill, and his work has been seen as a key element in igniting the user movement of today.[161]

---

[159] Clare, A. (1997). 'Anthony Clare'. In Mullan, B. (ed.) *R.D. Laing. Creative Destroyer*. Cassell, London, pp. 1–3.

[160] Tantam, D. (1999). 'R.D. Laing and anti-psychiatry'. In Freeman, H. (ed.). *A Century of Psychiatry*, Mosby, London, pp. 202–7.

[161] Crossley, .N (1998). 'R.D. Laing and the British anti-psychiatry movement: a socio-historical analysis'. *Social Science and Medicine*, **47**, 877–89.

References

Primary sources

Glasgow University Archive. DC81. Ferguson Rodger 295. *The impact of existential philosophy on psychology by* J. Schorstein.

Glasgow University Archive. DC81. Ferguson Rodger 450–2. W.R. Bion: *Experiences in Groups Parts* 1–3.

Glasgow University Library Special Collections. Laing's personal library.

Glasgow University Library Special Collections. Laing's personal library. 14. *The Divided Self.*

Glasgow University Library Special Collections. Laing's personal library. 351. Joyce, J. (1942). *Portrait of the Artist as a Young Man.* Jonathan Cape, London.

Glasgow University Library Special Collection. Laing's personal library. 621. Canetti, E. (1946). *Auto Da Fe.* (trans. Wedgwood, C.V.) Jonathan Cape, London.

Glasgow University Library Special Collection. Laing's personal library. 646. Macleod, G. (1958). *Only One Way Left.* Iona Community, Glasgow.

Glasgow University Library Special Collections. Laing's personal library. 1448. Hart, B. (1946). *The Psychology of Insanity.* Cambridge University Press, Cambridge.

Glasgow University Library Special Collections. Laing's personal library. 1892–1894. Whitten, W. (ed.) (1924–1925). *The World's Library of Best Books.* G. Newnes, London.

Glasgow University Library Special Collections. Laing's personal library. 1902. Gardner, H.M. (ed.) (1948). *Poems of Gerard Manley Hopkins.* Oxford University Press, London.

Greater Glasgow Health Board Archive HB74/1/1. Professor Stanley Alstead interviewed by Dr McKenzie.

MS Laing A64. R.D. Laing. Health and happiness, student essay prize Glasgow University, 1948.

MS Laing A112. R.D. Laing. An Examination of Tillich's Theory of Anxiety and Neurosis (1954).

MS Laing A112. Letter from J.D. Sutherland to Laing, 15 July 1954.

MS Laing A113. R.D. Laing (1954). Reflections on the Ontology of Human Relations.

MS Laing A114. R.D. Laing. Review of *The Undiscovered Self* by C.G. Jung, *Journal of Analytical Psychology* (1959).

MS Laing A116–7 R.D. Laing (1960). The Development of Existential Analysis. A paper submitted to RMPA, December 1960.

MS Laing A150/1–2. Cameron, J.L., Laing, R.D. and McGhie, A. Chronic Schizophrenic Patients and their Nurses: A Study in the Essentials of Environment. Glasgow, 1955.

MS Laing A153. R.D. Laing. The Rumpus Room, 1954–1955, Glasgow, 1956.

MS Laing A154. R.D. Laing. Notes for a lecture at Trinity, Dublin, 1955.

MS Laing A230. R.D. Laing. A critique of Binswanger's 'Ellen West'.

MS Laing A233. R.D. Laing. Draft entitled 'Love and Nihilism'.

MS Laing A229/A. R.D. Laing. The Case of Ellen West.

MS Laing A258. R.D. Laing. Dilthey.

MS Laing A258. R.D. Laing: Notes and drafts on Eugene Minkowski, c. 1960.

MS Laing A260. R.D. Laing. Notes on depression and mania, c. 1960.

MS Laing A343. R.D. Laing. A Diary: A Personal Journey: Conception to Birth.

MS Laing A408. R.D. Laing. Draft of an article entitled 'Philosophy and Medical Psychology' (1948).

MS Laing A410. R.D. Laing: Analytical notes on the poetry of Gerard Manley Hopkins. 21.5.54.

MS Laing A505. R.D. Laing. Draft entitled 'Glasgow past and present. a personal memoir'. London, November 29, 1976.

MS Laing 511/2. R.D. Laing. Drafts of a review for the New Scientist of 'Psychoanalysis and beyond' by Charles Rycroft, 1985.

MS Laing A514/1. R.D. Laing. Galley proofs of article for the *Times Literary Supplement* entitled 'God and DSM III'.

MS Laing A518. Lieutenant Murray Brookes and Captain Ronald D. Laing. On the Recognition of Simulated and Functional Deafness. Unpublished manuscript.

MS Laing A519. R.D. Laing. Draft entitled 'Impressions of a second-year medical student': a paper delivered to the Glasgow University Medico-Chirurgical Society, January 1947.

MS Laing A522. R.D. Laing. Draft entitled 'Autobiographical sketches'. London. November 1977.

MS Laing A531/2. R.D. Laing. *Biographical notes on Joe Schorstein*. London, 11–13 December 1978.

MS Laing A535. Cameron, J.L., Laing, R.D. and McGhie, A. (1955). Patient and Nurse. Effects of Environmental Changes in the Care of Chronic Schizophrenics. *The Lancet*, 1384–6. Offprint with manuscript.

MS Laing A580 (i). C.G. Jung (1906). *The Psychology of Dementia Praecox* (trans. Brill, A.A., 1936). Nervous and Mental Disease Publishing Company, USA.

MS Laing A590/1. R.D. Laing. Draft of 'The Divided Self'.

MS Laing A617. Proposal for Active Treatment Unit for Deteriorating Psychotics.

MS Laing A662. R.D. Laing. Draft notes.

MS Laing A685. R.D. Laing. Draft notes, 1950–61.

MS Laing A689. R.D. Laing. Handwritten extracts.

MS Laing A694. R.D. Laing. Typed and handwritten extracts.

MS Laing A708. R.D. Laing. Handwritten notes on Jung.

MS Laing A713. R.D. Laing. A Critique of Binswanger's Ellen West.

MS Laing B33. Letter from Laing to Victor Gollancz, 3 September 1959.

MS Laing B43. Letter from Laing to Dr Winnicott, 30 May 1958.

MS Laing B44. Letter from Dr Winnicott to Laing, 28 July 1958.

MS Laing B45. Letter from Ferguson Rodger to Laing, 30 June 1958.

MS Laing B46. Letter from Henry Chalk to Laing, 9 September 1958.

MS Laing B47. Letter from Karl Abenheimer to Laing, 10 September 1958.

MS Laing B48. Letter from Karl Abenheimer to Laing, 15 September 1958.

MS Laing B49–50. Letters between Laing and patient.

MS Laing B53. Reader's report on *The Divided Self*.

MS Laing B54. Reader's report on *The Divided Self*.

MS Laing DA23. Patient transcript.

MS Laing DB22. R.D. Laing. Patient notes.

MS Laing DB85. R.D. Laing. Patient notes.

MS Laing DB86. R.D. Laing. Patient notes.

MS Laing DB87. R.D. Laing. Patient notes.

MS Laing DD31. R.D. Laing. Patient notes.

MS Laing DE5. Letter from patient's mother to Laing.

MS Laing DF66. Parents' Group, 1955–1956.

MS Laing DF67. R.D. Laing's Tuesday group, 1957–1959.

MS Laing DF69. R.D. Laing. Patient notes.

MS Laing DF70. Patient's letters to Laing.

MS Laing DG53. Clinical notes by R.D. Laing, 1953–1954.

MS Laing DG57. R.D. Laing. Some comments on 'The Mental Hospital'.

MS Laing DG57. R.D. Laing. Doctor–Nurse–Patient Relations, 1954–1955.

MS Laing DG63. Staff Problem Discussion Group at Gartnavel, 1954–1955.

MS Laing DG64. L.E. 6 Dayroom.

MS Laing DH 67. Letter about patient to Laing.

MS Laing DJ27. Psychiatric report on patient.

MS Laing DL36. R.D. Laing. Patient report.

MS Laing DM41. R.D. Laing. Patient report.

MS Laing DM101. R.D. Laing. Patient notes.

MS Laing DM102. R.D. Laing. Patient notes.

MS Laing DM103. R.D. Laing. Patient notes.

MS Laing DN3. R.D. Laing. Patient notes.

MS Laing DR13. Patient letter to Laing.

MS Laing DS90. Ministers' Group, 1956.

MS Laing DS91. R.D. Laing. Clinical notes. Southern General Hospital, 1955–1956.

MS Laing DS92. R.D. Laing. Patient notes.

MS Laing GD42/20. Letter from Ferguson Rodger to Laing, 4 June 1960.

MS Laing GD42/50. Letter from Laing to S.A. Barnett, Zoology Department, University of Glasgow, 7 September 1960.

MS Laing K1. R.D. Laing. Elements for an Autobiography. 29 July 1968.

MS Laing K4. R.D. Laing. Autobiographical notes, c. 1970.

MS Laing K12. R.D. Laing. Notebook, 1951–1952.

MS Laing K13. R.D. Laing: Notebook, 1951–1960.

MS Laing K14. R.D. Laing. Notebook and diary covering Laing's stay at the military hospitals at Netley and Catterick, January 1952 to June 1953.

MS Laing K15. R.D. Laing. Notebook begun 12 March 1953.

MS Laing K16. R.D. Laing. Notebook, July 1953 to August 1962.

MS Laing K45. R.D. Laing. Reflections on his medical training and the Psychiatric Unit, Stobhill Hospital, Glasgow, c. 1970.

MS Laing R34. University of Glasgow, Faculty of Medicine. Certificate on Laing.

Secondary sources

Abrahamson, D. (2007). 'R.D. Laing and long-stay patients: discrepant accounts of the refractory ward and 'rumpus room' at Gartnavel Royal Hospital'. *History of Psychiatry*, **18**, 203–15.

Ackerknecht, E.H. (1967). 'A plea for a "Behaviourist" approach in writing the history of medicine'. *Journal of the History of Medicine and Allied Sciences*, **22**, 211–14.

Ackroyd, P. (1995). *Blake.* Sinclair-Stevenson, London.

A.C.M. (1983). 'Obituary of J L Halliday'. *British Medical Journal*, **28**, 697.

Anderson, B. (2006). *Imagined Communities. Reflections on the Origin and Spread of Nationalism* (revised edn). Verso, London.

Anderson, R. (1983). *Education and Opportunity in Victorian Scotland.* Edinburgh University Press, Edinburgh.

Andrews, J. (1998). 'R.D. Laing in Scotland: facts and fictions of the 'Rumpus Room' and interpersonal psychiatry'. In Gijswijt-Hofstra, M. and Porter, R. (eds), *Culture of Psychiatry and Mental Health Care in Postwar Britain and the Netherlands.* Rodopi, Amsterdam, pp. 121–50.

Andrews, J. and Smith, I. (1993). *'Let there be light again'. A History of Gartnavel Royal Hospital from its Beginnings to the Present Day.* Gartnavel Royal Hospital Press, Glasgow.

Anon (1947). *The Philosophy of Insanity. By a Late Inmate of the Glasgow Royal Asylum for Lunatics at Gartnavel.* With an introduction by Frieda Fromm-Reichmann M.D. The Fireside Press, London and New York.

Anon (2000). *The Story of a Community. Dingleton Hospital Melrose.* Chiefswood Publications, Melrose.

Appignanesi, L. (2008). *Mad, Bad and Sad. A History of Women and the Mind Doctors from 1800 to the Present.* Virago, London.

Arieti, S. (1955). *Interpretation of Schizophrenia.* Robert Brunner, New York.

Askay, R. (2001). 'Heidegger's philosophy and its implications for psychology, Freud, and existential psychoanalysis'. In Heidegger, M. (2001). *Zollikon Seminars. Protocols, Conversations, Letters.* (Boss, M. ed.) (trans. Mayr, F. and Askay, R.), Northwestern University Press, Evanston, Illinois, pp. 301–16.

Bakhtin, M. (1984). *Problems of Dostoyevsky's Poetics.* Manchester University Press, Manchester.

Batchelor, I. (1958). 'Schizophrenia—a psychotherapeutic approach'. In Ferguson Roger, T., Mowbray, R.M. and Roy, J.R. (eds), *Topics in Psychiatry.* Cassell, London, pp. 57–64.

Bateson, G., Jackson, D.D., Haley, J. and Weakland, J. (1956). 'Towards a theory of schizophrenia'. *Behavioural Science*, **1**, 251–64.

Behler, E. (1996). 'Nietzsche in the twentieth century'. In Magnus, B. and Higgins, K.M. (eds), *The Cambridge Companion to Nietzsche.* Cambridge University Press, Cambridge, pp. 281–322.

Bennett, M.R. and Hacker, P.M.S. (2003). *Philosophical Foundations of Neuroscience.* Blackwell, Oxford.

Bentall, R. (1992). 'A proposal to classify happiness as a psychiatric disorder'. *Journal of Medical Ethics*, **18**, 94–8.

Bentall, R.P. (2005). 'R.D. Laing: An appraisal in the light of recent research'. In Raschid, S. (ed.) *R.D. Laing. Contemporary Perspectives.* Free Association Books, London, pp. 222–45.

Berke, J. (1990). 'R.D. Laing'. *British Journal of Psychotherapy*, **7**, 175–7.

Berkenkotter, C. (2008). *Patient Tales. Case Histories and the Uses of Narrative in Psychiatry.* The University of South Carolina Press, South Carolina.

Berrios, G. (1987). '1911. Eugen Bleuler. The fundamental symptoms in dementia praecox or the group of schizophrenias'. In Thompson, C. (ed.) *The Origins of Modern Psychiatry.* John Wiley & sons, Chichester, pp. 165–210.

Berrios, G.E. (1987). 'Historical aspects of psychoses: 19th century issues'. *British Medical Bulletin*, **43**, 484–98.

Berrios, G.E. (2000). 'Schizophrenia: a conceptual history'. In Gelder, M.G., Lopez-Ibor, J.J. and Andreasen, N. (eds) *New Oxford Textbook of Psychiatry. Vol 1*. Oxford University Press, Oxford, pp. 567–571.

Berrios, G.E. and Markova, I. (2003) 'The self and psychiatry: a conceptual history', In Kircher, T. and David, A. (eds), *The Self in Neuroscience and Psychiatry*. Cambridge University Press, Cambridge, pp. 9–39.

Beveridge, A. (1996). 'R.D. Laing Revisited'. *Psychiatric Bulletin*, **22**, 452–6.

Beveridge, A. (2009). 'The benefits of reading literature'. In Oyebode, F. (ed.), *Mindreadings. Literature and Psychiatry*. RCPsych Publications, London, pp. 1–14.

Beveridge, C. and Turnbull, R. (1989). *The Eclipse of Scottish Culture. Inferiorism and the Intellectuals*. Polygon, Edinburgh.

Beveridge, C. and Turnbull, R. (1997). *Scotland After Enlightenment. Image and Tradition in Modern Scottish Culture*. Polygon, Edinburgh.

Beveridge, C. and Turnbull, R. (1998). 'Introduction to Laing RD'. *Wisdom, Madness and Folly*. Canongate, Edinburgh (originally published in 1985).

Bortle, S. (2001). 'Laing as a negative thinker'. *Janus Head*, **4**, 130–58.

Boston, J.R. (1976). 'The Divided Self'. *The Guardian*, 3 August 1976.

Bracken, P.J. (1999). 'Phenomenology and psychiatry'. *Current Opinion in Psychiatry*, **12**, 593–6.

Bracken, P. and Thomas, P. (2005). *Postpsychiatry*. Oxford University Press, Oxford.

Brierley, M. (1961). 'Review of The Divided Self'. *International Journal of Psychoanalysis*, **42**, 228–9.

Brody, E.B. and Redlich, F.C. (eds) (1952). *Psychotherapy with Schizophrenics*. International Universities Press, New York.

Brody, E.B. (1952). 'The treatment of schizophrenia: a review'. In Brody, E.B. and Redlich, F.C. (eds), *Psychotherapy with Schizophrenic*. International Press, New York, pp. 39–88.

Broome, M.R. and Borlotti (eds) (2009). *Psychiatry as Cognitive Neuroscience. Philosophical Perspectives*. Oxford University Press, Oxford.

Brown, C. (1987). *The Social History of Religion in Scotland since 1730*. Methuen, London.

Brown, D. (2004). *Gerard Manley Hopkins*. Northcote House, Horndon.

Brown, J.A.C. (1964). *Freud and the Post-Freudians*. Penguin, Harmondsworth.

Bronowski, J. (1958). *William Blake. A Selection of Poems and Letters*. Penguin Books, London.

Bryce, T.G.K. and Humes, W.M. (2003) *Scottish Education: Post-devolution*. Edinburgh University Press, Edinburgh.

Bullock, A. and Woodings, R.B. (eds) (1983). *The New Fontana Dictionary of Modern Thought*. Fontana Press, London.

Burston, D. (1996). *The Wing of Madness*. Harvard University Press, Cambridge, Massachusetts.

Burston, D. (2000). *The Crucible of Experience. R.D. Laing and the Crisis of Psychotherapy*. Harvard University Press, Cambridge, Massachusetts.

Burston, D. and Frie, R. (2006). *Psychotherapy as a Human Science*. Duquesne University Press, Pittsburg.

Busfield, J. (1996). *Men, Women and Madness. Understanding Gender and Mental Disorder*. Macmillan Press, London.

Calder, R. (1978–1979). 'Abenheimer and Laing—some notes'. *Edinburgh Review*, **32**, 108–16.

Cameron, J.L., Laing, R.D. and McGhie, A. (1955). 'Patient and nurse. Effects of environmental changes in the care of chronic schizophrenics'. *The Lancet*, **266**, 1384–6.

Camus, A. (1960). *The Plague* (trans. Gilbert, S.). Penguin Books, London (originally published in French, 1947).

Carman, T. (2007). 'Authenticity', In Dreyfus, H.L. and Wrathall, M.A. (eds) *A Companion to Heidegger*. Blackwell Publishing, London, pp. 285–96.

Carruthers, G. (2009). *Scottish Literature*. Edinburgh University Press, Edinburgh.

Carthy, I. (2008). 'Book Review: Gavin Miller, R.D. Laing'. *History of Psychiatry*, 19(2), 237–9.

Charlesworth, M. (1976). *The Existentialists and Jean-Paul Sartre*. George Prior, London.

Chekhov, A. (2002). *Ward No. 6 and Other Stories, 1892–1895*. Penguin Books, London.

Clare, A. (1980). *Psychiatry in Dissent. Controversial Issues in Thought and Practice* (2nd edn). Tavistock, London.

Clare, A. (1985). 'Freud's cases: the clinical basis of psychoanalysis'. In Bynum, W.F., Porter, R. and Shepherd, M. (eds), *The Anatomy of Madness. Essays in the History of Madness*. Vol. 1, London: Tavistock Publications, pp. 271–88.

Clare, A. (1993). *In the Psychiatrist's Chair*, Mandarin, London.

Clare, A. (1997). 'Anthony Clare'. In Mullan, B. (ed.) *R.D. Laing. Creative Destroyer*. Cassell, London, pp. 1–3.

Clark, R.W. (1982). *Freud. The Man and the Cause*. Granada, Frogmore, St Albans.

Clay, J. (1996). *R.D. Laing. A Divided Self*. Hodder & Stoughton, London.

Cohen-Solal, A. (2005). *Jean-Paul Sartre. A Life*. The New Press, New York.

Collier, A. (1977). *R.D. Laing: The Philosophy and Politics of Psychotherapy*. The Harvester Press, Hassocks, Sussex.

Collins, K. (1985). 'Angus MacNiven and the Austrian psychoanalysts'. *Glasgow Medicine*, 2, 18–19.

Collins, K. (1998). *Go and Learn–the International Story of the Jews and Medicine in Scotland 1739–1945*. Aberdeen University Press, Aberdeen.

Collins, K. (2008). 'Joseph Schorstein: R.D. Laing's "rabbi"'. *History of Psychiatry*, 19 (2), 185–201.

Condrua, G. (1991). 'Obituary of Medard Boss'. *Journal of the Society for Existential Analysis*, 2, 60–1.

Cramond, W.A. (1958). 'Clinical experience of tranquillising drugs in the psychoses'. In Ferguson Roger, T., Mowbray, R.M. and Roy, J.R. (eds), *Topics in Psychiatry*. Cassell and Company, London, pp. 176–86.

Crews, F.C. (ed.) (1998). *Unauthorized Freud. Doubters Confront a Legend*. Viking Books, New York.

Crichton Smith, I. (1987). *In the Middle of the Wood*. Victor Gollancz, London.

Critchley, S. and Schroeder, W.R. (ed.) (1999). *A Companion to Continental Philosophy*. Blackwell Publishing, Oxford.

Crossley, N. (1998). 'R.D. Laing and the British anti-psychiatry movement: a socio-historical analysis.' *Social Science and Medicine*, 47, 877–89.

Cybulska, E.M. (2000). 'The madness of Nietzsche: a misdiagnosis of the millennium?' *Hospital Medicine*, 61, 571–5.

Davie, G.E. (1961). *The Democratic Intellect. Scotland and her Universities in the Nineteenth Century*. Edinburgh University Press, Edinburgh.

Davie, G.E. (1986). *The Crisis of the Democratic Intellect*. Polygon, Edinburgh.

Dicks, H.V. (1970). *Fifty Years of the Tavistock Clinic*. Routledge & Kegan Paul, London.

Diski, J. (2010). *The Sixties*. Profile Books, London.

Dostoyevsky, F.M. (1947). *A Raw Youth* (trans. Garnett, C.). Dial Press, New York.

Dostoyevsky, F.M. (1984). *The Diary of a Writer* (trans. Brasol, B.). Ianmead, Haslemere.

Dostoyevsky, F.M. (1985). *The House of the Dead* (trans. McDuff, D.). Penguin, London.

Dostoyevsky, F.M. (1992). *Crime and Punishment* (trans. Pevear, R. and Volokhonsky, L.). Vintage, London.

Dostoyevsky, F. (2003). *Notes from the Underground and The Double* (trans. Coulson, J.). Penguin Books, London.

Drabble, M. (ed.) (2000). *The Oxford Companion to English Literature*. Oxford University Press, Oxford.

Dreyfus, H.L. (2009). 'The roots of existentialism'. In Dreyfus, H.L. and Wrathall, M.A. (eds), *A Companion to Phenomenology and Existentialism*. Wiley-Blackwell, Oxford, pp. 137–61.

Dreyfus, H.L. and Wrathall, M.A. (eds) (2007). *A Companion to Heidegger*. Blackwell Publishing, London.

Dreyfus, H.L. and Wrathall, M.A. (eds) (2009). *A Companion to Phenomenology and Existentialism*. Wiley-Blackwell, Oxford.

Dru, A. (ed.) (1938). *The Journals of Soren Kierkegaard*. Oxford University Press, London.

Earnshaw, S. (2006). *Existentialism*. Continuum, London.

Ellenberger, F.H. (1970). *The Discovery of the Unconscious. The History and Evolution of Dynamic Psychiatry*. Basic Books, New York.

Engstrom, E.J. and Weber, M.W. (1999). 'Emil Kraepelin (1856–1926)'. In Freeman, H. (ed.), *A Century of Psychiatry*. Mosby, London, pp. 49–51.

Esslin, M. (1976). *Artaud*. Fontana/Collins, Glasgow.

Evans, R.I. (ed.) (1976). *R.D. Laing. The Man and his Ideas*. E.P. Dutton & Co., New York.

Fairbairn, W.R.D. (1957). 'Freud: the psychoanalytic method and mental health'. *British Journal of Medical Psychology*, **30**, 53–62.

Ferdern, P. (1953). *Ego psychology and the psychoses*. Imago, London.

Ferguson, R. (1990). *George MacLeod. Founder of the Iona Community*. Collins, London.

Ferm, V. (ed) (1958). *A History of Philosophical Systems*. Rider, New York.

Fish, F. (1964). *Outline of Psychiatry*. Wright, Bristol.

Fisher, S. and Greenberg, R. (1985). *The Scientific Credibility of Freud's Theories and Therapies*. Columbia University Press, Columbia.

Foucault, M. (1965). *Madness and Civilisation. A History of Insanity in the Age of Reason* (trans. Howard, R.). Tavistock, London (originally published in French in 1961).

Foucault, M. (2006). *History of Madness* (trans. Murphy, J. and Khalfa, J.). Routledge, London.

Frank, J. (1977). *Dostoyevsky: The Seeds of Revolt, 1821–1849*. Robson Books, London.

Freeman, T. (1961). 'Review of The Divided Self'. In British *Journal of Medical Psychology*, **34**, 79–80.

Freeman, T., Cameron, J.L. and McGhie, A. (1958). *Chronic Schizophrenia*. Tavistock, London.

Freud, S. (1961). 'Dostoevsky and parricide'. In *Complete Psychological Works*, Vol. 21. Hogarth Press, London, pp. 177–94.

Freud, S. (2002). *Civilization and its Discontents* (trans. McLintock, D.) Penguin Books, London (originally published in 1930).

Friedenberg, E.Z. (1973). *Laing*. Fontana/Collins, London.

Fromm-Reichmann, F. (1952). 'Some Aspects of Psychoanalytic Psychotherapy with Schizophrenics'. In Brody, E.B. and Redlich, F.C. (eds), *Psychotherapy with Schizophrenics*. International Universities Press, New York, pp. 89–111.

Fromm-Reichmann, F. and Moreno, J.L. (1956). *Progress in Psychotherapy*. Grune & Stratton, New York.

Fulford, B., Morris, K., Sadler, J. and Stanghellini (eds) (2003). *Nature and Narrative. An Introduction to the New Philosophy of Psychiatry*. Oxford University Press, Oxford.

Fulford, K.W.M., Thornton, T. and Graham, G. (2006). *Oxford Textbook of Philosophy and Psychiatry*. Oxford University Press, Oxford.

Gardiner, M. (2006). *From Trocchi to Trainspotting. Scottish Critical Theory since 1960*. Edinburgh University Press, Edinburgh.

Gardiner, P. (1988). *Kierkegaard*. Oxford University Press, Oxford.

Gardner, H.M. (ed.) (1948). *Poems of Gerard Manley Hopkins*. Oxford University Press, London.

Garff, J. (2005). *Soren Kierkegaard. A Biography*. (trans. Kirmmse, B.H.) Princeton University Press, Princeton.

Gay, P. (1988). *Freud. A Life for Our Time*. Dent, Cambridge.

Gelder, M. (1991). 'Adolf Meyer and his influence on British psychiatry'. In Berrios, G.E. and Freeman, H. (eds), *150 Years of British Psychiatry 1841–1991*. Gaskell, London, pp. 419–35.

Gellner, E. (1992). *The Psychoanalytic Movement. The Cunning of Unreason* (second edn). Fontana, London.

Gide, A. (1967). *Dostoyevsky*. Peregrine Books, London.

Goldstein, J. (2001). *Console and Classify. The French Psychiatric Profession in the Nineteenth Century*. University of Chicago Press, Chicago and London.

Gomes, P.J. (2000). 'Introduction to Tillich P (1952). *The Courage to Be*'. (2nd edn.). Yale University Press, New Haven and London, pp. xi–xxxiii.

Gomez, L. (1997). *An Introduction to Object Relations*. Free Association Press, London.

Greenberg, J.R. and Mitchell, S.A. (1983). *Object Relations in Psychoanalytic Theory*. Harvard University Press, Massachusetts, Cambridge.

Gregory, R. (ed.) (1987). *The Oxford Companion to Mind*. Oxford University Press, Oxford.

Gregory Smith, G. (1919). *Scottish Literature: Character and Influence*. Macmillan, London.

Grieder, A. (1991). 'On the existential-phenomenological background of R.D. Laing's The Divided Self'. *Journal of the Society for Existential Analysis*, **2**, 8–15.

Guntrip, H. (1952). 'A study of Fairbairn's theory of schizoid reactions'. *British Journal of Medical Psychology*. **25**, 86–103.

Guntrip, H. (1961). *Personality Structure and Human Interaction: the Developing Synthesis of Psychodynamic Theory*. International Universities Press, New York.

Hacker, P.M.S. (2007). *Human Nature: the Categorical Framework*. Blackwell, Oxford.

Haeckel, E. (1992). *The Riddle of the Universe* (trans. McCabe, J.). Prometheus Books, New York.

Halliday, J.L. (1949). *Psychological Medicine. A Study of the Sick Society*. William Heinemann, London.

Halling, S. and Dearborn Nill, J. (1995). 'A brief history of existential-phenomenological psychiatry and psychotherapy'. *Journal of Phenomenological Psychology*, **26**(1), 1–45.

Hare, B. and Bielecka, P. (eds) (2006). *Divided Selves. The Scottish Self-Portrait from the 17th Century to the Present*. The Fleming-Wyfold Art Foundation, London.

Hayward, M.L. and Taylor, J.E. (1956). 'A schizophrenic patient describes the action of intensive psychotherapy'. *Psychiatric Quarterly*, **30**, 211–48.

Hayward, R. (2007). 'Recovering R.D. Laing'. *Metascience*, **16**, 525–7.

Healy, D. (2002). *The Creation of Psychopharmacology*. Harvard University Press, Cambridge MA.

Heaton, J. (1991). 'The Divided Self: Kierkegaard or Winnicott?' *Journal of the Society for Existential Analysis*, **2**, 30–7.

Heaton, J. (2000). 'On R.D. Laing: style, sorcery, alienation'. *The Psychoanalytic Review*, **87**, 511–26.

Heaton, J.M. (2005). 'Laing and psychotherapy'. In Raschid, S. (ed.) *R.D. Laing. Contemporary Perspectives*. Free Association Book, London, pp. 313–25.

Heidegger, M. (1949). 'On the essence of truth'. In Heidegger, M., *Existence and Being*. (introduction by Brock, W.). Gateway, South Bend, Indiana, pp. 292–324.

Heidegger, M. (1962). *Being and Time* (trans. Macquarrie, J. and Robinson, E.). Blackwell, Oxford.

Heidegger, M. (2001). *Zollikon Seminars. Protocols, Conversations, Letters* (Boss, M., ed,) (trans. Mayr, F. and Askay, R.). Northwestern University Press, Evanston, Illinois.

Henderson, D.K. (1964). *The Evolution of Psychiatry in Scotland*. E. & S. Livingstone, Edinburgh.

Henderson, D.K. and Gillespie, R.D. (1940). *A Textbook of Psychiatry for Students and Practitioners* (fifth edn). Oxford University Press, London.

Hirschman, J. (1965). *Antonin Artaud Anthology*. City Lights Books, San Francisco.

Hoare, P. (2002). *Spike Island. The Memory of a Military Hospital*. Fourth Estate, London.

Hoenig, J. (1995). 'Schizophrenia'. In Berrios, G. and Porter, R. (eds), *A History of Clinical Psychiatry*, Athlone, London, pp. 336–48.

Hoff, P. (1995) 'Kraepelin'. In Berrios, G. and Porter, R. (eds), *A History of Clinical Psychiatry*. Athlone, London, pp. 261–79.

Hollingdale, R.J. (1996). 'The hero as outsider'. In Magnus, B. and Higgins, K.M. (eds), *The Cambridge Companion to Nietzsche*. Cambridge University Press, Cambridge, pp. 71–89.

Holmes, R. (2008). *The Age of Wonder. How the Romantic Generation Discovered the Beauty and Terror of Science*. Harper Press, London.

Honderich, T. (ed.) (1995). *The Oxford Companion to Philosophy*. Oxford University Press, Oxford.

Hood, J. (2001). 'The Young R.D. Laing: A Personal Memoir And Some Hypotheses.' In Steiner, R., Johns, J. (eds), *Within Time & Beyond Time. A Festschrift for Pearl King*. Karnac, London, pp. 39–53.

Hopkins, G.M. (1996). *The Complete Poems with Selected Prose of Gerard Manley Hopkins*. Fount, London.

Hornstein, G.A. (2005). *To Redeem One Person is to Redeem the World. The Life of Frieda Fromm-Reichmann*. Others Press, New York.

Howarth-Williams, M. (1977). *R.D. Laing. His Work and its Relevance for Sociology*. Routledge and Kegan Paul, London.

Hunter-Brown, I. (2007). *R.D. Laing and Psychodynamic Psychiatry in 1950s Glasgow: A Reappraisal*. Free Association Books, London.

Hunter, R. and Macalpine, I. (1963). *Three Hundred Years of Psychiatry 1535–1860*. Oxford University Press, London.

Huxley, J. (1940). *Religion without Revelation*. Watts & co., London.

Ingleby, D. (1998). 'The view from the North Sea'. In Gijswijt-Hofstra, M., Porter, R. (eds), *Cultures of Psychiatry and Mental Health Care in Postwar Britain and the Netherlands*. Rodopi, Amsterdam, pp. 295–314.

James, W. (1902). *The Varieties of Religious Experience*. Longmans, Green, and Co, London.

Jaspers, K. (1950). *The Perennial Scope of Philosophy*. Routledge Kegan, London.

Jaspers, K. (1963). *General Psychopathology* (trans. Hoenig, J. and Hamilton, M.). Manchester University Press, Manchester.

Jaspers, J. (2000). 'Philosophical memoir'. In Ehrlich, E., Ehrlich, L.H. and Pepper, G.B. (eds), *Karl Jaspers: Basic Philosophical Writings*. Humanity Books, New York.

Jones, E. and Wessely, S. (2005). *Shell Shock to PTSD. Military Psychiatry from 1900 to the Gulf War*. Psychology Press, Hove and New York.

Jones, C. (1998). 'Raising the anti: Jan Foudraine, Ronald Laing and Anti-Psychiatry'. In Gijswijt, M. and Porter, R. (eds), *Cultures of Psychiatry and Mental Health Care in Postwar Britain and the Netherlands*. Rodopi, Amsterdam, pp. 283–94.

Jones, M. (ed.) (1952). *Social Psychiatry: A Study of Therapeutic Communities*. Tavistock, London.

Kafka, F. (1953). *Wedding Preparations in the Country and Other Stories*. Penguin Books, London.

Kaufmann, W. (1958). *Existentialism from Dostoyevsky to Sartre*. Meridian Books, Cleveland and New York.

Kaufmann, W. (1974). *Nietzsche. Philosopher, Psychologist, Antichrist* (fourth edn). Princeton University Press, Princeton.

Kierkegaard, S. (2004). *The Sickness unto Death*. Penguin Books, London.

Kirkbright, S. (2004). *Karl Jaspers. A Biography. Navigations in Truth*. Yale University Press, New Haven and London.

Kirsner, D. (1976). *The Schizoid World of Jean-Paul Sartre and R.D. Laing*. University of Queensland Press, Queensland.

Kirsner, D. (1990). 'An abyss of difference: Laing, Sartre and Jaspers'. *Journal of the British Society for Phenomenology*, **21**, 209–15.

Kirsner, D. (2005). 'Laing and philosophy'. In Raschid, S. (ed.) *R.D. Laing. Contemporary Perspectives*. Free Association Books, London, pp. 154–74.

Kotowicz, Z. (1997). *R.D. Laing and the Paths of Anti-Psychiatry*. Routledge, London.

Kraepelin, E. (1913). *Lectures on Clinical Psychiatry*. Bailliére, Tindall and Cox, London.

Lafont, C. (2007). 'Hermeneutics'. In Dreyfus, H.L. and Wrathall, M.A. (eds), *A Companion to Heidegger*. Blackwell Publishing, London, pp. 265–84.

Laing, A. (1991). 'R.D. Laing. The first five years'. *Journal of the Society for Existential Analysis*, **2**, 24–9.

Laing, A. (1994). *R.D. Laing. A Biography*. Peter Owen, London.

Laing, A. (2006). *R.D. Laing. A Life* (2nd edn. with new introduction). Sutton Publishing, Thrupp.

Laing, R.D. (1949). 'Philosophy and medicine'. *Surgo*, June, 134–5.

Laing, R.D. (1950). 'Health and society'. *Surgo*, Candlemas, 91–2.

Laing, R.D. (1953). 'An instance of the Ganser Syndrome'. *Journal of the Royal Army Medical Corps*, **99**, 169–72.

Laing, R.D. (1957). 'An examination of Tillich's theory of anxiety and neurosis'. *The British Journal of Medical Psychology*, **30**, 88–91.

Laing, R.D. (1960). *The Divided Self. A Study of Sanity and Madness*. Tavistock Publications, London.

Laing, R.D. (1961). *The Self and Others*. Tavistock, London.

Laing, R.D. (1963). 'Minkowski and schizophrenia'. *Review of Existential Psychology and Psychiatry*, **3**, 195–207.

Laing, R.D. (1964). 'Review of Karl Jasper's general psychopathology'. *International Journal of Psychoanalysis*, **45**, 590–3.

Laing, R.D. (1965) *The Divided Self*. Pelican, London.

Laing, R.D. (1967). *The Politics of Experience and The Bird of Paradise*. Penguin, Harmondsworth.

Laing, R.D. (1969). *Self and Others*. Penguin Books, Harmondsworth.

Laing, R.D. (1970). 'Religious Sensibility.' *The Listener*, 23 April 1970, pp. 536–7.

Laing, R.D. (1970). *Knots*. Tavistock, London.

Laing, R.D. (1976). *The Facts of Life*. Penguin, London.

Laing, R.D. (1979). *Sonnets*. Michael Joseph, London.

Laing, R.D. (1980). 'What is the matter with mind?' In Kumar, S. (ed.) *The Schumacher Lectures*. Blond & Briggs, London, pp. 1–19.

Laing, R.D. (1982). *The Voice of Experience*. Allen Lane, London.

Laing, R.D. (1985). *Wisdom, Madness and Folly. The Making of a Psychiatrist 1927–1957*, 1998 reprint. Canongate, Edinburgh.

Laing, R.D. (1987). 'Laing's understanding of interpersonal experience'. In Gregory, R. (ed.), *The Oxford Companion to Mind*. Oxford University Press, Oxford, pp. 417–18.

Laing, R.D. (1996). 'The invention of madness'. In Smart, B. (ed.) *Michel Foucault. Critical Assessments*. Vol. IV. Routledge, London. Originally published in *New Statesman*, 1987, 16 June, p. 843. pp. 76–9.

Laing, R.D. and Cooper, D. (1964). *Reason and Violence. A Decade of Sartre's Philosophy 1950–1960*. Tavistock, London.

Laing, R.D. and Esterson, A. (1958). 'The collusive function of pairing in analytic groups'. *British Journal of Medical Psychology*, **31**, 117–23.

Laing, R.D. and Esterson, A. (1964). *Sanity, Madness and the Family*. Penguin Books, London.

Laing, R.D., Phillipson, H. and Lee, R.A. (1966). *Interpersonal Perception*. Tavistock, London.

Lidz, T. (1972). 'Schizophrenia, R.D. Laing and the contemporary treatment of psychosis'. In Boyers, R. and Orrill, R. (eds), *Laing and Anti-Psychiatry*. London: Penguin, London, pp. 123–56.

Lomas, P. (1968). 'Psychoanalysis—Freudian or existential'. In Rycroft, C. (ed.), *Psychoanalysis Observed*. Constable, London, pp. 119–48.

Lomas, P. (1973). *True and False Experience*. Allen Lane, London.

Lunt, A. (1990). *Apollo Versus the Echomaker. A Laingian approach to Psychotherapy, Dreams and Shamanism*. Element Books, Longmead.

Lynch, M. (ed.) (2001). *The Oxford Companion to Scottish History*. Oxford University Press, Oxford.

Macalpine, I. and Hunter, R.A. (1955) *Daniel Paul Schreber. Memoirs of My Nervous Illness*. Dawson & Sons, London.

Macdonald, C.M.M. (2009). *Whaur Extremes Meet. Scotland's Twentieth Century*. John Donald, Edinburgh.

Mackey, L. (1971). *Kierkegaard. A Kind of Poet*. University of Pennsylvania Press, Philadelphia.

MacLeod, G. (1944). *We Shall Rebuild*. Iona Community, Glasgow.

MacLeod, G. (1958). *Only One Way Left*. Iona Community, Glasgow.

Macmurray, J. (1957). *The Self as Agent*. Faber & Faber, London.

Macmurray, J. (1961). *Persons in Relation*. Faber & Faber, London.

Macquarrie, J. (1973). *Existentialism*. Pelican Books, London.

Macquarrie, J. (1999). *On Being a Theologian*. SCM Press, London.

Magnus, B. and Higgins, K.M. (eds) (1996). *The Cambridge Companion to Nietzsche*. Cambridge University Press, Cambridge.

Makari, G. (2008). *Revolution in the Mind. The Creation of Psychoanalysis*. Duckworth, London.

Mann, T. (1958). *Confessions of Felix Krull, Confidence Man*. (trans. Lindley, D.). Penguin Books, London.

Massie, A. (2009). *Surviving*. Vagabond Voices, An Rubha.

Masson, J. (1992). *Against Therapy*. Fontana, London.

Matthews, E. (1996). *Twentieth Century French Philosophy*. Oxford University Press, Oxford.

Matthews, E. (2002). *The Philosophy of Merleau-Ponty*. Acumen, Chesam.

Matthews, E. (2005). 'Laing and Merleau-Ponty'. In Raschid, S. (ed.) *R.D. Laing. Contemporary Perspectives*. Free Association Books, London, pp. 79–98.

Matthews, E. (2006). *Merleau-Ponty*. Continuum, London.

Matthews, E. (2009) *Broken Brains and Broken Minds*. Talk to Scottish Psychiatry and Philosophy Group, 30 September, 2009.

Mautner, T. (2005). *A Dictionary of Philosophy*. Penguin, London.

May, R., Angel, E. and Ellenberger, H.F. (eds) (1958). *Existence. A New Dimension in Psychiatry and Psychology*. Basic Books, New York.

McCrone, D. (1992). *Understanding Scotland. The Sociology of a Stateless Nation*. Routledge, London.

McGhie, A. (1958). 'Psychological aspects of schizophrenia'. In Ferguson Roger, T., Mowbray, R.M. and Roy, J.R. (eds), *Topics in Psychiatry*. Cassell, London, pp. 35–46.

Mezan, P. (1972). 'After Freud and Jung, Now Comes R.D. Laing'. *Esquire*, **77**, 92–7; 160–78.

Mezan, P. (1976). 'Portrait of a twentieth-century sceptic'. In Evans, R.I. (ed.) *R.D. Laing. The Man and his Ideas*. E.P. Dutton & Co., New York, pp. xxii–lxxv.

Micale, M. (2007). 'Two cultures revisited: the case of the fin de siecle'. In Bivins, R. and Pickstone, J.V. (eds), *Medicine, Madness and Social History. Essays in Honour of Roy Porter*. Palgrave, London, pp. 210–33.

Millard, D.W. (1996). 'Maxwell Jones and the therapeutic community'. In Freeman, H. and Berrios, G.E. (eds), *150 Years of British Psychiatry. Volume II: the Aftermath*. Athlone, London, pp. 581–604.

Miller, G. (2001). 'Cognition and community: The Scottish philosophical context of the 'divided self'. *Janus Head*, **4**, 104–29.

Miller, G. (2004). *R.D. Laing*. Edinburgh University Press, Edinburgh.

Miller, G. (2005). *Alasdair Gray. The Fiction of Communion*. Rodopi, Amsterdam.

Miller, G. (2008). 'Scottish psychoanalysis. A rational religion'. *Journal of the History of the Behavioural Sciences*, **44**(1), 38–58.

Miller, G. (2008). 'Psychiatry as hermeneutics: Laing's argument with natural science'. *Journal of Humanistic Psychology*, **48**, 42–60.

Miller, G. (2009). 'How Scottish was R.D. Laing?' *History of Psychiatry*, **20**(2), 226–32.

Miller, G. (2009). 'R.D. Laing and theology: the influence of Christian existentialism on *The Divided Self*'. *History of the Human Sciences*, **22**, 1–21.

Miller, G. (2009). 'Scotland's authentic plurality: The New Essentialism in Scottish studies'. *Scottish Literary Review*, **1/1**, 157–74.

Mischler, E.G. (1973). 'Man, Morality, and Madness: Critical Perspectives on the Work of R.D. Laing'. In Rubinstein, B.B. (ed.), *Psychoanalysis and Contemporary Science*, Vol. 2. Macmillan, New York, pp. 369–94.

Mitchell, J. (1974). *Psychoanalysis and Feminism*. Penguin Books, Harmondsworth. Reprinted with a new introduction, 2000.

Momus (2010). *The Book of Scotlands*. Sternberg Press (place of publication not given).

Mullan, B. (1995). *Mad to be Normal. Conversations with R.D. Laing*. Free Association Books, London.

Mullan, B. (1997). *R.D. Laing. Creative Destroyer*. Cassell, London.

Mullan, B. (1999). *R.D. Laing. A Personal View*. Duckworth, London.

Neeleman, J. (1990). (trans. and introduction). 'Classic Texts No 3. The nuclear symptoms of schizophrenia and the praecox feeling. By H.C. Rumke'. *History of Psychiatry*, **1**, 331–41.

Nehamas, A. (1985). *Nietzsche. Life as Literature*. Harvard University Press, Cambridge, Massachusetts.

Nietzsche, F. (1979). *Ecce Homo* (trans. Hollingdale, R.J.). Penguin Books, London.

Nietzsche, F. (1995). *The Birth of Tragedy* (trans. Fadiman, C.P.). Dover Publications, New York.

Nietzsche, F. (2000). *The Antichrist* (trans. Lodovici, A.M.). Prometheus Books, New York.

Nietzsche, F. (2006). *The Gay Science*. Dover Publications, New York.

Orth, M. and Trimble, M.R. (2006). 'Friedrich Nietzsche's mental illness—general paralysis of the insane vs. frontotemporal dementia'. *Acta Psychiatrica Scandanavica*, **114**, 439–45.

Ott, H. (1994). *Martin Heidegger. A Political Life* (trans. Blunden, A.). Fontana Press, London (originally published in Germany in 1988).

Palinurs (1944). *The Unquiet Grave*. First published by Horizon, London in 1944, Revised edn. 1945. Published in London by Penguin, 1967.

Phillips, A. (1988). *Winnicott*. Fontana Press, London.

Pines, M. (1991). 'The development of the psychodynamic movement'. In Berrios, G.E. and Freeman, H. (eds), *150 Years of Psychiatry 1841–1991*. Gaskell, London, pp. 206–301.

Podach, E.F. (1974). *The Madness of Nietzsche*. (trans. Voight, F.A.) Gordon Press, New York.

Poole, R. (1998). 'The unknown Kierkegaard: twentieth century receptions'. In Hannay, A. and Munro, G. (eds), *The Cambridge Companion to Kierkegaard*. Cambridge University Press, Cambridge, pp. 48–75.

Poole, R. (2005). 'R.D. Laing's reading of Kierkegaard'. In Raschid, S. (ed.) *R.D. Laing. Contemporary Perspectives*. Free Association Book, London, pp. 99–112.

Porter, R. (ed.) (1997). *Rewriting the Self. Histories from the Renaissance to the Present*. Routledge, London.

Rank, O. (1959). *The Myth of the Birth of the Hero and Other Writings*. Alfred A. Knopf, New York.

Ratcliffe, M. (2008). *Feelings of Being. Phenomenology, Psychiatry and the Sense of Reality*. Oxford University Press, Oxford.

Ratcliffe, M. (2009). 'Understanding existential changes in psychiatric illness: the indispensability of phenomenology'. In Broome, M.R. and Borlotti (eds), *Psychiatry as Cognitive Neuroscience. Philosophical Perspectives*. Oxford University Press, Oxford, pp. 223–45.

Redlich, F.C. (1952). 'The Concept of Schizophrenia and Its Implications for Therapy'. In Brody, E.B. and Redlich, F.C. (eds), *Psychotherapy with Schizophrenics*, International Universities Press, New York, pp. 18–38.

Rice, J.L. (1985). *Dostoyevsky and the Healing Art: An Essay in Literary and Medical History.* Ardis, Ann Arbor.

Rillie, J. (1988). 'The Abenheimer/Schorstein Group.' *Edinburgh Review,* **78–9**, 104–07.

Roazen, P. (1976). *Freud and his Followers.* Allen Lane, London.

Robinson, D., Zarate, O. (2003). *Introducing Kierkegaard.* Icon Books, Cambridge.

Rodman, F.R. (2003). *Winnicott. Life and Work.* Perseus Publishing, Cambridge.

Rosen, J. (1953). *Direct Analysis. Selected Papers.* Grune Stratton, New York.

Rycroft, C. (1995). *Critical Dictionary of Psychoanalysis.* Penguin Books, London.

Safranski, R. (1999). *Martin Heidegger. Between Good and Evil.* (trans. Oser,s E.) Harvard University Press, Harvard (originally published in German in 1994).

Sartre, J.P. (1958). 'Existentialism is a Humanism'. In Kaufmann, W. (ed.) (1958). *Existentialism from Dostoyevsky to Sartre.* Meridian Books, Cleveland and New York, pp. 287–311.

Sartre, J.P. (1969). *Introduction to Being and Nothingness.* (trans. Barnes, H.E.) Metheun, London.

Sartre, J.P. (1972). *The Psychology of the Imagination.* Methuen, London.

Sartre, J.P. (1973). *Existentialism and Humanism.* Eyre Methuen, London.

Sartre, J.P. (1974). *Foreword* (trans. Sheridan Smith, A.M.) to Laing, R.D., Cooper, D.G. *Reason and Violence. A Decade of Sartre's Philosophy1950–1960.* Pantheon Books, New York.

Sassi, C. (2005). *Why Scottish Literature Matters.* The Saltire Society, Edinburgh.

Sechahaye, M.A. (1950). *Autobiography of a Schizophrenic Girl.* Grune & Stratton, New York.

Sechahaye, M.A. (1951). *Symbolic Realization—a New Method of Psychotherapy applied to a Case of Schizophrenia.* International University Press, New York.

Sechehaye, M.A. (1956). *A New Psychotherapy in Schizophrenia.* Grune & Stratton, New York.

Schatzi, T.R. (2007). 'Early Heidegger on Sociality'. In Dreyfus, H.L. and Wrathall, M.A. (eds), *A Companion to Heidegger.* Blackwell Publishing, London, pp. 233–47.

Schneider, K.J. (2000). 'R.D. Laing's existential-humanistic practice: what was he actually doing?' *Psychoanalytic Review,* **87**, 591–9.

Schweitzer, A. (1975). *The Psychiatric Study of Jesus. Exposition and Criticism* (trans. Joy, C.R.) Peter Smith, Gloucester, Mass. (originally published in German in 1913).

Schorstein, J. (1960). *The Present State of Consciousness.* Penguin Science Survey B, London.

Schorstein, J. (1961). 'The story of Nan: a case of severe head injury'. *Physiotherapy,* **47**, 335–6.

Schorstein, J. (1964). 'The metaphysics of the atom bomb'. *The Philosophical Journal,* **1**, 33–46.

Sedgwick, P. (1982). *Psychopolitics.* Pluto Press, London.

Shamdasani, S. (2003). *Jung and the Making of Modern Psychology. The Dream of a Science.* Cambridge University Press, Cambridge.

Shorter, E. (1997). *A History of Psychiatry. From the Era of the Asylum to the Age of Prozac.* John Wiley and sons, New York.

Shorter, E. (2005). *A Historical Dictionary of Psychiatry.* Oxford University Press, New York.

Showalter, E. (1987). *The Female Malady. Women, Madness and English Culture, 1830–1980.* Virago Press, London.

Siegler, M., Osmond, H. and Mann, H. (1972). 'Laing's models of madness'. In Boyers, R. and Orrill, R. (eds), *Laing and Anti-Psychiatry.* Penguin Books, London, pp. 99–122.

Sigal, C. (2005). *Zone of the Interior.* Pomona Books, Hebden Bridge (first published in 1976).

Smith, I.D. and Swann, A. (1993) 'In praise of the asylum—the writings of two nineteenth century Glasgow patients'. In Goie, L.D. and Vijselaar, J. (eds) *Proceedings of the 1st European Congress on the History of Psychiatry and Mental Health Care*. Erasmus Publishing, Rotterdam, pp. 90–5.

Smith, R. (1997). *The Fontana History of the Human Sciences*. Fontana Press, London.

Snow, C.P. (1959). *The Two Cultures and the Scientific Revolution*. Cambridge University Press, Cambridge.

Spiegelberg, H. (1972). *Phenomenology in Psychology and Psychiatry*. Northwestern University Press, Evanston.

Starkie, E. (1961). *Arthur Rimbaud*. Faber & Faber, London.

Staunton, A.H. and Schwartz, H.S. (1954). *The Mental Hospital*. Basic Books, New York.

Steiner, G. (1992). *Heidegger* (2nd edn.). Fontana Press, London.

Stern, P.J. (1979). 'Introduction to the English translation'. In Boss, M., *Existential Foundations of Medicine and Psychology* (trans. Conway, S. and Cleaves, A.). Jason Aronson, Northvale, pp. ix–xxii.

Stewart, J. (2006). 'An "enigma to their parents": the founding and aims of the Notre Dame Child Guidance Clinic, Glasgow'. *The Innes Review*, **57**, 54–76.

Storr, A. (1973). *Jung*. Fontana, Glasgow.

Sulloway, F.J. (1980). *Freud. Biologist of the Mind. Beyond the Psychoanalytic Legend*. Fontana, London.

Sutcliffe, S. (2010). 'After 'The Religion of My Fathers': The quest for composure in the 'Post-Presbyterian' Self'. In Abrams, L. and Brown, C.G. (eds), *A History of Everyday Life in Twentieth-Century Scotland*. Edinburgh University Press, Edinburgh, pp. 181–205.

Suzuki, A. (2006). *Madness at Home. The Psychiatrist, the Patient, and the Family in England, 1820–1860*. University of California Press, Berkeley and Los Angeles.

Tantam, D. (1996). 'Fairbairn'. In Freeman, H. and Berrios, G.E. (eds), *150 Years of British Psychiatry. Volume II: the Aftermath*, Athlone, London, pp. 549–64.

Tantam, D. (2000). 'R.D. Laing and anti-psychiatry'. In Freeman, H. (ed.), *A Century of Psychiatry*. Mosby, London, pp. 202–07.

Thompson, D.O. (2002). 'Dostoyevsky and science'. In Leatherbarrow, W.J. (ed.) *The Cambridge Companion to Dostoyevsky*. Cambridge University Press, Cambridge, pp. 191–211.

Thompson, J. (1974). *Kierkegaard*. Gollancz, London.

Thompson. M.G. (1998). 'Existential psychoanalysis: A Laingian perspective'. In Marcus, P. and Rosenberg, A. (eds), *Psychoanalytic Versions of the Human Condition*. New York University Press, New York, pp. 332–61.

Thompson, M.G. (2000). 'The heart of the matter. R.D. Laing's enigmatic relationship with psychoanalysis'. *Psychoanalytic Review*, **87**, 483–509.

Thornton, T. (2007). *Essential Philosophy of Psychiatry*. Oxford University Press, Oxford.

Tomes, N. (1994). 'Feminist histories of psychiatry'. In Micale, M.S. and Porter, R. (eds), *Discovering the History of Psychiatry*. Oxford University Press, Oxford, pp. 348–84.

Torrey, E.F. (1992). *Freudian Fraud. The Malignant Effect of Freud's Theory on American Culture and Thought*. Harper-Collins, New York.

Toynbee, P. (1960). 'Review of *The Divided Self*'. In *The Observer*, quoted on the back cover of *The Self and Others*.

Trilling, L. (1955). *The Opposing Self*. Harcourt Brace Jovanich, New York and London.

Turnbull, R. and Beveridge, C. (1988). 'Laing and Scottish Philosophy'. *Edinburgh Review*, **78**(7), 119–128.

Tyson, A. (1971). 'Homage to Catatonia'. *New York Review of Books*, **16**, 3–6.

Warnock, M. (1969). *Introduction to Being and Nothingness* by Jean-Paul Sartre (trans. Barnes, H.E.) Metheun, London.

Warnock, M. (1970). *Existentialism*. Oxford University Press, Oxford.

Webster, R. (1996). *Why Freud was Wrong. Sin, Science and Psychoanalysis*. Fontana, London.

Weigert, E. (1949). 'Existentialism and its relation to psychotherapy.' *Psychiatry*, **21**, 399–412.

Westphal, M. (1999). 'Kierkegaard'. In Critchtley, S. and Schroeder, W.R. (eds). *A Companion to Continental Philosophy*, Blackwell, Oxford, pp. 128–38.

White, N. (2004). 'Hopkins, Gerard Manley (1844–1889)'. In *Oxford Dictionary of National Biography*. Oxford University Press, Oxford. http://www.oxforddnb.com/view/article/37565

Winnicott, D.W. (1958). *Collected Papers*. Tavistock, London.

Van Derzen-Smith, E. (1991). 'Ontological insecurity revisited'. *Journal of the Society for Existential Analysis*, **2**, 38–48.

Van Deurzen, E. and Arnold-Baker, C. (2005). *Existential Perspectives on Human Issues. A Handbook for Therapeutic Practice*. Palgrave Macmillan, London.

Van de Weyer, R. (1996). 'Introduction'. In Gerard Manley Hopkins (1996). *The Complete Poems with Selected Prose of Gerard Manley Hopkins*. Fount, London, pp. vii–x.

Zilboorg, G. (1941). *A History of Medical Psychology*. (in collaboration with Henry, G.W.) W.W. Norton & Co., New York.

Unarchived sources

Application by Laing for post of registrar at the Royal Mental Hospital, Glasgow, 23 September 1953.

Case Conference Note-Book from 9-2-54 to 13-1-58. Unarchived document recently donated to Glasgow University Archive by Professor Sir Michael Bond.

Letter to The Secretary Western Regional Hospital Board from J. Eric Paterson on Laing, 30 September 1953.

Letter to the Secretary, Western Regional Health Board about Laing from Ivy Mackenzie, 6 October 1953.

Letter to The Secretary of the Western Regional Health board on Laing by J.F.D. Murphy, 29 September 1953.

Letter from Laing to Dr MacNiven, 11 June 1956.

Letter to Secretary of the Paddington Group Hospital Management Committee about Laing from Angus MacNiven, 12 June 1956.

Letter to Dr Max M. Levin, Foundations' Fund for Research in Psychiatry, New Haven, Connecticut from Dr MacNiven, 30 March 1960.

Letter to Dr MacNiven from Laing, 12 May 1964.

Letter from Laing to Dr MacNiven, 18 May 1965.

Letter to Dr Laing from Dr McClatchey, 15 May 1964.

Research Fellowship Application by Laing to Foundations' Fund for Research in Psychiatry, 21 March 1960.

Index